A Colour Atlas of the

BRAIN & SPINAL CORD

AN INTRODUCTION TO NORMAL NEUROANATOMY

MARJORIE A. ENGLAND

Senior Lecturer in Anatomy
Medical Sciences
University of Leicester
and
Lately Honorary Senior Research Fellow,
Royal College of Surgeons
of England

JENNIFER WAKELY

Lecturer in Anatomy
Medical Sciences
University of Leicester

N⌀ Mosby-Wolfe

Copyright © Marjorie A. England and Jennifer Wakely, 1991
Published in 1991 by Mosby–Wolfe, an imprint of Times Mirror International Publishers Limited.
Printed by BPC Books Limited, Aylesbury, England.
ISBN 0 7234 0870 X (Hardcover); ISBN 0 7234 1696 6 (Soft cover)

Reprinted 1993 and 1996.

A CIP catalogue record for this book is available from the British Library.

For full details of all Times Mirror International Publishers Limited titles please write to Times Mirror International Publishers Limited, Lynton House, 7–12 Tavistock Square, London WC1H 9LB, England.

Contents

To
Mr K. Garfield
on his retirement,
Our photographer and friend

Acknowledgements

Many of the illustrations in this book show our own preparations. In addition, the authors are deeply grateful to many people who generously contributed to this book with their advice and time, and who often provided access to their personal collections of materials or those prepared for their institutions. Their enthusiasm for this subject was both a delight and an encouragement to us.

In particular we are grateful to Professor T.W.A. Glenister, CBE, Charing Cross and Westminster Hospital Medical School, London (CXWMS) and to the Anatomy Department for allowing us to photograph some of the specimens in their collection.

Professor B.A. Wood, Middlesex Hospital Medical School, London (MHMS) also allowed us to photograph materials from the departmental collection.

Professor R.E. Coupland, University of Nottingham Medical School (UN) generously allowed us to photograph specimens from his departmental collection.

We are also indebted to Professor N. Gluhbegovic, University of Utrecht, The Netherlands, who advised us on many occasions on the preparation of frozen dissected brains. He also allowed us to use one of his preparations (see page **97**).

Professor V. Chan-Palay, Neurology Institute, University Hospital of Zurich, generously supplied two photomicrographs of neuropeptide Y neurons from her research studies. Professor Dr Eva Braak, Klinikum der Johann Wolfgang Goethe-Universitat Frankfurt, West Germany, kindly supplied micrographs of somatostatin-immunoreactive neurons.

Dr N.A. Lassen, Department of Clinical Physiology, Bispebjerg Hospital, Copenhagen, Denmark, provided Xenon-133 intracarotid technique photographs of the auditory cortex.

Dr E. Motti, Instituto Di Neurochirurgia, Milano, Italy, provided scanning electron micrographs of the blood vessels of the choroid plexus.

Professor H.M. Duvernoy, Université de Franche-Comte, Besançon, Cedex, France, generously allowed us to use a preparation from his book, *Human Brainstem Vessels*.

Professor F. Walker and Professor I. Lauder, Department of Pathology, University of Leicester provided some materials for this book.

Professor John Marshall, Institute of Ophthalmology, London, provided two histological sections of the retina.

Dr G.H. Wright, University of Cambridge, advised one of us about the materials available in the Anatomy Department collection.

Miss E. Allen, Qvist Curator, The Hunterian Museum, The Royal College of Surgeons of England (RCS) kindly allowed us to photograph specimens in the museum. She was ably assisted by Miss A. Serrant.

Dr V. Navaratnam and Dr E. Ford, Department of Anatomy, University of Cambridge (CAM), very kindly provided materials from the departmental collection. Mr B. Logan generously advised and assisted us with some preparations for which we are very grateful.

Dr M.R. Matthews, Department of Human Anatomy, University of Oxford (OXF), generously allowed us to photograph materials in the department.

Dr G. Batcup, Consultant Pathologist, University of Leeds, provided and prepared fetal materials and we are very grateful for her generosity and to Dr M.O. Mohamdee, her Senior Registrar for her help.

Dr E.C. Blenkinsopp, Consultant Pathologist, and Dr W.K. Blenkinsopp, Consultant Pathologist, Watford General Hospital, both very generously provided specimens.

Dr J. Lowe, Department of Pathology, University of Nottingham, prepared electron micrographs of a synapse, nerve fibres and immunocytochemical preparations for us.

Dr M. Ingle Wright, University of Manchester, kindly provided her own special preparations of the ear.

Dr J. Southgate, Leicester Royal Infirmary, generously provided three histological sections of the eye.

Dr B. Bracegirdle, Wellcome Museum of the History of Medicine kindly allowed one of us to examine and photograph histological sections of the nervous system prepared in the 19th century. These included preparations by Martin Cole from the 1890's; Dr Needham's collection amassed in the 1870's; specimens prepared in the 1860's for Smith, Beck and Beck Co., and Martin Cole in 1884.

Dr D.C. Bouch, Consultant Histopathologist, Leicester Royal Infirmary, generously provided facilities for sectioning half-brains. We are very grateful for this privilege and to his staff for their advice.

Dr N. Messios, Consultant Radiologist, Leicester Royal Infirmary, assisted greatly with photographs from the CT scanner.

Dr A. Fletcher, Consultant Pathologist, Leicester

Royal Infirmary, kindly provided immunocyto-chemical preparations of nervous tissue.

Dr D. James, Consultant Radiologist, Leicester Royal Infirmary, kindly assisted us on several films.

Professor A.R. Fielder, Birmingham University and Mr H. Harris, Leicester Royal Infirmary, generously donated images of the retina.

Nuclear magnetic resonance figures were provided by Dr G. Bydder, Senior Lecturer, Royal Postgraduate Medical School, London.

The colour-enhanced magnetic resonance image (MRI) was provided through the courtesy of Dr M.W. Vannier, Associate Professor of Radiology, Mallinckrodt Institute of Radiology at Washington University Medical Center, St. Louis, Missouri, USA.

Elscint Ltd., Watford, provided CT scans and NMR images.

Dr I. Talbot, Reader in Pathology, Dr M. Levene, Reader in Child Health, Dr A. Fletcher, Consultant Histopathologist, and Mrs L. Palmer and Mr R. Stewart, Mr R. Cullen and Mrs G. Hayward, Leicester Royal Infirmary, also advised us on materials. Dr Fletcher additionally gave us immunocytochemical and silver-stained preparations.

Mr G.A. Bell, Principal, Schools of Radio-graphy, Leicester Royal Infirmary, assisted us with a special brain preparation, as did Dr M.A. Goodwin, University of Leicester.

We are also grateful to Mr P.A. Runnicles, Chief Technician, and to Mr C. Syms, The Middlesex Hospital School of Medicine who assisted greatly. Mr R. Watts, Chief Technician, and Mr P.A. Ryan, Charing Cross Hospital Medical School; Mr E.T. Williams, University of Cambridge; and Mr R. White, University of Oxford; Mr B. Logan, Prosector, Department of Anatomy, The University of Cambridge, and Miss M. Hudson, Charing Cross and Westminster Hospital School of Medicine all advised and generously assisted us.

Assistance and advice were also received from Mr J.E. Cartledge, Leicester General Hospital; Mr F. Young, Chief Technician, Nottingham University Medical School; and from Mr G. Bottomley, Chief Technician; Mr G.L.C. McTurk, Chief Technician; Mr C.R. de'Lacey, Mrs A. Lea, Mrs C. Libetta, Mrs B. Hayward, Miss S. Uppal, Mr I.

Indans, Mr S. Byrne, Mr I. Paterson, Mr C. Brooks, and Mr H. Kowalski, University of Leicester.

Mr D. Adams, University of Leicester, generously advised us on the preparation of materials and prepared some of the histological specimens.

Professor A.R. Lieberman, Dean, University College, London, generously assumed the task of reading the final manuscript and we are deeply indebted to him for all his work and for his suggestions on Golgi staining.

We are also grateful to Mr G. Tresidder, Consultant Surgeon and Anatomist, to Dr L. Howard, University of Leicester and Dr A. Lawson, University of Ghana, who very generously read the manuscript and commented upon the book. Miss S. Pattani, a medical student, assisted us in some photographs. We are deeply grateful for all their constructive suggestions and interest.

The authors are very grateful to Dr J.M. England, Consultant Haematologist, Watford General Hospital, and to Mr R.H. Wakely, Photographer, who kindly assisted us and encouraged us throughout the preparation, writing and production of this book.

We are also grateful to J.B. Lippincott Company for permission to reproduce one figure from *The Human Brain: a photographic guide* by Gluhbegovic and Williams, 1980.

Springer-Verlag Publishers gave permission to use one figure from *Human Brainstem Vessels* by Professor H.M. Duvernoy. Dr M.B. Carpenter gave permission to reproduce an illustration from his book, *Core Text of Neuroanatomy*. The original photograph was produced by Dr Harry A. Kaplan. The publishers Williams and Wilkins also gave permission for us to use this picture.

An especial acknowledgement is made to Mr K. Garfield, Chief Technician, Central Photographic Unit, University of Leicester, who produced many of the photographs in this book. His expertise and interest have contributed greatly.

The authors are deeply grateful for all the work contributed by Mr Anton Lawrencepulle and Lara Last, Wolfe Publishing, towards the production of this book.

Preface

This Atlas is intended to illustrate those aspects of the normal human brain and spinal cord which are of importance in the study of neuroanatomy. Neuroanatomy is a very difficult subject for the student of medicine or nursing and is often even for the postgraduate, not only because of the three-dimensional nature of the material but because of its complexity and associated vocabulary. However, once knowledge of the vocabulary is acquired, then the functional aspects may be better appreciated; we have designed this book to reflect this approach to learning.

The book is divided into two parts. In the first part the morphology of the brain and spinal cord is presented and the second part illustrates their functional relationships. All of the illustrations in this book are from human material and it is our intention to limit the text wherever possible to the central nervous system. The student should be aware, however, that this separation is an artificial one and that the central nervous system is integrated with the peripheral system. It is suggested that the reader consult the textbooks listed in 'Suggestions for Further Reading' and use them in conjunction with this Atlas.

The descriptions accompanying the photographs are intended to link them and to indicate the relevant features or orientation. It is not the intention to label every structure present on a specimen. Photographs illustrating more than one feature may be used on more than one occasion. In general, the terminology used is based on the 6th edition of the *Nomina Anatomica*. Several older names have been retained, however, because of their current usage in texts and in the medical profession.

Points of historical, physiological or clinical interest have been presented as footnotes marked by a spot. Important terminology appears on grey-coloured pages.

A guide for a student examination of the brain has been included. The pages should be followed sequentially to illustrate the main morphological features of the brain.

This Atlas has been written both as an introduction to neuroanatomy for medical, nursing and paramedical students and as a review for those familiar with this subject. It is our sincere hope that having completed his or her study the reader will have not only an understanding of a very complex and difficult subject, but also an appreciation of the three-dimensional beauty and mystery of the human brain and spinal cord.

STRUCTURAL FEATURES OF THE CENTRAL NERVOUS SYSTEM

AN INTRODUCTION TO THE HUMAN NERVOUS SYSTEM

Central and Peripheral Systems

The brain is an active controller of the body. It receives and processes information from the various sense organs about its external and internal environments. The brain then selects from several possible courses of action and generates and controls the body's responses. The information received from the sense organs may also be stored as a 'memory' to integrate past history and present experience.

The main centres of nervous correlation and integration are the brain and spinal cord. Together they are called the central nervous system (or CNS). Information is transmitted to and from the brain and spinal cord by the peripheral nervous system composed of the cranial and spinal nerves and their associated ganglia. Nerves which carry impulses toward the central nervous system are called afferent (or sensory) and those which carry nerve impulses away from the central nervous system are called efferent (or motor). Afferent or efferent nerves supplying the body wall or extremities are also referred to as *somatic*; and those supplying the smooth muscles of internal organs, the blood vessels, and cardiac muscle are called *visceral*; those supplying glands are called *secretor*.

The brain and spinal cord lie protected in the bony skull and vertebral column. They are bathed and suspended in cerebrospinal fluid which is also found in a series of interconnected cavities inside the brain called the ventricles. The peripheral nervous system, however, usually lies outside the bones and so is not protected by them.

The brain and spinal cord are composed of nerve cells (neurons) supported by specialised cells called neuroglia. Each neuron has a cell body (perikaryon) and several processes. Neurons have traditionally been classified by their size, and by the number, length, and branching of their processes. These processes are classified as axons or dendrites.

An axon is a long process, usually single, that is clearly demarcated from the cell's body at its point of origin from the cell. It generally, but not exclusively, conducts impulses (action potentials) away from the cell body. Axons greater than 1 μm in diameter in the peripheral nervous system and 0.25 μm diameter in the CNS are myelinated. Axons tend to be of a uniform diameter along their length. A distinctive ultrastructural feature of the axon hillock (site of origin from the cell body) and initial segment of the axon is that the microtubules are grouped into bundles and linked by side-arms. In the initial segment, but not in the axon hillock, and also at nodes of Ranvier, an undercoating of dense material underlies the membrane (axolemma) of the axon. Dendrites merge with the contours of the cell body where they arise from it. They are usually multiple, shorter than axons and branch extensively. They form the receptor sites of the cells and so tend to conduct information towards the cell body.

A nerve fibre consists of an axon and its supporting cells. A surrounding basal lamina is present in the peripheral nervous system. Neurons are functionally connected by synapses, specialised sites where information is transmitted across a small gap between one neuron and another by chemical messengers, the neurotransmitters.

Neurotransmitters interact with receptors on the cell body or processes and this interaction leads to a change in a cell function. Neurotransmitters are classified into three groups: excitatory, inhibitory, and those which play a modulatory role in neuronal function. The commonest excitatory neurotransmitter in the central nervous system is glutamic acid (glutamate), an amino acid. The most widespread inhibitory neurotransmitter in the brain is gamma-aminobutyric acid (GABA), and for the spinal cord is glycine. Neurotransmitters that play a modulatory role do not directly excite or inhibit neurons but may, for example, alter their response or sensitivity to an excitatory or inhibitory neurotransmitter. Other common neurotransmitters in the CNS are acetylcholine, dopamine, noradrenaline and the neuropeptides. A further complicating factor is that a given transmitter substance may have either excitatory or inhibitory effects depending on the nature and response of receptors on the post-synaptic membrane of the cell concerned.

A textbook of physiology or pharmacology should be consulted for further detailed information.

The brain and spinal cord are organized into two tissues: grey matter and white matter. The grey matter is composed of neuropil, an intermingling of axons and dendrites where they establish synaptic contact. Grey matter also contains neuronal cell bodies and neuroglia. The white matter is composed of nerve fibres and the surrounding neuroglia. Bundles of nerve fibres in the central nervous system with a common origin and destination are called nerve tracts. In the peripheral nervous system bundles of nerve fibres form peripheral nerves and nerve roots. A pathway is a chain of functionally interconnected neurons.

Additionally, the nerve fibres present in the central and peripheral nervous system may be described as myelinated or unmyelinated fibres. Myelinated nerve fibres are those axons surrounded by an insulating myelin sheath. This myelin sheath is produced by supporting neurological cells called oligodendrocytes in the CNS and by Schwann cells in the peripheral nervous system; the latter facilitate the regeneration of injured fibres.

Autonomic System

This system, a component of both the central and peripheral systems, is responsible, with the endocrine system, for the stability and maintenance of the internal environment. For the most part the autonomic system functions at the subconscious level i.e. structures supplied by the autonomic system have an involuntary innervation. The autonomic system contains both afferent (sensory) and efferent (motor or secretor) fibres, myelinated and unmyelinated fibres, and ganglia. Its activities are, however, integrated with those of the endocrine glands. Nerves pass to involuntary (i.e. smooth or cardiac) muscles in organs of the gastrointestinal tract, bladder, heart, etc., and to exocrine glands e.g. salivary glands, sweat glands, etc.

The autonomic system is further divided into two parts: the sympathetic and parasympathetic parts. The sympathetic part prepares the body for emergencies i.e. fear, rage, strenuous exercise. The heart rate increases and a relative redistribution of the circulation occurs. Blood vessels are constricted in the skin and intestines and blood leaves these areas. The blood pressure rises and the increased supply of blood is made available to the brain, heart and skeletal muscles. Intestinal peristalsis is inhibited and the rectal and bladder sphincters closed. The pupils of the eyes dilate and the body is ready for a 'fight or flight' response.

The parasympathetic part of the autonomic nervous system is responsible for conserving energy and the routine maintenance of bodily activities. It promotes digestion by stimulating peristalsis and the secretions of the glands of the gastrointestinal tract. Stimulation of the parasympathetic system also constricts the pupil, decreases the heart rate and relaxes the rectal and bladder sphincters.

It is characteristic of the autonomic nervous system that the pathway from the central nervous system to the organ supplied is always interrupted by a ganglion. It, therefore, has two components: preganglionic, between the CNS and the ganglion, and postganglionic, between the ganglion and the organ.

While many viscera have both sympathetic and parasympathetic supplies, by which a functional 'balance' is effected, some only have one supply. Equally important is the fact that some viscera are constantly inhibited by one or other of the two components of the autonomic nervous system e.g. the heart.

The classical concept of autonomic nervous system function includes only two neurotransmitters: acetylcholine and noradrenaline (norepinephrine). Acetylcholine occurs throughout the parasympathetic system and in the synapses between preganglionic sympathetic fibres and postganglionic cells in sympathetic ganglia. Noradrenalin occurs in postganglionic sympathetic innervation.

Recent studies on this system have identified other autonomic neurotransmitters. For example, some cells in the ganglia supplying postganglionic sympathetic fibres to the gut contain peptide transmitters (somatostatin, substance P, enkephalin). Similar non-adrenergic, non-cholinergic nerves are present in the wall of the bladder. Their cell bodies lie in the pelvic ganglia.

Nervous Tissue

All nervous tissue consists of nerve cells (neurons), supporting cells (glial cells or neuroglia) and blood vessels.

A neuron consists of the cell body or perikaryon, which contains the nucleus and other organelles, and one or more cell processes. The cell bodies are concentrated in areas of grey matter. A neuronal process together with its sheathing cells, constitutes a nerve fibre. Fibres in the peripheral nervous system have an additional covering of basal lamina. Nerve fibres are concentrated in areas of white matter. Cytoplasmic components and neurotransmitters are synthesized in the cell body and can be transported along the processes by cytoplasmic flow. This mechanism is best understood in axons (axoplasmic flow).

Listed below are the stains and injection media used to prepare specimens illustrated in this Atlas, and the purpose for which they were used.

1 Stains for thick brain slices
With Mulligan's stain the grey matter is blue and the white matter remains unstained.

2 Myelin stains, distinguishing grey matter from white matter by selectively staining myelin sheaths of nerve fibres
Weigert stain
Weigert-Pal stain
Weil's stain
Luxol fast blue stain
Solochrome cyanin stain

3 Stains to show the shape and structure of individual nerve cells or fibres
Cresyl violet stain
Toluidine blue stain
Thionin stain
Golgi Cox stain
Most silver stains including Bodian and Palmgren's stain
Stains for glial cells, including Holtzer's stain

4 Stains to show the general structure and organisation of tissues
Haematoxylin and eosin stain
Phosphotungstic acid and haematoxylin stain
Van Gieson's stain
Light green and orange G stain
De Castro stain (embryos)
Masson's trichrome stain
Carmine stain

5 Counterstains, used to provide a background contrasting colour to the major stain
Nuclear fast red stain
Haematoxylin stain
Light green stain
Fuchsin stains
Neutral red stain

For example, a section stained with Luxol fast blue might be counterstained with acid fuchsin.

6 Specific immunocytochemical stains for particular components of tissues
Neurofilament antigen stain
Glial fibrillary acidic protein stain
Stains for neuropeptides e.g. neuropeptide Y and somatostatin

7 Other stains identifying particular tissue components
Elastin stain for elastic tissue
Osmium tetroxide for lipids
Block staining with silver nitrate for connective tissue

8 Injection media used to demonstrate the distribution of blood vessels at tissue level
Gelatine and carmine
Gelatine and India Ink

9 Stains for transmission electron microscopy to make the tissue electron dense
Lead citrate stain
Uranyl acetate stain

● *In some cases the precise identity of the stain in a loaned section was not known because of the age of the specimen. These sections have been indicated as 'myelin stain' or 'silver stain'. The general nature of the stain is apparent from an examination of the structures displayed in the section.*

● *The depth and colour of Weigert and Weigert-Pal staining may vary according to the staining and the section-mounting conditions, or may fade with time. It is normally a shade of brown, but may fade to a golden or purplish tone.*

A–D

Histological preparations to show neurons and nerve fibres.

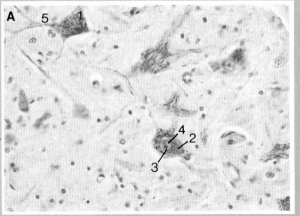

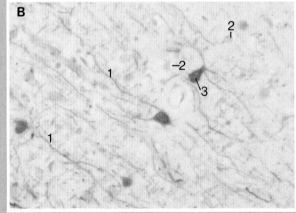

A An histological section showing the parts of a neuron. Cresyl violet stain. x669

1 Cell body
2 Nissl substance
3 Nucleolus
4 Nucleus
5 Process

● *Chromatolysis is the disappearance of Nissl substance staining when the cell's axon is cut.*

B A section of cerebellar cortex stained immuno-cytochemically for the presence of neurofilament antigen, to show the presence of nerve fibres, cell bodies and the nuclei of the unstained neuroglial cells. Haematoxylin counterstain for nuclei. x558.

1 Nerve fibre
2 Neuroglial nucleus
3 Neuronal cell body

Mrs G. Hayward

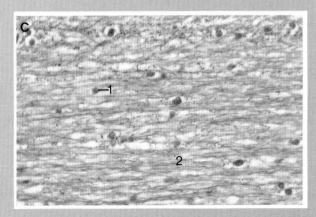

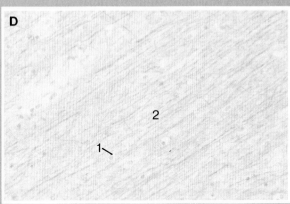

C An area of white matter in the cerebrum, showing nerve fibres in longitudinal section. Palmgren's stain. x558

1 Glial cell nucleus
2 Nerve fibres

Dr A. Fletcher

D An area of white matter from the cerebellum showing nerve fibres in longitudinal section. Neurofilament antigen stain. x335.

1 Glial cell nucleus
2 Nerve fibres

Dr A. Fletcher

13

Neurons are classified according to their shape. This is determined by the number of processes arising from the cell body. Most are multipolar, with many processes. Bipolar cells, found in developing neural tissue and in the retina, have two processes. Unipolar cells, with only one process, are found in the dorsal root ganglia of the spinal cord.

E-G Histological sections to show neuronal shapes.

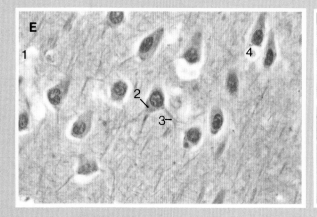

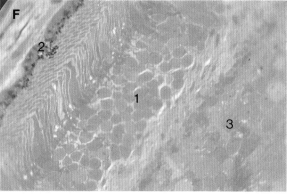

E A group of multipolar neurons in the hippocampus. Silver stain. x558
1 Blood vessel
2 Cell body
3 Cell process of neuron
4 Neuroglial nucleus

F Bipolar cells in the retina. Their lemon-like shape is due to the presence of only one process at each end (pole) of the cell. Toluidine blue stain. x669
1 Bipolar neurons
2 Pigment epithelium
3 Retina

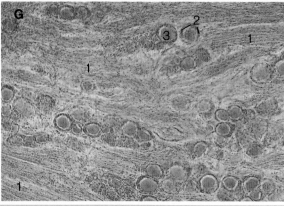

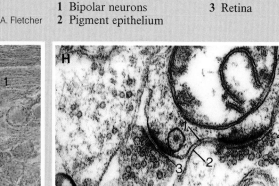

G Unipolar neurons appear circular in section, having only one process. They are usually surrounded by glial cells, the satellite cells. An histological section showing a group of unipolar neurons in a dorsal root ganglion. Unknown stain. x112
1 Nerve fibres
2 Satellite cells
3 Unipolar neuron

H A transmission electron micrograph showing a synapse in the cerebral cortex of a 4-month-old infant. Lead citrate stain. x47,500
1 Post-synaptic membrane
2 Pre-synaptic membrane
3 Synaptic cleft
4 Synaptic vesicles

Information is transferred from one neuron to another at specialised regions of the cell known as synapses.

Synaptic vesicles contain the substances known as neurotransmitters by which means neurons communicate.

- Brain tissues have no sensations. Pain or pressure on non-nervous tissue (e.g. blood vessels, meninges) produces sensations (e.g. headache).

- Santiago Ramón y Cajal (1852–1934), one of the founders of modern neurohistology, made extensive use of silver stains to demonstrate neuronal shapes and connections. These studies led him to develop and defend the Neuronal Theory of neural organization, now known to be correct. This states that nerve cells are separate entities which contact each other, and are not continuous with each other.

- Camillo Golgi (1843–1926) introduced a silver staining method which led to significant advances in the histological study of nervous tissue. He was awarded the Nobel Prize jointly with S. Ramon y Cajal in 1906 for his many contributions to histology.

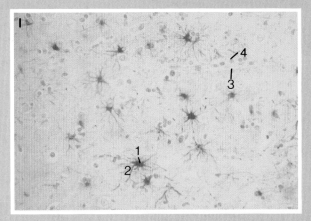

I A section to show astrocytes in grey matter. GFAP stain, haematoxylin counterstain for nuclei. x446
1 Astrocyte
2 Astrocyte process
3 Blood vessel
4 Nucleus of unstained oligodendrocyte

Dr J. Lowe

Astrocytes frequently contact blood vessels. They control the permeability of the vessels by determining that the endothelial cells of the vessels develop tight junctions. They may also have a role in nutrition of the nervous tissue.

Glial Cells

The supporting tissues of the central nervous system are called glial cells. There are three basic types of glial cells: astrocytes which have many processes; oligodendrocytes which have few processes; and microglia which are irregular in shape. Astrocytes and oligodendrocytes are often referred to together as macroglia.

Macroglia: Astrocytes

Astrocytes have many functions; they can take up potassium released during neuronal activity, store glycogen, and phagocytose degenerating synaptic terminals. They can also retrieve GABA and glutamate after these transmitters have been released at nerve terminals.

Astrocytes have many long processes. They may be identified by immunocytochemical staining to demonstrate glial fibrillary acidic protein in the cell (GFAP staining).

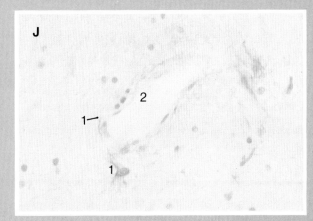

J A section showing astrocyte processes (feet) around a blood vessel in the cerebellar cortex, GFAP stain, haematoxylin counterstain for nuclei. x446
1 Astrocyte processes
2 Blood vessel

Mrs G. Hayward

On the outer surface of the brain astrocyte processes interweave to form a limiting layer. Together with the basal lamina the astrocytic processes form a surface layer, the glia limitans.

K The glia limitans on the outside of the midbrain. GFAP stain. x279

1 Astrocytes
2 Glia limitans
3 Neural tissue
4 Subarachnoid space

Dr A. Fletcher

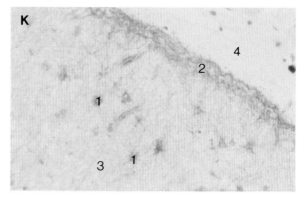

Macroglia: Oligodendrocytes

Oligodendrocytes form the myelin sheaths of myelinated nerve fibres in the central nervous system. Myelin is formed when the oligodendrocyte extends a flap of cell membrane around one or more axons and wraps the membrane many times around the axon. Because of their association with nerve fibres, oligodendrocytes are more prevalent in white matter than in grey matter. Their nuclei are commonly seen in rows between the nerve fibres.

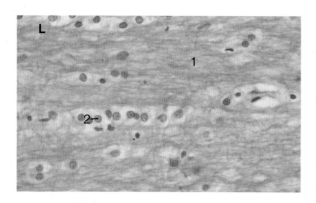

L Oligodendrocyte nuclei and nerve fibres in the white matter of the pons. Haematoxylin and eosin stain. x625

1 Nerve fibres
2 Oligodendrocyte nuclei

M A myelinated nerve fibre from the cerebral cortex showing the relationship between the oligodendrocyte, the myelin sheath and the axon as seen by transmission electron microscopy. Lead citrate stain. x67,250

1 Axon
2 Microtubules
3 Mitochondrion
4 Myelin
5 Oligodendrocyte cytoplasm

Dr J. Lowe

N Detail of the myelin sheath as seen by transmission electron microscopy. Lead citrate stain. x94,150

1 Myelin lamellae
2 Oligodendrocyte cytoplasm

Dr J. Lowe

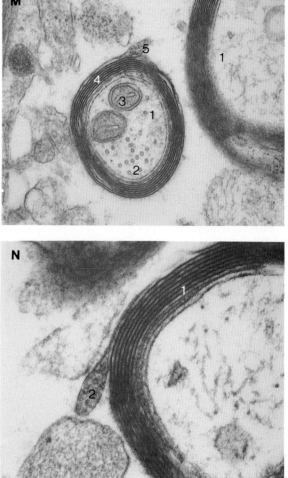

Microglia

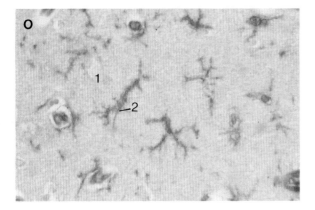

O Microglia in white matter stained by Lectin Ricinus communis Agglutinin-1 (Biotinylated) and detected by avidin-biotin complex with DAB (diamino benzidine). x558
1 Blood vessel
2 Microglial cell

Dr J. Lowe and Mr D. Powe

● *Microglia are macrophages.*

● *Astrocytes retain their ability to divide throughout life.*

● *The commonest origin of cerebral tumours is from the glial cells. Specific staining methods are used to identify the cell type giving rise to the tumour.*

TERMINOLOGY

In topographical anatomy the directional terms used are based on the standing human body and are described as **superior** (towards the head), **inferior** (towards the feet), **anterior** (ventral or abdominal surface of the body) and **posterior** (dorsal or back of the body). In neuroanatomy this terminology remains applicable to the spinal cord, but not to the brain.

The brain is bent across the vertical axis and is too convoluted to employ usefully the same terminology as that for the upright body. Imagine the human body as a straight cylinder, like an earthworm's body, and the central nervous system inside it is stretched out straight. The parts of the central nervous system then lie behind one another in a straight line. This line is the neuraxis. The following terminology can be applied: **rostral** (towards the nose) and **caudal** (towards the tail) and these terms are still used when the neuraxis is bent as in the developing and adult human brain.

An alternative terminology is used in relation to the brain inside the head. **Anterior** is towards the face, **posterior** towards the occipital region, **superior** towards the top of the head, and **inferior** towards the base of the skull.

Another set of terms is used in relation to the spinal cord. Imagine a dog, the spinal cord would have a **dorsal** surface running along its back and a **ventral** surface towards the belly. If the dog stands on its hind legs to imitate the human upright posture these surfaces become **posterior** and **anterior** respectively. These two pairs of terms may be used interchangeably in relation to the spinal cord.

If the brain is sectioned along the neuraxis in the median plane, the section is termed **sagittal** or **median**. Those sections parallel to the sagittal (median) plane are called **paramedian**. Brain sections at right angles to the neuraxis of the forebrain are termed **coronal** while those cut parallel with its superior and inferior margins are **horizontal**. Sections at right angles to the axis of the brain stem are **transverse**; those parallel with its long axis are **longitudinal**.

In association with these spatial terms are the words used to describe the direction of nerve fibres, i.e. **ascending** (running in a rostral direction) and **descending** (running in a caudal direction). If a fibre remains on the same side of the body it is **ipsilateral** to the parent cell body and if it crosses the midline it is said to **decussate** and then it becomes **contralateral** (on the opposite side to the parent cell body).

External structures can be seen on the surface of the brain or spinal cord without cutting it. **Internal** features do not appear on the surface and so can only be seen in sections.

Terminology

Terminology used to indicate directions of the brain.

A An external and lateral view of the brain (left side). x.7
1 Anterior
2 Inferior
3 Lateral
4 Medial (curved arrow at top)
5 Posterior
6 Superior

Because the brain bends during development the orientation is described in relation to two axes.

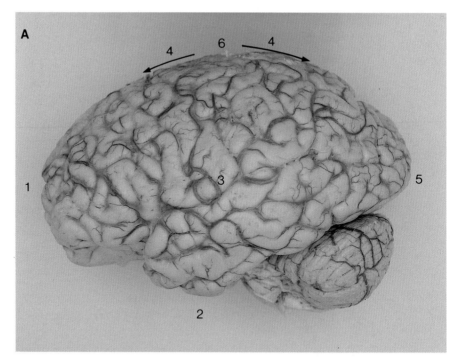

B Orientation of the cerebral hemispheres. x.7
1 Anterior
2 Caudal
3 Inferior
4 Neuraxis (dotted line)
5 Posterior
6 Rostral
7 Superior

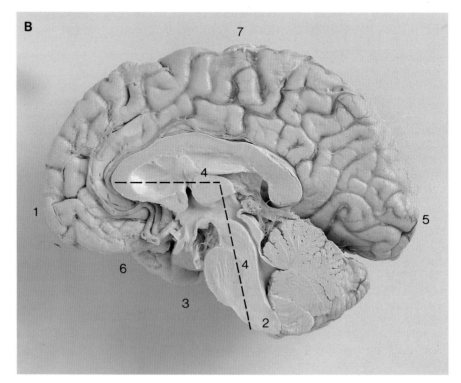

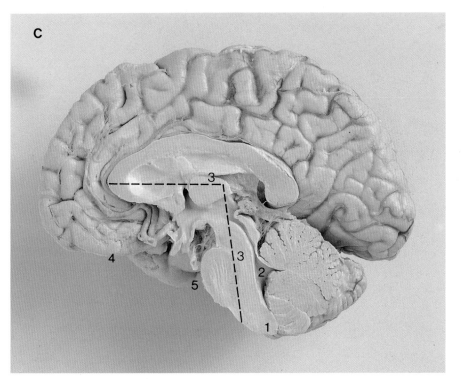

C The longitudinal axis of the brainstem and spinal cord. x.7
1 Caudal
2 Dorsal (posterior)
3 Neuraxis (dotted line)
4 Rostral
5 Ventral (anterior)

Planes of Section

A brain is usually sectioned in the following planes:

A A sagittal or median section through the brain. x.49
1 Caudal
2 Lateral
3 Medial
4 Posterior
5 Rostral (anterior)

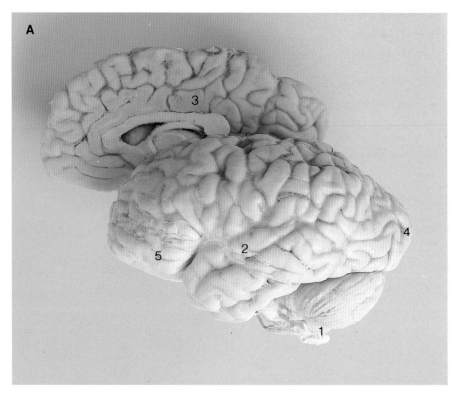

B A sagittal section parallel to the median plane of the brain (paramedian section). x.63
1 Anterior (rostral)
2 Dorsal or superior
3 Lateral
4 Medial
5 Posterior
6 Ventral or inferior

● *The term 'parasagittal' is becoming redundant and 'sagittal' refers to all sections parallel to the median plane*[*]. *Many authors, however, still use 'paramedian' to refer to these sections.*

[*] O'Rahilly, R. *Acta Anat.*, **131**, 1-2: 1988

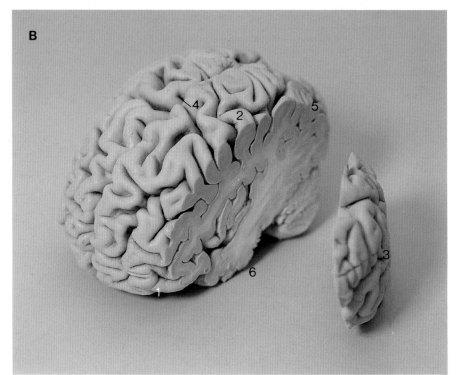

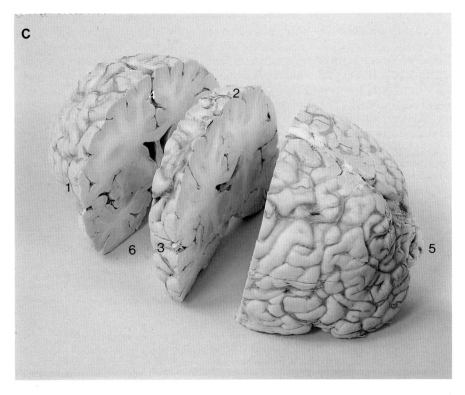

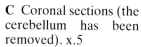

C Coronal sections (the cerebellum has been removed). x.5
1 Anterior (rostral)
2 Dorsal or superior
3 Lateral
4 Medial
5 Posterior
6 Ventral or inferior

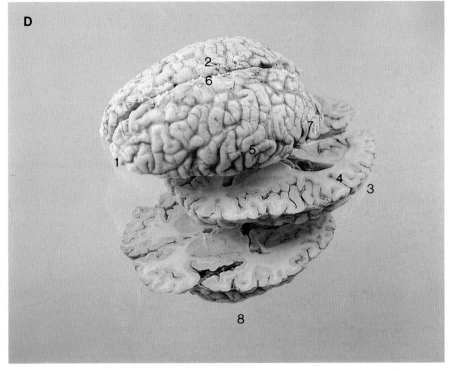

D Horizontal sections. x.42
1 Anterior (rostral)
2 Dorsal or superior
3 External
4 Internal
5 Lateral
6 Medial aspect of brain
7 Posterior
8 Ventral or inferior

21

EMBRYOLOGY

Early Development

The central nervous system develops from a midline ectoderm neural plate (Stage 8, Week 2). Neural folds form, rise and fuse to form a neural tube. Initially, fusion is in the caudal hindbrain and proceeds cranially and caudally until only the two ends of the tube remain open (neuropores). The rostral and caudal neuropores eventually close. When the rostral neuropore closes, this region is known as the lamina terminalis.

The cranial end of the neural tube expands and the main divisions of the central nervous system are established (Week 4); these are the forebrain (prosencephalon), midbrain (mesencephalon), hindbrain (rhombencephalon), and spinal cord. The optic cup is an outgrowth of the forebrain. The midbrain and part of the hindbrain become the brainstem. The cerebellum is also an hindbrain derivative.

In Week 5 the three areas of the brain subdivide to form five regions.

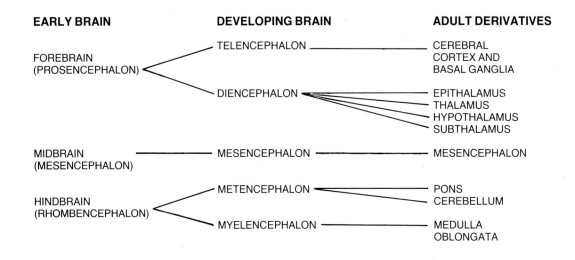

EARLY BRAIN	DEVELOPING BRAIN	ADULT DERIVATIVES
FOREBRAIN (PROSENCEPHALON)	TELENCEPHALON	CEREBRAL CORTEX AND BASAL GANGLIA
	DIENCEPHALON	EPITHALAMUS THALAMUS HYPOTHALAMUS SUBTHALAMUS
MIDBRAIN (MESENCEPHALON)	MESENCEPHALON	MESENCEPHALON
HINDBRAIN (RHOMBENCEPHALON)	METENCEPHALON	PONS CEREBELLUM
	MYELENCEPHALON	MEDULLA OBLONGATA

● *Midbrain and hindbrain derivatives may be defined as forming the brainstem in the adult. Some alternative definitions of brainstem also include the diencephalon.*

Flexures of the Brain

The brain flexures appear early in development. The first, the midbrain flexure, occurs in Week 3 between the forebrain and midbrain. At this flexure the forebrain bends in a ventral direction. During Week 4 the second flexure, the cervical or neck flexure, occurs between the hindbrain and spinal cord. This flexure disappears after the head extends during Week 8. The third flexure, the pontine flexure, occurs during Week 5 in the region of the pons. The appearance of this flexure causes the roof of the rhombencephalon to splay and form a diamond-shape.

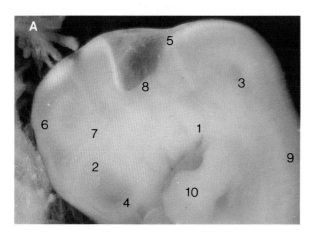

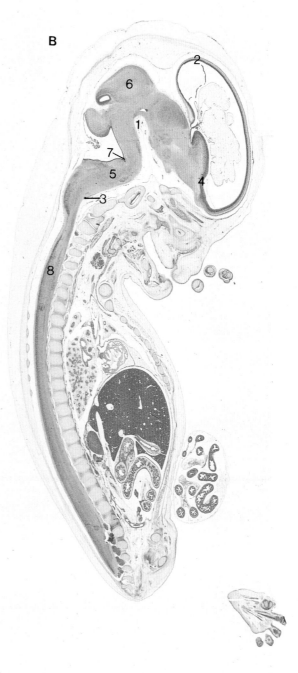

A The early brain flexures of a 12 mmCR (Stage 16) embryo viewed from the side. x13

  1 Branchial arches
  2 Cerebral hemisphere
  3 Cervical flexure
  4 Forebrain
  5 Hindbrain
  6 Midbrain
  7 Midbrain flexure
  8 Pontine flexure
  9 Spinal cord
 10 Upper limb and handplate

B The primary brain flexures illustrated on a 27 mmCR embryo. Haematoxylin and eosin stain. x5

  1 Cephalic (midbrain) flexure
  2 Cerebral hemispheres
  3 Cervical flexure
  4 Forebrain
  5 Hindbrain
  6 Midbrain
  7 Pontine flexure
  8 Spinal cord

MHMS

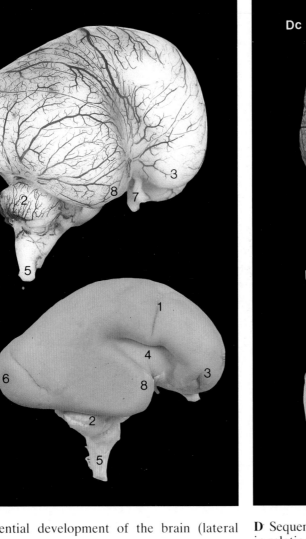

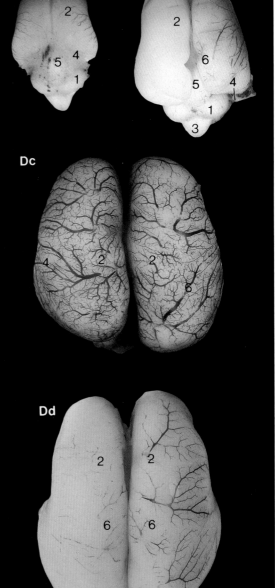

C Sequential development of the brain (lateral view).

a Week 11-12 x1.4
b Week 13-14 x1.4
c Week 17-18 x2.3
d Months 6-7 x1

1 Central sulcus
2 Cerebellum
3 Frontal lobe
4 Insula
5 Medulla oblongata
6 Occipital lobe
7 Olfactory bulb
8 Temporal lobe

a-c Dr G. Batcup **d** RCS

D Sequential expansion of the cerebral hemispheres in relation to the midbrain viewed from above. The meninges have been removed on one side in **b** and **d.**

a Week 11-12 x1.4
b Week 13-14 x1.4
c Week 15 x1.4
d Week 17-18 x1.4

1 Cerebellum
2 Cerebral hemispheres
3 Medulla oblongata
4 Meninges
5 Midbrain
6 Parietal lobe

a-c Dr G. Batcup

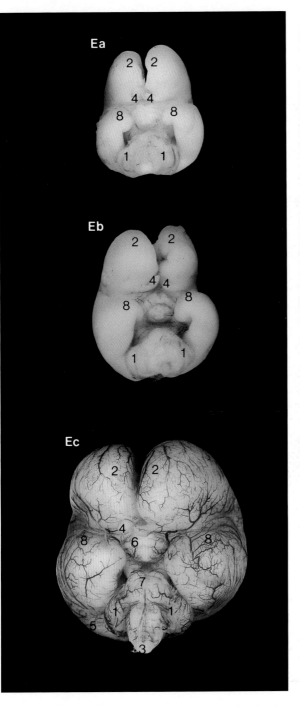

E Sequential series of development of the brain viewed from below.

a Week 13-14 x1.67   **c** Week 17-18 x1.3
b Week 15 x1.67

1 Cerebellum	**5** Occipital lobe
2 Frontal lobe	**6** Optic nerve
3 Medulla oblongata	**7** Pons
4 Olfactory bulb	**8** Temporal lobe

F Sagittal sections of fetal brain to illustrate sequential development.

a Week 8 x1.4   **c** Months 6-7 x1
b Week 13-14 x1.2

1 Cerebellum	**5** Occipital lobe
2 Cerebral hemispheres	**6** Parietal lobe
3 Frontal lobe	**7** Temporal lobe
4 Medulla oblongata	

a-c Dr G. Batcup

b Dr G. Batcup **c** RCS

Cavities of the Brain

The lumen of the early neural tube is retained in the adult brain and spinal cord.

Two balloon-like cerebral vesicles grow out at the rostral end of the forebrain (telencephalon). The hollow space inside each hemisphere is called the lateral ventricle and is continuous through the interventricular foramen with the original space in the forebrain (diencephalon) which becomes the third ventricle. The third ventricle is continuous with the lumen of the midbrain (cerebral aqueduct) which, in turn, is continuous with the lumen of the hindbrain (fourth ventricle). At the boundary between the midbrain and hindbrain is a distinct constriction, or isthmus. The diamond-shaped hindbrain's fourth ventricle and the central canal of the spinal cord merge without a distinct boundary. The floor of the fourth ventricle is diamond-shaped.

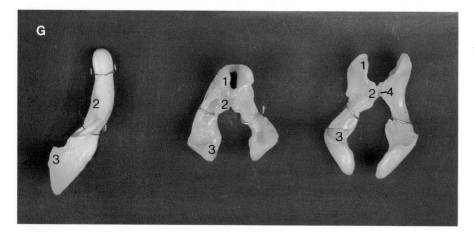

G Plastic casts of the developing ventricles in Weeks 12-24. x1.01
1 Anterior horn of the lateral ventricle
2 Body of lateral ventricle
3 Inferior horn of the lateral ventricle
4 Third ventricle

RCS

H Ventricular cast superimposed on the base of the brain (130 mmCR fetus) to show its position in relation to the external features of the brain. x1.9
1 Anterior horn of the lateral ventricle
2 Body of lateral ventricle
3 Cerebellum
4 Frontal lobe
5 Inferior horn of the lateral ventricle
6 Occipital lobe
7 Spinal cord
8 Temporal lobe

RCS

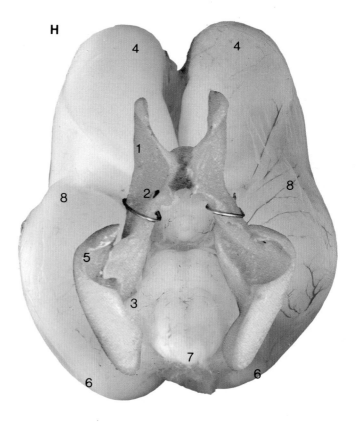

Choroid Plexus

The choroid plexus forms when blood vessels and pia mater invaginate the thin, ependymal medial wall of the cerebral hemispheres (choroidal fissure), and the thin, ependymal roofs of the thalamus and hindbrain. These plexuses form the choroid plexuses of the lateral, third and fourth ventricles.

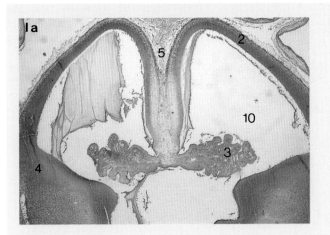

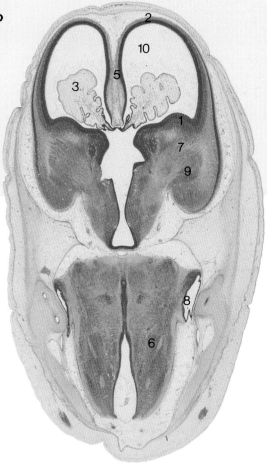

I The developing choroid plexus.

a A coronal paraffin wax section through the lateral ventricles of a 22 mmCR embryo. De Castro stain. x21
b A Week 10 (57 mmCR) fetus sectioned through the midbrain. Haematoxylin and eosin stain. x8.8

  1 Caudate nucleus
  2 Cerebral hemisphere
  3 Choroid plexus
  4 Corpus striatum
  5 Forebrain
  6 Hindbrain
  7 Internal capsule
  8 Lateral recess
  9 Lentiform nucleus
10 Ventricle (lateral)

MHMS

Corpus Striatum

As the two cerebral hemispheres (telencephalon) expand they develop a C-shape, with the formation of the temporal lobe. The lateral ventricle inside each hemisphere similarly becomes C-shaped.

A swelling, the corpus striatum, develops in the floor of each lateral ventricle. As the ventricle becomes C-shaped the caudal end of the corpus striatum becomes drawn out with it, forming the tail of the caudate nucleus and the amygdaloid nucleus on its distal end. Thus the caudate nucleus assumes the C-shaped conformation seen in the adult brain.

Expansion of the cerebral hemisphere brings the medial aspect of the hemisphere into contact with the lateral side of the diencephalon, in the region of the future thalamus. The surfaces adhere and tissue continuity is established, with the thalamus and corpus striatum adjacent to each other.

Projection fibres begin to form to link the cerebral hemisphere with the diencephalon and brainstem. These split the corpus striatum into two parts, the caudate nucleus medially and the lentiform nucleus laterally. They grow through the region between the corpus striatum and the thalamus, forming the internal capsule.

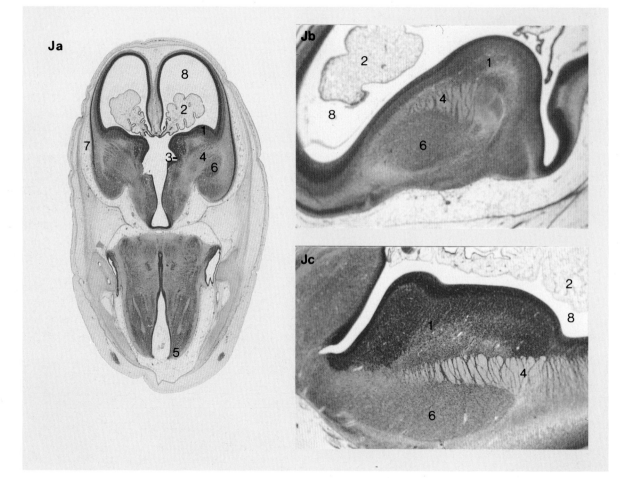

J The development of the corpus striatum, internal capsule, caudate and lentiform nuclei. Haematoxylin and eosin stain.
a A Week 10 (57 mmCR) fetus sectioned through the basal ganglia. Haematoxylin and eosin stain. x6.8
b A paraffin wax section through the basal ganglia of a 35 mmCR fetus. Haematoxylin and eosin stain. x22
c A paraffin wax section through the basal ganglia of a 3 month fetus. Haematoxylin and eosin stain. x22

1 Caudate nucleus
2 Choroid plexus
3 Hypothalamic sulcus
4 Internal capsule
5 Hindbrain
6 Lentiform nucleus
7 Meninx
8 Ventricle (lateral)

MHMS

Histological development of the Cerebral Cortex

Four fundamental layers are formed in the embryonic CNS. From them all the adult components develop. Initially there is one pseudostratified layer of neuroepithelial cells, the ventricular zone. A second zone is formed when the nuclei of these cells congregate around the lumen of the neural tube, leaving an outer layer made up mainly of cell processes, the marginal zone. Cells then migrate out of the ventricular zone to create a third layer between the ventricular and marginal zones; this is the intermediate zone. The fourth layer is the subventricular zone, lying between the ventricular and the intermediate zones (Boulder Committee terminology, *Anat. Rec.* **166**: 257-262, 1970). In the developing cerebral cortex,

cells migrate out from the intermediate zone to form an extra layer, the cortical plate, between the intermediate and marginal zones. Cell rearrangement within the cortical plate creates the layers of mature neocortex. Nerve fibres, the corticopetal fibres, entering the developing cortex from other parts of the brain are a trigger for neuronal maturation.

Most of the adult cortex is called neocortex and has six layers numbered I to VI. Layer I forms first in the marginal layer. Layers II to VI form in the cortical plate from the inside outwards. Successive waves of cells migrate into the cortical plate across the intermediate zone.

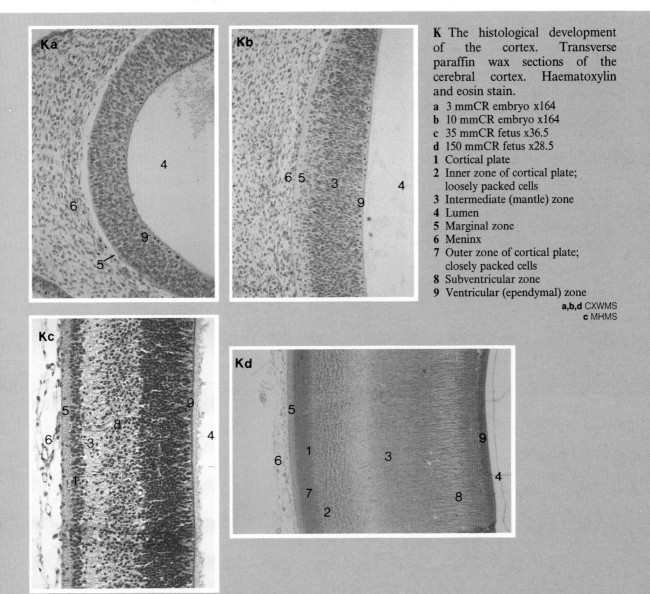

K The histological development of the cortex. Transverse paraffin wax sections of the cerebral cortex. Haematoxylin and eosin stain.

a 3 mmCR embryo x164
b 10 mmCR embryo x164
c 35 mmCR fetus x36.5
d 150 mmCR fetus x28.5
1 Cortical plate
2 Inner zone of cortical plate; loosely packed cells
3 Intermediate (mantle) zone
4 Lumen
5 Marginal zone
6 Meninx
7 Outer zone of cortical plate; closely packed cells
8 Subventricular zone
9 Ventricular (ependymal) zone

a,b,d CXWMS
c MHMS

Cerebellum

The cerebellum forms from cells in the rhombic lip and dorsal part of the alar lamina of the metencephalon. Initially they then enlarge and overgrow the rostral half of the fourth ventricle. The pons and medulla oblongata are overlapped in this process.

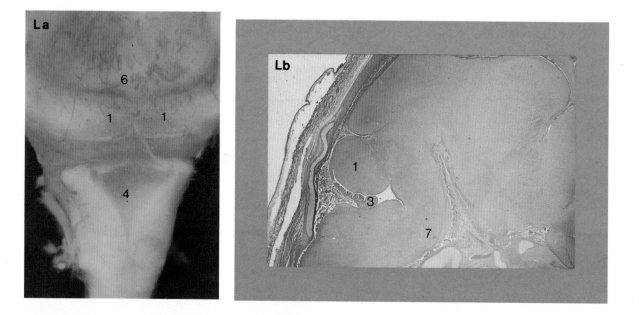

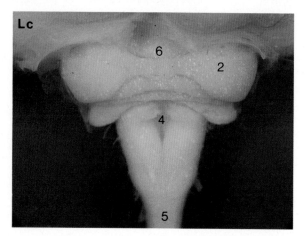

L Development of the cerebellum
a Week 10 57 mmCR fetus x14.6
b Week 10 57 mmCR fetus De Castro stain. x7.1
c Week 15 123 mmCR fetus x3.7
1 Cerebellum
2 Cerebellar hemisphere
3 Choroid plexus in fourth ventricle
4 Fourth ventricle with roof removed
5 Medulla oblongata
6 Mesencephalon
7 Pontine flexure

b CXWMS

• *The cerebellar cortex forms by cell migration in a different manner to the cerebral cortex. Stellate and granular cells are formed from a superficial secondary germinal layer, the outer granular layer from which cells migrate inwards to populate the cortex. The Purkinje cells are formed from the ventricular zone.*

Cranial nerves

The olfactory nerves (I) are processes of bipolar neurons in the olfactory epithelium. The optic nerve (II) is a brain pathway. The remaining cranial nerves (III-XII) can be divided into those without ganglia (III, IV, VI, XI, XII) and those which possess ganglia (V, VII, VIII, IX, X). Those with ganglia contain sensory or autonomic components or both. The ganglia are formed by a combination of neural crest cells and cells derived from a thickening (placode) of the ectoderm. In this they differ from dorsal root (sensory) ganglia of the spinal cord and the autonomic ganglia of the sympathetic chain which do not have a placodal component.

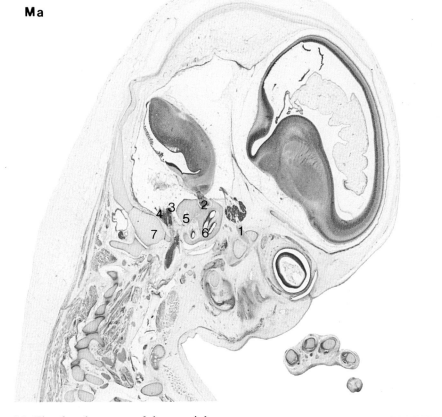

Ma

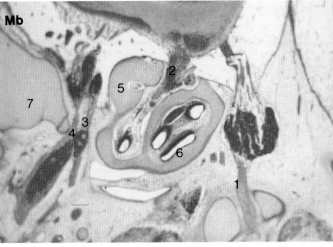

Mb

M The development of the cranial nerves.
a A longitudinal paraffin wax section of a 35 mmCR fetus. Haematoxylin and eosin stain. x6.2
b A close-up of the brainstem showing the emergence of nerves V, VIII, IX, and X and their associated ganglia. Haematoxylin and eosin stain. x9
1 V nerve and ganglion
2 VIII nerve
3 IX nerve and ganglia
4 X nerve and ganglia
5 Petrous temporal cartilage
6 Semicircular canals
7 Skull base

MHMS

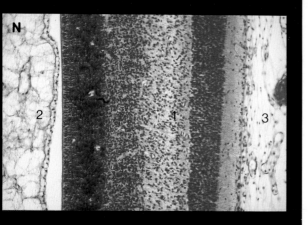

Meninges

The meninges form from mesoderm condensing around the neural tube to form the primitive meninx. The outer part of the meninx forms dura mater, and the inner forms pià-arachnoid. The neural crest contributes to the latter layer. The subarachnoid space forms as fluid accumulates in the pia-arachnoid layer. A layer of cells on the outside of the arachnoid acts as a barrier to the fluid. This fluid is the cerebrospinal fluid and it is produced by the choroid plexus (see page **71**).

N Medial side of the cerebral hemisphere with meninx of a three month fetus. Haematoxylin and eosin stain. x45
1 Brain
2 Choroid plexus
3 Meninx

MHMS

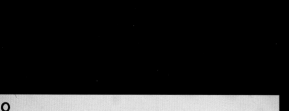

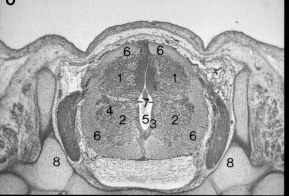

Alar and Basal Plates

Cell bodies of developing neurons collect around the lumen of the neural tube forming the intermediate zone, while their processes (nerve fibres) form the marginal layer on the outside. The cross-sectional profile of the lumen becomes diamond-shaped. The sulcus limitans in the side wall of the lumen divides the mantle layer into alar plate above and basal plate below. Structures which are derived from the alar plate will have sensory functions and those from the basal plate will be motor.

O A transverse paraffin wax section through the thoracic level of the spinal cord in a 22 mmCR embryo. The alar and basal plates are shown. De Castro stain. x22
1 Alar plate
2 Basal plate
3 Ependyma
4 Intermediate zone
5 Lumen
6 Marginal layer
7 Sulcus limitans
8 Vertebra

MHMS

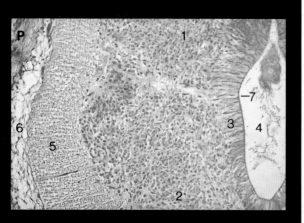

P A higher magnification of Figure **O** to show the alar and basal plates. The alar plate becomes the dorsal (posterior) horn and the basal plate becomes the ventral (anterior) horn and the lateral horn. The marginal layer becomes the white matter. De Castro stain. x89
1 Alar plate
2 Basal plate
3 Ependyma
4 Lumen
5 Marginal layer
6 Meninx
7 Sulcus limitans

MHMS

Q-S Sequential stages in the development of the brainstem to show the fate of the alar and basal plates.

Q A paraffin wax section through the head of a 22 mmCR embryo passing through the hindbrain (myelencephalon) and forebrain (diencephalon and telencephalon), to show the formation of the lateral, third and fourth ventricles and the alar and basal plates. De Castro stain. x6.8

• *The diencephalon has no basal plate; the alar plate forms both thalamus and hypothalamus.*

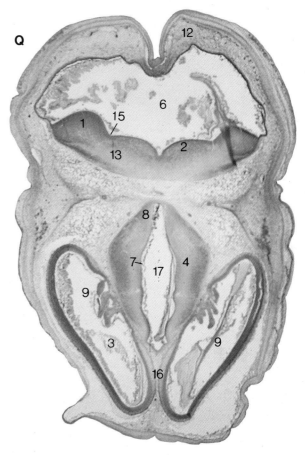

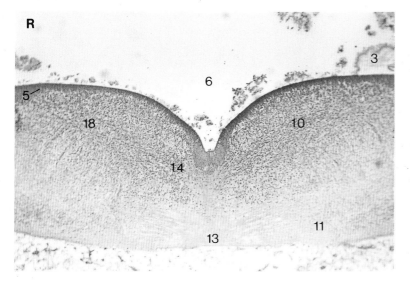

R Transverse histological section through the basal plate of the myelencephalon to show the formation of cell columns which will become motor cranial nerve nuclei. Cell columns in the alar plate become sensory nuclei. De Castro stain. x30

 1 Alar plate
 2 Basal plate
 3 Choroid plexus
 4 Diencephalon
 5 Ependyma
 6 Fourth ventricle
 7 Hypothalamic sulcus
 8 Hypothalamus
 9 Lateral ventricle
 10 Mantle (intermediate) layer
 11 Marginal layer
 12 Meninx
 13 Myelencephalon
 14 Somatic motor cell column
 15 Sulcus limitans
 16 Telencephalon
 17 Third ventricle
 18 Visceral motor cell column

S A coronal paraffin wax section through the head and neck of a three months fetus to show the formation of nuclei in the midbrain and medulla. Haematoxylin and eosin stain. x3.5

  1 Alar plate
  2 Basal plate
  3 Base of skull
  4 Cerebral aqueduct
  5 Cerebral hemispheres
  6 Cerebral peduncle
  7 Choroid plexus
  8 Dorsal root ganglion
  9 Epiphysis
 10 External ear
 11 First cervical nerve root
 12 Humerus
 13 Hypoglossal nerve
 14 Hypoglossal nucleus
 15 Inferior olivary nucleus
 16 Inner ear
 17 Internal jugular vein
 18 Jugular foramen
 19 Lateral ventricle
 20 Medulla oblongata
 21 Meninx
 22 Mesencephalic trigeminal nucleus
 23 Midbrain
 24 Nuclei of vestibulocochlear nerve
 25 Oculomotor nucleus
 26 Pyramid of medulla oblongata
 27 Red nucleus
 28 Shoulder
 29 Solitary nucleus
 30 Spinal cord
 31 Spinal trigeminal nucleus
 32 Substantia nigra
 33 Sulcus limitans
 34 Tectum
 35 Vertebral artery
 36 Vertebral column
 37 Vestibulocochlear nerve

MHMS

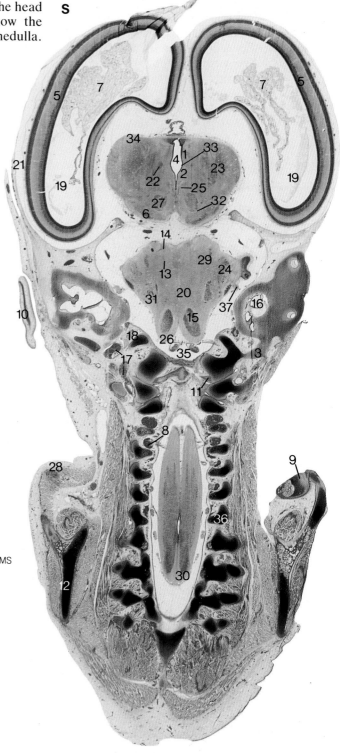

● *The presence of cervical, pontine and midbrain flexures between the divisions of the developing central nervous system explains why forebrain,* *midbrain, hindbrain and spinal cord are all cut in the same coronal section.*

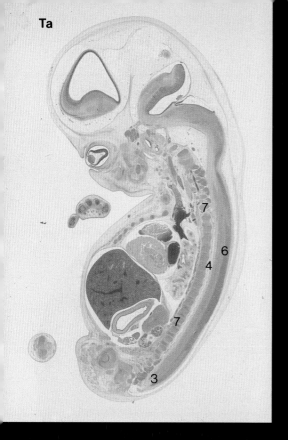

Ta

Spinal Cord

T The sequential changes in spinal cord development showing its change in relative length compared with the vertebral column.

a The spinal cord occupies the length of the spinal column. 25 mmCR embryo. Haematoxylin and eosin stain. x3.9

b The spinal cord in a 40 mmCR fetus in a longitudinal histological section. Haematoxylin and eosin stain. x.2.4

c A dissection of the spinal cord in a fetus. x1.1

1 Cervical expansion
2 Lumbar expansion
3 Sacral cord
4 Spinal canal
5 Spinal nerves
6 Thoracic cord
7 Vertebral column

a,b CXWMS
c RCS

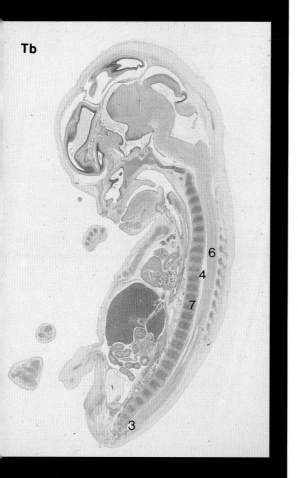

Tb

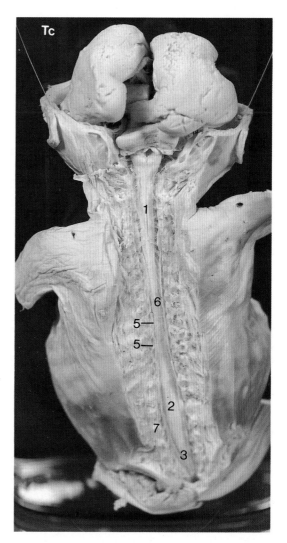

Tc

CRANIAL CAVITY

The brain lies within the cranial cavity of the skull and is continuous with the spinal cord lying within the vertebral canal. The brain and spinal cord are covered with three protective layers called the meninges (see Meninges page **41**).

The floor of the cranial cavity is divided into three regions separated by two descending steps. These regions are the anterior, middle and posterior cranial fossae.

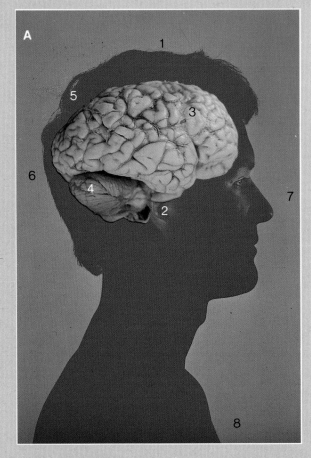

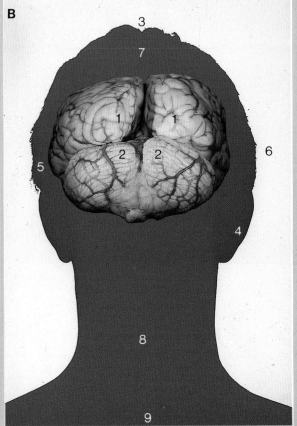

A Position of the brain *in situ* (viewed from the right side). x.33
1 Dorsal or superior
2 External acoustic meatus
3 Cerebral hemisphere
4 Cerebellum
5 Hair
6 Posterior
7 Rostral or anterior
8 Ventral or inferior

B Position of the brain *in situ* (viewed from the back). x.4
1 Cerebral hemisphere
2 Cerebellum
3 Dorsal or superior
4 Ear
5 Hair
6 Lateral
7 Medial
8 Neck
9 Ventral or inferior

C A transilluminated view of the base of the skull (internal aspect). x.62
1 Anterior cranial fossa
2 Body of sphenoid bone
3 Carotid canal
4 Foramen magnum
5 Frontal bone
6 Middle cranial fossa
7 Occipital bone
8 Parietal bone
9 Petrous temporal bone
10 Posterior cranial fossa

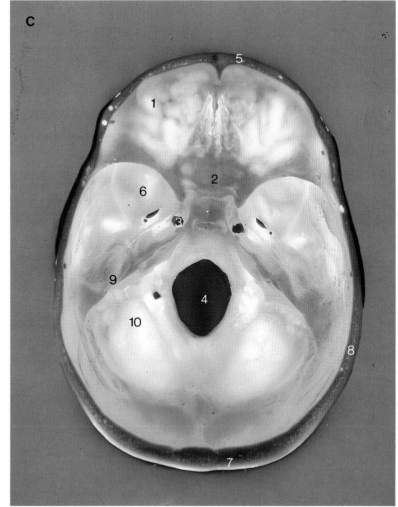

D Sagittal radiographic image electronically reconstructed from computerized tomography (CT) scans to show the cranial cavity in relation to the external features of the head.
1 Anterior cranial fossa
2 External auditory meatus
3 Hypophyseal fossa
4 Larynx
5 Middle cranial fossa
6 Nasal cavity
7 Oral cavity
8 Orbit
9 Posterior cranial fossa
10 Skull vault
11 Vertebral column

Elscint Ltd

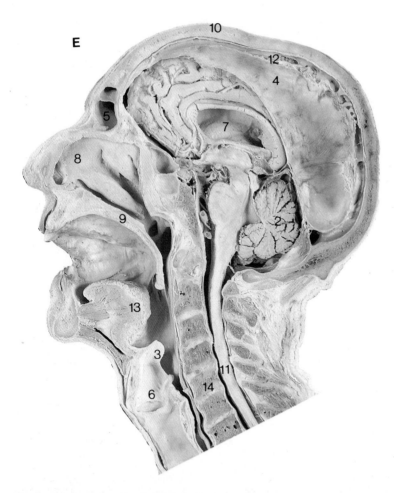

E The brain and meninges within the cranial cavity. The left half of a sagittal section. x.44

1 Cerebral hemisphere
2 Cerebellum
3 Epiglottis
4 Falx cerebri
5 Frontal sinus
6 Larynx
7 Lateral ventricle
8 Nasal cavity
9 Palate
10 Skull
11 Spinal cord
12 Superior sagittal sinus
13 Tongue
14 Vertebral column

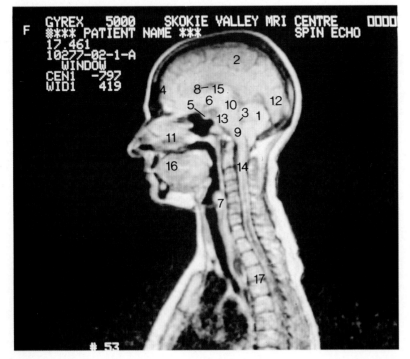

F Nuclear magnetic resonance (NMR) image of a sagittal section through the head and neck.

1 Cerebellum
2 Cerebral hemisphere
3 Fourth ventricle
4 Frontal lobe
5 Hypophysis
6 Hypothalamus
7 Larynx
8 Lateral ventricle
9 Medulla oblongata
10 Midbrain
11 Nasal cavity
12 Occipital lobe
13 Pons
14 Spinal cord
15 Thalamus
16 Tongue
17 Vertebral column

Elscint Ltd

EXTERNAL FEATURES OF THE BRAIN

The major regions of the brain are based upon their position in the skull.

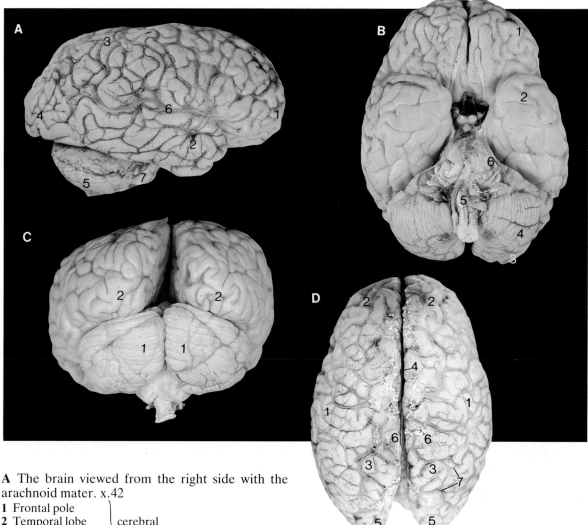

A The brain viewed from the right side with the arachnoid mater. x.42

1 Frontal pole ⎫
2 Temporal lobe ⎬ cerebral
3 Parietal lobe ⎭ hemisphere
4 Occipital lobe
5 Cerebellar hemisphere
6 Lateral sulcus
7 Medulla oblongata

B The base of the brain viewed from below. Most of the arachnoid mater and minor blood vessels have been removed. x.5

1 Frontal lobe ⎫
2 Temporal lobe ⎬ cerebral hemisphere
3 Occipital pole ⎭
4 Cerebellar hemisphere
5 Medulla oblongata
6 Pons

C The back (posterior poles) of the cerebral hemispheres and cerebellum. x.42

1 Cerebellar hemisphere
2 Occipital lobe of cerebral hemisphere

D The brain viewed from above. x.5

1 Cerebral hemisphere
2 Frontal lobe of cerebral hemisphere
3 Gyri
4 Longitudinal fissure
5 Occipital lobe of cerebral hemisphere
6 Parietal lobe of cerebral hemisphere
7 Sulci

● *Lobe refers to an entire area, while pole refers to its extremity.*

INTERNAL FEATURES OF THE BRAIN

Most brainstem structures are not visible externally. They can be seen in a sagittal section.

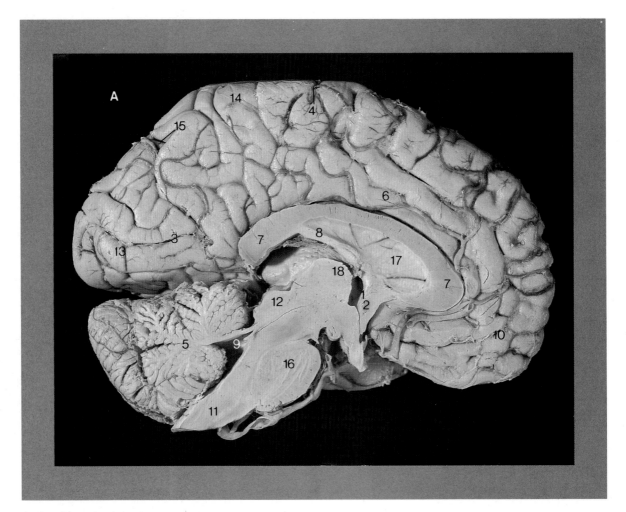

A A mid-sagittal section of the brain. x1

1 Anterior column of the fornix	**7** Corpus callosum
2 Anterior commissure	**8** Fornix (body)
3 Calcarine sulcus	**9** Fourth ventricle
4 Central sulcus	**10** Frontal lobe
5 Cerebellum	**11** Medulla oblongata
6 Cingulate gyrus	**12** Midbrain

13 Occipital lobe
14 Parietal lobe
15 Parieto-occipital sulcus
16 Pons
17 Septum pellucidum
18 Thalamus

● *The pineal gland and the cerebral aqueduct (of Sylvius) are not shown on this specimen, see Cerebral Hemispheres D on page 83.*

● *The brainstem comprises the midbrain, pons, and medulla oblongata.*

● *The fornix and corpus callosum are 'arched' in shape, and the different parts have different names.*

● *For a more detailed nomenclature see the individual regions.*

● *The terms 'medulla oblongata' and the commonly used shortened form 'medulla' may be used interchangeably.*

MENINGES

The brain and spinal cord are protected by three membranes called meninges. The outermost is the dura mater, the middle one the arachnoid mater, and the inner one next to the nervous tissue is the pia mater. These layers have a protective function; they enclose the central nervous system and anchor it against sudden movements. They also enclose the cerebrospinal fluid, which forms a fluid cushion to protect the brain from trauma and is an intermediary in the exchange of substances between the brain and the rest of the body. The arachnoid mater is an important component of the blood-brain barrier (see page **69**) by means of which an optimal environment is created and maintained for the cells of the central nervous system.

The cranial dura mater is a double layer of tough connective tissue. Its outer layer adheres to the bones of the skull and forms their periosteum. Its inner layer, the true dura mater, lines the skull and forms sheets of tissue which dip between the cerebral hemispheres (falx cerebri), between the cerebellar hemispheres (falx cerebelli) and between the cerebellum and the cerebrum (tentorium cerebelli). The dura mater forms a pathway for the cranial venous sinuses. The spinal dura mater does not form the periosteum of the vertebral canal, only the true dura mater is present.

The arachnoid mater is composed of connective tissue with flat interdigitating cells on its surface. A narrow potential space, the subdural space, lies between the arachnoid and the dura mater. It contains only a little serous lubricating fluid. A wider space, the subarachnoid space, separates the arachnoid from the pia mater. It is crossed by connections, the arachnoid trabeculations, which run between the arachnoid mater and the pia mater. It contains the arteries and veins of the brain and spinal cord and the cerebrospinal fluid. The subarachnoid space is sealed off by the interdigitations and tight junctions between the cells on the arachnoid surface known as mesothelial cells. In the region of the superior sagittal sinus (see veins page **63**) the arachnoid mater projects through small openings in the dura mater. These projections resemble granules (arachnoid granulations). Their function is to return cerebrospinal fluid (CSF) to the blood in the superior sagittal sinus in the process of CSF circulation.

The pia mater is very thin and rich in capillaries. It is attached to the brain, closely following the contours of its folds (gyri) and fissures (sulci). It is also closely bound to the spinal cord. Additionally the spinal pia mater forms an anchoring sheet, the denticulate ligament. Within the brain, the tela choroidea are thin areas in the roof of the third and fourth ventricles and the wall of the lateral ventricle. They consist of an adherent layer of pia mater and ependyma and give rise to the choroid plexus.

● *The arachnoid and pia mater are collectively referred to as leptomeninges.*

● *Blood haemorrhaging between the dura mater and the skull forms an epidural (extradural) haematoma. Blood haemorrhaging between the dura mater and arachnoid mater forms a subdural haematoma, while haemorrhaging below the arachnoid is a subarachnoid haemorrhage.*

● *An epidural or extradural space is normally found around the spinal cord. It contains fat and veins, the epidural venous plexus, which drains the marrow spaces of the vertebral bodies and empties into the segmental veins.*

● *Meningitis is an infection of the meninges. Usually the arachnoid and pia mater are involved (lepromeningitis).*

A-D The dura mater and its blood supply.

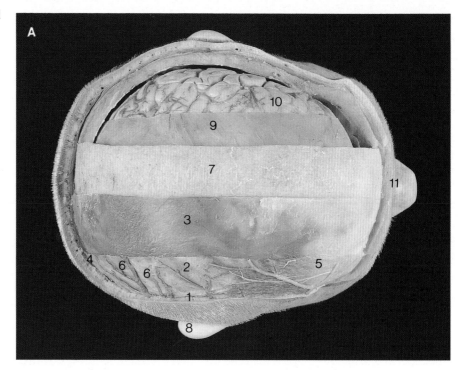

A Layered dissection of the scalp, cranial vault and its coverings viewed from above. x.54

1 Skin and dense subcutaneous tissue ⎱
2 Epicranial aponeurosis   ⎱ Five
3 Loose connective tissue and   ⎰ layers
   pericranium   of
4 Occipital belly of   scalp
   occipitofrontalis muscle ⎰
5 Frontal belly of
   occipitofrontalis muscle

6 Branches of superficial temporal artery
7 Cranial vault bone
8 External ear
9 Dura mater   ⎱ Meninges
10 Pia-arachnoid mater ⎰
11 Nose

Dissection by: Bari M. Logan

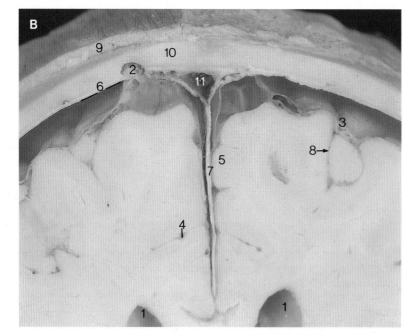

B A coronal section through the superior sagittal sinus. x1.35

1 Anterior horns of lateral ventricles
2 Arachnoid granulation
3 Arachnoid mater
4 Blood vessel
5 Cerebral cortex
6 Dura mater
7 Falx cerebri
8 Pia mater (arrow)
9 Scalp
10 Skull
11 Superior sagittal sinus

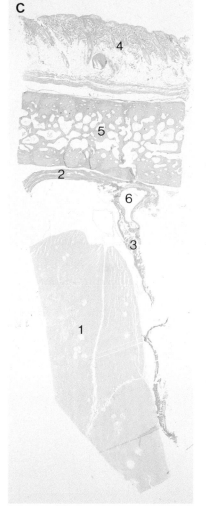

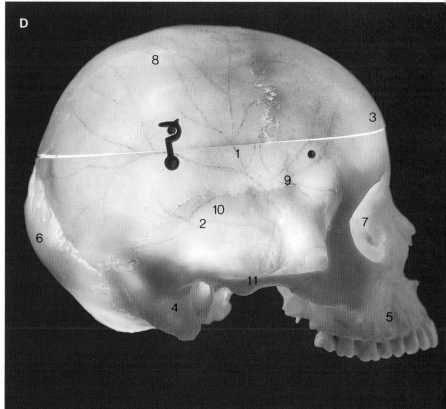

C Coronal section of the skull and meninges. Orange G and light green stain. x4.2

1 Cerebral hemisphere
2 Dura mater
3 Falx cerebri
4 Scalp (with hair-roots)
5 Skull bone
6 Superior sagittal sinus

D A transilluminated adult skull to illustrate the course of the middle meningeal artery in relation to the pterion. x.72

1 Course of the anterior branch of the middle meningeal artery and its branches
2 Course of the posterior branch of the middle meningeal artery and its branches
3 Frontal bone
4 Mastoid process
5 Maxilla
6 Occipital bone
7 Orbit
8 Parietal bone
9 Pterion
10 Squamous temporal bone
11 Zygomatic arch

E-H Histological sections of the meninges.

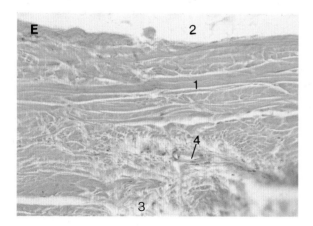

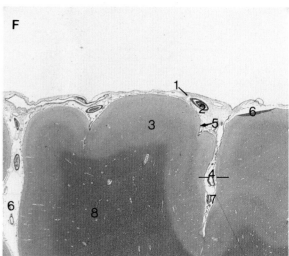

F

E The dura mater is composed of numerous collagen bundles. It has a rich blood supply and innervation. Haematoxylin and eosin stain. x279
1 Collagen bundles
2 External aspect
3 Internal aspect
4 Small blood vessel

F Histological section to show the arachnoid mater bridging the sulci of the cerebral hemisphere, stained with phosphotungstic acid and haematoxylin. x4
1 Arachnoid mater
2 Blood vessel
3 Cerebral cortex
4 Gyri
5 Pia mater (arrow)
6 Subarachnoid space
7 Sulcus
8 White matter

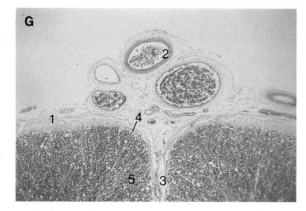

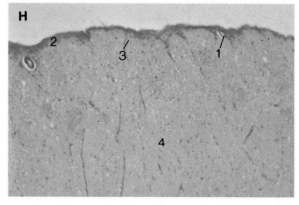

G Histological section to show the leptomeninges (the arachnoid and pia maters) investing the spinal cord. Weigert-Pal stain. x56
1 Arachnoid mater
2 Blood vessel
3 Median fissure (of the spinal cord)
4 Pia mater
5 White matter (of spinal cord)

H Histological section showing prolongations of the pia mater with capillaries, entering the white matter of the midbrain. Van Gieson stain. x89
1 Capillary
2 Pia mater
3 Prolongation of pia mater
4 White matter

Mr D. Adams

CAM

I-R Specialisations of the meninges.

I-J Specialisations of the dura mater.

I

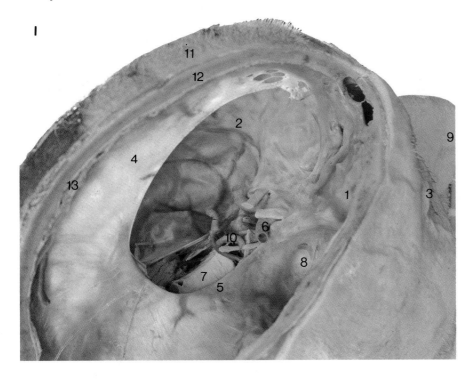

I Cranial cavity viewed from the right side and above, with the falx cerebri and tentorium cerebelli. The midbrain is *in situ*. x.74

1 Anterior cranial fossa
2 Branches of middle meningeal artery
3 Eyelid
4 Falx cerebri
5 Free margin of tentorium cerebelli
6 Internal carotid artery
7 Midbrain
8 Middle cranial fossa
9 Nose
10 Posterior cerebral artery
11 Scalp
12 Skull bone
13 Superior sagittal sinus

J

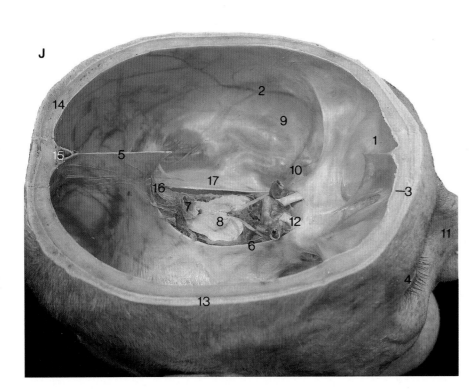

J The interior of the cranial cavity viewed from above to display the arrangement of the dura mater. Both cerebral hemispheres have been removed and the brainstem severed through the midbrain. x.6

1 Anterior cranial fossa
2 Branches of middle meningeal artery
3 Dura mater
4 Eyelid
5 Falx cerebri
6 Free edge of tentorium cerebelli
7 Great vein (of Galen)
8 Midbrain
9 Middle cranial fossa
10 Middle meningeal artery
11 Nose
12 Optic nerve
13 Scalp
14 Skull bone
15 Superior sagittal sinus
16 Tentorial notch
17 Tentorium cerebelli

K-N Specialisations of the arachnoid mater.

K

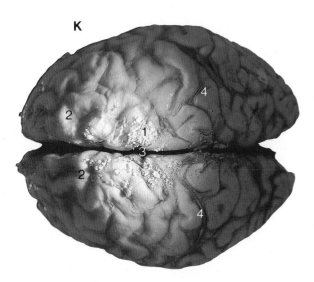

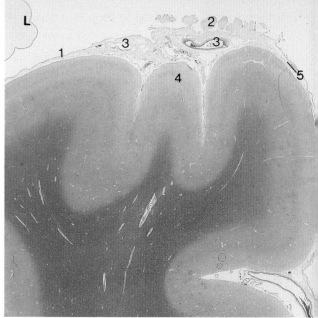

K Arachnoid granulations *in situ* on the parietal lobes of the cerebral hemispheres. x.5
1 Arachnoid granulations
2 Frontal lobes
3 Longitudinal cerebral fissure
4 Parietal lobes

L Low power view of an histological section to show an arachnoid granulation, stained with solochrome cyanin and nuclear fast red. x3.4
1 Arachnoid mater
2 Arachnoid granulation
3 Blood vessels
4 Cerebral cortex
5 Subarachnoid space

● *Arachnoid granulations consist of a group of arachnoid villi which project into the superior sagittal sinus or into venous lacunae which drain into the sinus.*

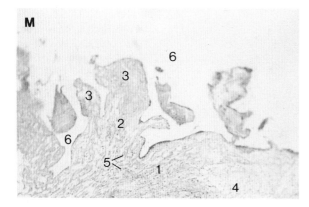

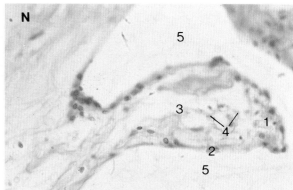

M Histological section to show the structure of an arachnoid granulation. Phosphotungstic acid and haematoxylin stain. x56
1 Arachnoid mater
2 Arachnoid granulation
3 Arachnoid villi
4 Subarachnoid space
5 Trabeculae
6 Venous lacunae

N High magnification photomicrograph to illustrate the histology of an individual arachnoid villus. Phosphotungstic acid and haematoxylin stain. x356
1 Arachnoid villus
2 Mesothelial cells
3 Subarachnoid space
4 Trabeculae
5 Venous lacunae

O-R Specialisations of the pia mater. (Also see Ventricles page **71**).

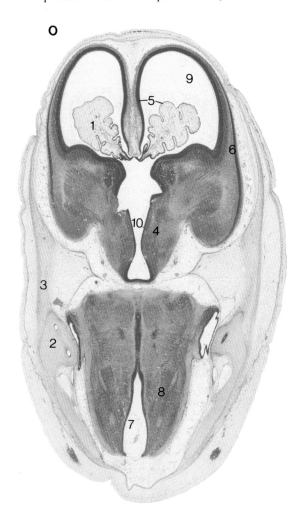

O The epithelium of the choroid plexus is a continuation of the ependymal lining of the ventricles. 27 mmCR embryo. Haematoxylin and eosin stain. x8.8

1 Choroid plexus
2 Developing ear
3 Developing skull
4 Diencephalon
5 Ependyma
6 Forebrain
7 Fourth ventricle
8 Hindbrain
9 Lateral ventricle
10 Third ventricle

MHMS

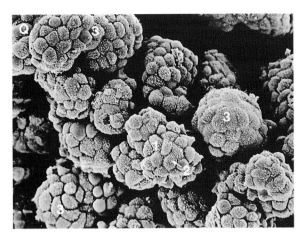

Q A scanning electron micrograph showing the surface of the choroid plexus of the fourth ventricle that is bathed by cerebrospinal fluid. x274

1 Epithelial cell
2 Microvilli (arrow)
3 Villi of choroid plexus

Mr G. McTurk

● *In some cases the pia mater is so closely apposed to the underlying foot-processes of the astrocytes that they are considered to be a single layer, the pia-glia.*

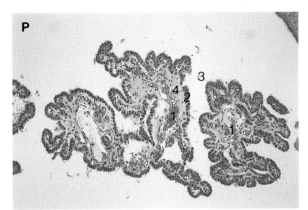

P A section of choroid plexus of the lateral ventricle. Haematoxylin and eosin stain. x111

1 Blood vessels
2 Ependyma of choroid plexus
3 Interior of the lateral ventricle
4 Pia mater

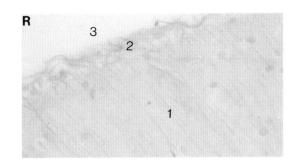

R Histological section of attachments between neurological processes (glial fibres) and the pia mater of the cerebellum. Holtzer's stain. x557

1 Neuroglial processes
2 Pia mater
3 Subarachnoid space

BLOOD SUPPLY TO THE BRAIN AND SPINAL CORD

Brain: Arteries

The arteries of the brain fall into five main groups:

1 Meningeal, ophthalmic and glandular branches

2 Cortical branches to the surface of the brain mostly supplying superficial grey matter

3 Central (basal, nuclear or medullary) branches into the brain substance that supply fibre tracts and nuclear masses

4 Choroidal branches to the choroid plexuses in the ventricles

5 Spinal branches

The brain tissue is supplied by two pairs of arteries lying in the subarachnoid space: the internal carotid and the vertebral arteries. The vertebral arteries join to form the basilar artery.

These vessels, their branches and those of the other half of the brain are linked together by communicating arteries, in an anastomotic ring at the base of the brain called the arterial circle (Circle of Willis). Large cortical branches (anterior, middle and posterior cerebral arteries), radiating from the circle, supply the surface and fine, penetrating branches for example, the striate arteries supply the interior of the brain. The cerebral arteries anastomose on the surface of the cerebral hemispheres. Once arteries have penetrated the brain substance they become end arteries, communicating only at capillary level.

The brainstem and cerebellum are supplied by the basilar and vertebral arteries.

The most powerful cerebral vasodilator is carbon dioxide. During sleep there is normally cerebral vasodilation but no increase in blood flow during anxiety or intellectual activity.

● *Brain tissue deprived of its blood supply quickly dies.*

● *A 'stroke' usually follows occlusion of, or haemorrhage from, a striate artery.*

● *The Circle of Willis is a frequent site of aneurysm.*

● *Thomas Willis (1621-1675). One of the founders of the Royal Society who made extensive studies of the human brain and its blood supply.*

A diagram showing the arterial circle (Circle of Willis).

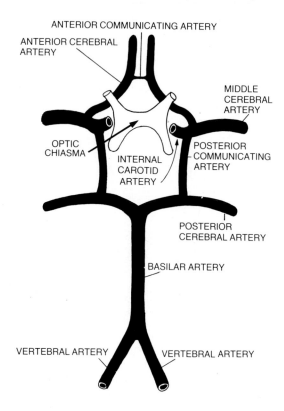

ANTERIOR COMMUNICATING ARTERY

ANTERIOR CEREBRAL ARTERY

MIDDLE CEREBRAL ARTERY

OPTIC CHIASMA

INTERNAL CAROTID ARTERY

POSTERIOR COMMUNICATING ARTERY

POSTERIOR CEREBRAL ARTERY

BASILAR ARTERY

VERTEBRAL ARTERY   VERTEBRAL ARTERY

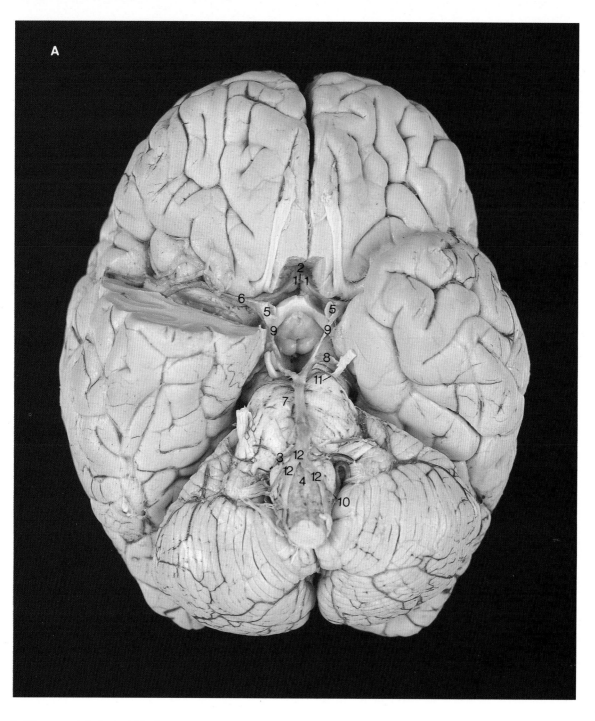

A The arterial circle (Circle of Willis) on the base of the brain. x1.02

1 Anterior cerebral artery
2 Anterior communicating artery
3 Anterior inferior cerebellar artery
4 Anterior spinal artery
5 Internal carotid artery
6 Middle cerebral artery
7 Pontine branches
8 Posterior cerebral artery
9 Posterior communicating artery
10 Posterior inferior cerebellar artery
11 Superior cerebellar artery
12 Vertebral arteries joining to form basilar artery

1 Meningeal, Ophthalmic and Glandular Branches

The meningeal branches are illustrated in the chapter on Meninges. The blood supply to the eye is illustrated in the chapter on the visual system. The glandular branches (e.g. hypophysis (pituitary)) are not within the scope of this book.

Superior hypophyseal branches of the internal carotid artery supply capillary beds in the hypothalamus and hypophyseal stalk. These capillary networks drain into long and short portal veins along the hypophyseal stalk. The portal veins form a second bed of sinusoidal capillaries between the endocrine cells of the adenohypophysis (anterior lobe of the pituitary gland, see Diencephalon page **112**). These in turn drain into the cavernous sinus (see Veins page **63**). Inferior hypophyseal arteries from the internal carotid artery supply the neurohypophysis (posterior or neural lobe of the pituitary gland).

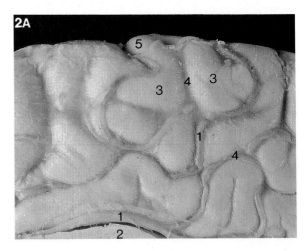

2 Cortical Branches

The cortical branches of the cerebrum and cerebellum arise from larger vessels. They pass along the sulci to penetrate the grey matter. They are covered by a sleeve of pia mater.

2A The superior cerebral arteries and veins supplying the substance of the hemispheres follow the gyri and sulci. x1.15
1 Blood vessels
2 Corpus callosum
3 Gyri
4 Sulci
5 Superior cerebral surface

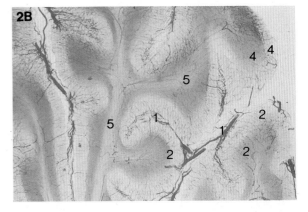

2B Carmine injected blood vessels on the surface of the cerebellum giving off fine branches into the substance of the grey matter. **c.** 1860 x5.6

2C Carmine injected specimen of the cerebral cortex to demonstrate that the grey matter has a richer blood supply than the white matter. **c.** 1860 x5.6
1 Blood vessels
2 Cerebellar cortex
3 Cerebral cortex
4 Grey matter
5 White matter

2B-2C Wellcome Museum

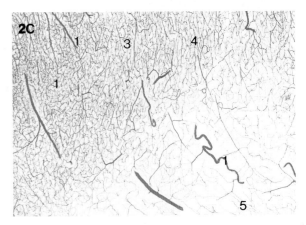

Cerebrum **2D-2E** The areas supplied by the anterior, middle and posterior cerebral arteries. Lateral view (**D**) and medial view (**E**).

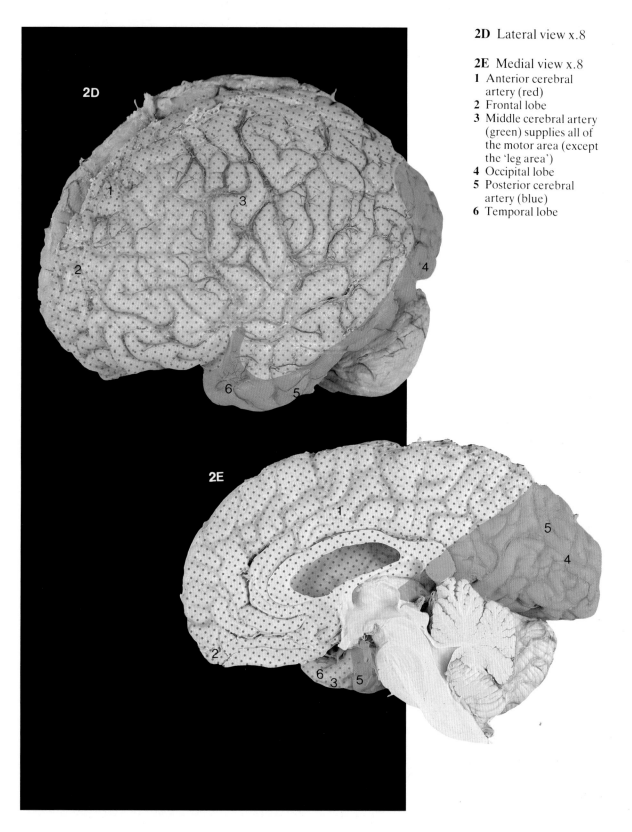

2D Lateral view x.8

2E Medial view x.8
1 Anterior cerebral artery (red)
2 Frontal lobe
3 Middle cerebral artery (green) supplies all of the motor area (except the 'leg area')
4 Occipital lobe
5 Posterior cerebral artery (blue)
6 Temporal lobe

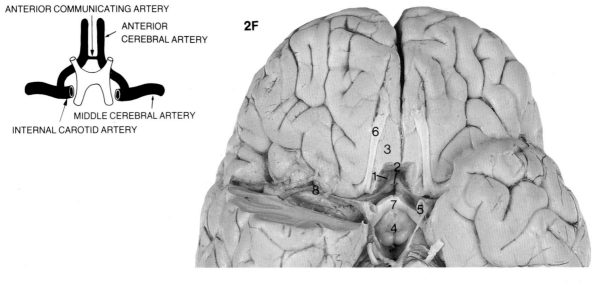

ANTERIOR COMMUNICATING ARTERY

ANTERIOR CEREBRAL ARTERY

2F

MIDDLE CEREBRAL ARTERY

INTERNAL CAROTID ARTERY

2F The anterior cerebral artery supplies the medial aspect of the frontal and parietal lobes (except the cuneus). Base of brain showing the anterior cerebral artery arising from the arterial circle (Circle of Willis). x.85

1 Anterior cerebral artery
2 Anterior communicating artery
3 Gyrus rectus
4 Hypothalamus

5 Internal carotid artery
6 Olfactory tract
7 Optic chiasma
8 Middle cerebral artery

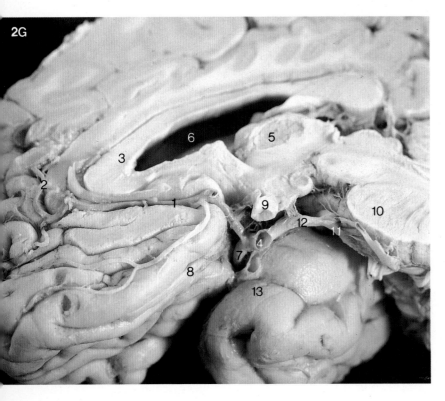

2G The anterior cerebral artery viewed from the medial surface of the frontal lobe. x1.1

1 Anterior cerebral artery
2 Branches of anterior cerebral artery
3 Corpus callosum
4 Internal carotid artery
5 Interthalamic connection
6 Lateral ventricle
7 Middle cerebral artery
8 Olfactory tract
9 Optic chiasma
10 Pons
11 Posterior cerebral artery
12 Posterior communicating artery
13 Temporal lobe

● *The anterior cerebral artery is a branch of the internal carotid artery.*

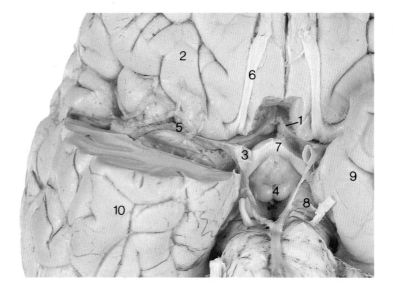

2Ha

INTERNAL CAROTID
ARTERY

MIDDLE
CEREBRAL
ARTERY

POSTERIOR
COMMUNICATING
ARTERY

A diagram illustrating this region.

2H The middle cerebral artery runs in the lateral sulcus. Inferior view of the cerebral hemispheres.

a x1.16

b x1.3
1 Anterior cerebral artery
2 Frontal lobe
3 Internal carotid artery
4 Mamillary bodies
5 Middle cerebral artery
6 Olfactory tract
7 Optic chiasma
8 Posterior cerebral artery
9 Temporal lobe
10 Temporal lobe (removed on the left side of photograph)

● *The middle cerebral artery is the largest branch of the internal carotid artery.*

● *The internal carotid artery is divided into four parts: cervical, intrapetrosal, intracavernous and supraclinoid. The latter two are referred to as the 'carotid siphon'.*

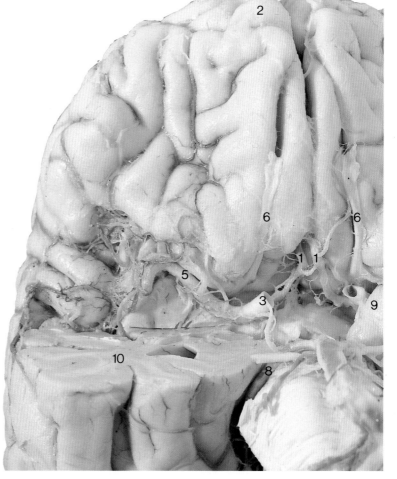

2Hb

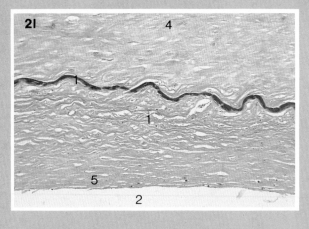

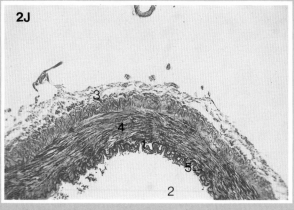

2I A transverse section of the internal carotid artery. Elastin stain. x223

2J A transverse section of the middle cerebral artery to show it contains a substantial amount of elastic tissue. Phosphotungstic acid and haematoxylin stain. x89

1 Elastin
2 Lumen of vessel
3 Tunica adventitia
4 Tunicica media
5 Tunica intima

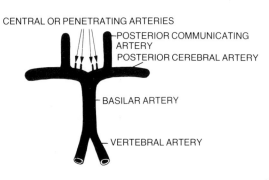

A diagram of the posterior cerebral artery, basilar artery and vertebral arteries.

2K The posterior cerebral artery supplies the occipital lobe and some of the inferior surface of the temporal lobe. x.7

1 Basal ganglia (temporal lobe removed)
2 Basilar artery
3 Cerebellum
4 Cerebellum (removed)
5 Frontal lobe
6 Gyrus rectus (partly removed)
7 Medulla oblongata
8 Occipital lobe
9 Oculomotor nerve
10 Olfactory bulb
11 Pons
12 Posterior cerebral artery
13 Posterior communicating artery
14 Temporal lobe
15 Temporal lobe (removed)

Cerebellum Each half of the cerebellum is supplied by three arteries: the superior cerebellar, anterior inferior cerebellar, and posterior inferior cerebellar. The posterior inferior cerebellar also supplies the adjacent portion of the medulla oblongata.

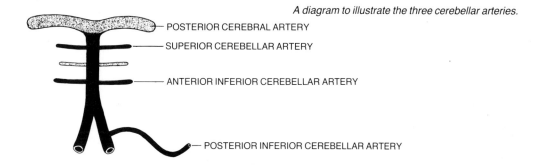

A diagram to illustrate the three cerebellar arteries.

POSTERIOR CEREBRAL ARTERY

SUPERIOR CEREBELLAR ARTERY

ANTERIOR INFERIOR CEREBELLAR ARTERY

POSTERIOR INFERIOR CEREBELLAR ARTERY

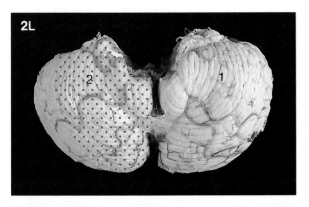

2L The superior cerebellar artery is on the superior surface of the cerebellar hemispheres (areas of supply in red). The brainstem has been removed. x.67
1 Cerebellum
2 Superior cerebellar artery

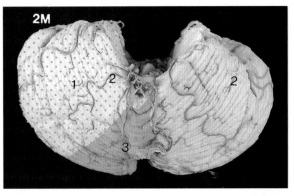

2M The anterior inferior cerebellar (area of supply in green) and posterior inferior cerebellar (area of supply in blue) arteries are on the inferior surface of the cerebellar hemispheres. The brainstem has been removed. x.73
1 Anterior inferior cerebellar artery
2 Cerebellum
3 Posterior inferior cerebellar artery

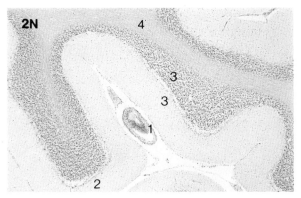

2N A small artery and vein on the cerebellar surface to show that they run between the folia. Bodian stain and neutral red stain. x33
1 Blood vessel
2 Folium
3 Grey matter
4 White matter

3 Central Branches

These small vessels are branches of larger vessels, and pass into the brain. Three areas with a very rich supply are: the anterior perforated substance (striate or lenticulostriate arteries); and the internal and external capsules (branches of the anterior and middle cerebral arteries and anterior and posterior communicating arteries); the posterior perforated substance (branches of basilar and posterior cerebral arteries). The central branches supply the basal ganglia, brain stem, cerebellum, thalamus and hypothalamus.

● *The striate arteries are frequently the site of cerebrovascular accidents (CVA).*

A diagram to illustrate the striate arteries.

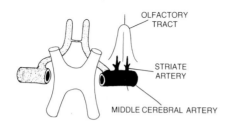

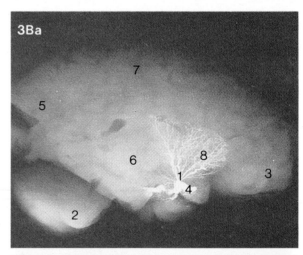

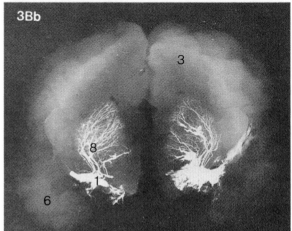

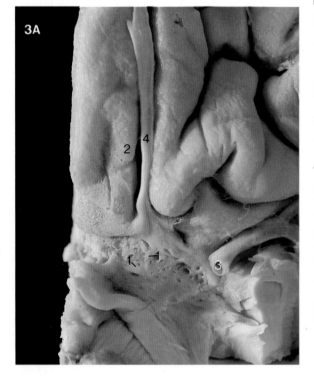

3A-3B Anterior perforated substance.

3A The frontal lobe viewed from below. The temporal lobe has been partially removed to show the anterior perforated substance. x5.7

1 Anterior perforated substance (with openings
   for striate arteries)
2 Gyrus rectus
3 Middle cerebral artery
4 Olfactory tract

● *The posterior perforated substance lies in the midbrain between the cerebral peduncles.*

3B Radiographs of fixed brain injected with radio-opaque material to show the deep branches of the middle cerebral artery supplying the basal ganglia.
a Lateral view
b Frontal view

1 Anterior perforated
   substance
2 Cerebellum
3 Frontal lobe
4 Middle cerebral artery

5 Occipital lobe
6 Temporal lobe
7 Parietal lobe
8 Position of basal ganglia
   and internal capsule

Dr Harry A. Kaplan and
Dr M.B. Carpenter

4 Choroidal Branches

The branches supplying the choroid plexus of the ventricles are:

LOCATION OF CHOROID PLEXUS	BLOOD SUPPLY
LATERAL VENTRICLE	Anterior choroidal (a branch of internal carotid artery) Posterior choroidal (a branch of posterior cerebral artery)
THIRD VENTRICLE	Posterior Choroidal
FOURTH VENTRICLE	A branch of posterior inferior cerebellar artery

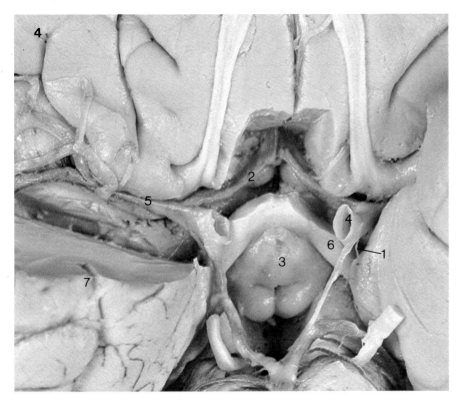

4 The origin of the anterior choroidal artery from the internal carotid artery. x2

1 Anterior choroidal artery
2 Anterior cerebral artery
3 Hypothalamus
4 Internal carotid artery
5 Middle cerebral artery
6 Optic tract
7 Temporal lobe

5 Brainstem and Spinal Branches

Brainstem The basilar artery supplies almost all of the brainstem and cerebellum. It bifurcates to form the posterior cerebral arteries supplying blood to the occipital lobe.

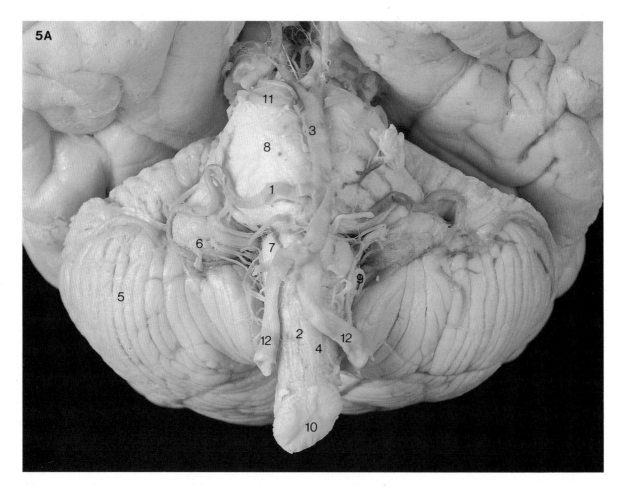

5A Blood supply to the brainstem. x1.6

1 Anterior inferior cerebellar artery
2 Anterior spinal artery
3 Basilar artery
4 Brainstem
5 Cerebellum
6 Choroid plexus in the lateral aperture of the fourth ventricle
7 Medulla oblongata
8 Pons
9 Posterior inferior cerebellar artery
10 Spinal cord
11 Superior cerebellar artery
12 Vertebral artery

• *Nuclei containing cell bodies have a greater density of blood supply than tracts which consist of fibres.*

• *The medial medullary syndrome is caused by interruption to the supply in the anterior group of arteries.*

• *The lateral medullary syndrome is caused by interruption to the supply in the lateral arteries.*

• *The posterior inferior cerebellar artery is one of the commonest sites for occlusion by thrombus.*

5B-5D Territories of arterial supply (shown by outlines) of the medulla oblongata and pons.

5B Pons. Weigert stain. x2.6

5C Medulla oblongata at the level of the inferior olivary nuclear complex. Mulligan stain. x2.4

5D Medulla oblongata at the level of the posterior column nuclei. Weigert stain. x2.1

1 Anterior inferior cerebellar artery
2 Anterior spinal artery
3 Long circumferential branches (basilar artery)
4 Medulla oblongata
5 Paramedian branches (basilar artery)
6 Posterior inferior cerebellar artery
7 Posterior spinal artery
8 Short circumferential branches (basilar artery)
9 Vertebral artery

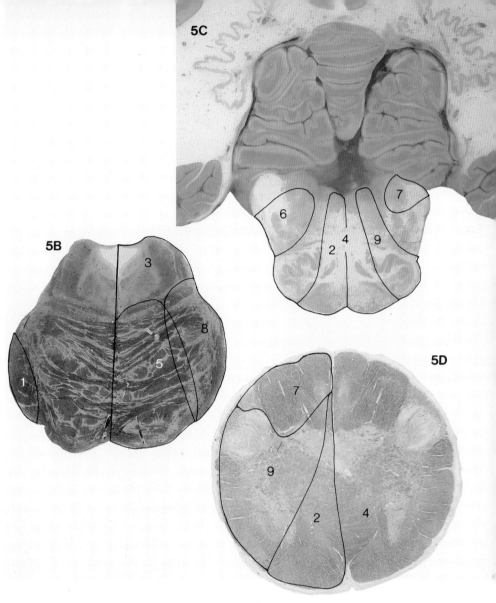

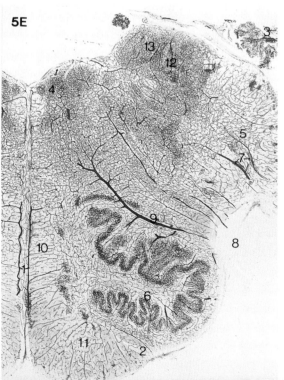

5E A cleared section of the medulla oblongata at the level of the inferior olivary nucleus. It was injected with a mixture of gelatine and India Ink to show the internal distribution of the anterior spinal, vertebral and posterior inferior cerebellar arteries. x7

1 Anterior group of arteries (from anterior spinal artery)
2 Anterolateral group of arteries (from vertebral artery)
3 Choroid plexus of the fourth ventricle
4 Hypoglossal nucleus
5 Inferior cerebellar peduncle
6 Inferior olivary nucleus
7 Lateral group of arteries (from vertebral and posterior inferior cerebellar arteries)
8 Lateral medullary fossa
9 Lateral medullary vein
10 Medial lemniscus
11 Medullary pyramid
12 Posterior group of arteries (from posterior inferior cerebellar artery)
13 Vestibular nuclei

Prof. H. Duvernoy

Spinal branches The spinal cord is supplied by two branches from each vertebral artery which descend to supply the cord. Additionally the cord receives an arterial supply from small branches (radicular arteries) which are derived from segmental branches of the aorta and from the vertebral arteries.

- *The posterior spinal artery may be a branch from the vertebral artery.*

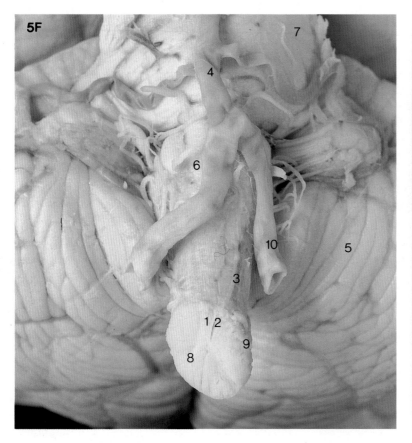

5F The anterior spinal artery descends in the anterior median fissure of the cord. View of the base of the brain and upper cervical cord. x1.85

  1 Anterior (ventral) horn
  2 Anterior median fissure
  3 Anterior spinal artery
  4 Basilar artery
  5 Cerebellum
  6 Medulla oblongata
  7 Pons
  8 Posterior (dorsal) horn
  9 Spinal cord
10 Vertebral artery

5G The posterior spinal artery descends in two branches one on each side of the posterior (dorsal) spinal nerve roots. View of part of the spinal cord from the posterior surface. x.86

1 Denticulate ligament
2 Dura mater
3 Pia mater
4 Posterior (dorsal) columns
5 Posterior (dorsal) spinal artery
6 Posterior spinal nerve roots
7 Radicular vessels

UN

Cerebral Angiography

A-D Cerebral angiograms demonstrating the blood supply to the brain and skull. An angiogram is produced by introducing a radio-opaque substance into a blood vessel. Angiograms of the carotid and vertebral arteries demonstrate their territories in the head, neck and brain.

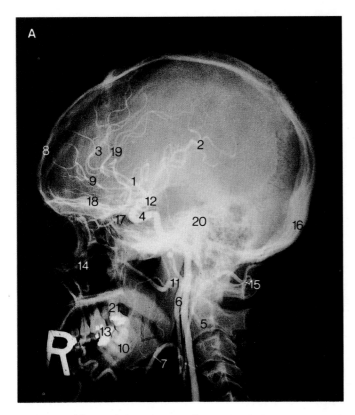

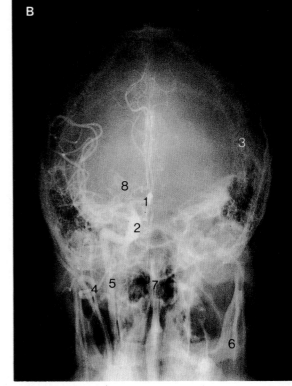

A A carotid arterial angiogram in a lateral view.
1 Anterior cerebral artery
2 Branches of middle cerebral artery
3 Callosomarginal artery
4 Carotid siphon
5 Cervical vertebra
6 External carotid artery
7 Facial artery
8 Frontal bone
9 Frontopolar arteries
10 Mandible
11 Maxillary artery
12 Middle cerebral artery
13 Mouth
14 Nasal cavity
15 Occipital artery
16 Occiput
17 Ophthalmic artery
18 Orbitofrontal arteries
19 Pericallosal artery
20 Petrous temporal bone
21 Teeth

B A frontal view of a carotid angiogram.
1 Anterior cerebral artery
2 Carotid siphon
3 Coronal suture
4 External carotid artery
5 Internal carotid artery
6 Mandible
7 Nose
8 Striate arteries

● *A tumour in the hypophyseal (pituitary) fossa may cause the curves of the carotid siphon to straighten.*

● *Branches of the middle cerebral artery crossing the insula form loops.*

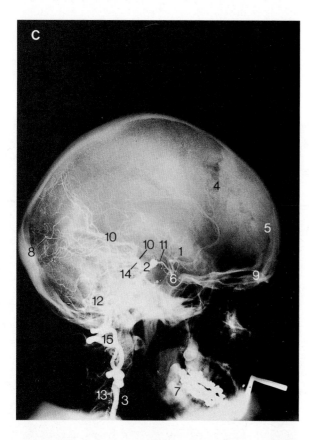

C A vertebral artery angiogram in lateral view.
1 Arteries to thalamus
2 Basilar artery
3 Body of a cervical vertebra
4 Coronal suture
5 Frontal bone
6 Hypophyseal fossa
7 Mandible
8 Occiput
9 Orbit
10 Posterior cerebral artery
11 Posterior communicating artery
12 Posterior inferior cerebellar artery
13 Spine of a cervical vertebra
14 Superior cerebellar artery
15 Vertebral artery

● *In this individual some filling of the posterior communicating and anterior cerebral arteries has occurred, showing the continuity of the arterial circle (Circle of Willis).*

D A frontal view of a vertebral artery angiogram.
1 Basilar artery
2 Nose
3 Petrous temporal bone
4 Posterior cerebral artery
5 Superior cerebellar artery
6 Vertebral artery

A-D Dr D. James

Brain: Veins

Cerebrum

Cerebral veins are unusual; they have no valves or muscular tissue. Blood drains from deep in the substance of the brain into large superficial veins which cross the subarachnoid space and drain into large venous sinuses of the dura mater.

The veins may be divided into two groups: those draining the cerebrum and those of the cerebellum and brainstem.

Those of the cerebrum are further divided into external and internal vessels. The external veins drain the surface of the cerebrum. The superolateral surface of each hemisphere is drained by 8-12 superior superficial veins which pass upward and forward to end in the superior sagittal sinus. Some veins from the medial aspect also drain into this sinus.

Other veins on the superolateral surface drain into the superficial middle cerebral vein, which lies in the lateral sulcus and joins the cavernous sinus. Anastomotic vessels drain from it inferolaterally into the transverse sinus and superiorly into the superior sagittal sinus.

The superficial middle cerebral vein is connected to the superior sagittal sinus by the superior anastomotic vein; and to the transverse sinus by the inferior anastomotic vein.

The surface of the insula is drained by the deep middle cerebral vein. The anterior cerebral vein accompanies the anterior cerebral artery and drains the territory supplied by the artery. The anterior cerebral and the deep middle cerebral vein join with striate veins (internal cerebral veins which emerge through the anterior perforated substance) to form the basal vein. The basal vein on each side ultimately joins the great cerebral vein (of Galen) which drains the inside of the brain. The great cerebral vein is formed by the union of two internal cerebral veins under the splenium of the corpus callosum. The internal cerebral veins receive the thalamostriate veins (also known as venae terminales) from the corpus striatum and the choroidal veins of each lateral ventricle.

The inferior surface of each cerebral hemisphere is drained by inferior superficial cerebral veins. They drain into the transverse sinus, inferior cerebral veins, superior petrosal sinus, cavernous sinus, middle cerebral veins and basal vein of their own side.

Cerebellum

There are two main groups of cerebellar veins: the superior and inferior veins. The superior veins drain into the straight sinus, the internal cerebral veins, and the transverse and superior petrosal sinuses.

The inferior veins drain into the inferior petrosal, sigmoid and occipital sinuses.

Brainstem

Veins of the brainstem form a superficial venous plexus, deep to the arteries, within which larger venous channels can be distinguished.

1 Midbrain. Veins from the midbrain drain into the great cerebral vein, and some, along with those of the area around the interpeduncular fossa, also drain into the basal veins.

2 Pons. The pontine veins drain into the basal vein, cerebellar veins, and the superior and inferior petrosal and transverse sinuses. Sometimes a median pontine vein is present, and a distinct lateral venous channel is usually present on either side.

3 Medulla Oblongata. Some veins on the anterior surface drain into a midline anterior median vein which is continuous with a vein of the same name on the anterior surface of the spinal cord. On the posterior surface the veins drain into a posterior median vein which is continuous with a vein of the same name on the posterior surface of the spinal cord. This vein drains into the inferior petrosal and basilar venous sinuses.

Radicular veins (associated with the last four cranial nerve rootlets) drain into the petrosal sinus, occipital sinuses or internal jugular vein.

A lateral vein similar to that found in the pons may be present on each side, draining into the petrosal or transverse sinus.

Venous Sinuses of the Dura Mater

There are several large sinuses lying externally to the brain in the dural folds. These are the superior sagittal sinus, inferior sagittal sinus, and straight sinus; the blood from these sinuses and from the great cerebral vein meets at the confluence of the sinuses, where venous blood then flows into the bilateral transverse sinuses. They eventually pass from the skull as the internal jugular veins through the jugular foramina.

The cavernous sinuses, lying on each side of the body of the sphenoid bone, connect with one another and with the other intracranial sinuses (for example, superior petrosal, sigmoid, occipital). Blood may flow in any direction in this sinus. It also connects with the superficial middle cerebral veins draining the lateral surfaces of the brain, and with veins in the pharyngeal, pterygoid and orbital regions.

Blood from the great cerebral vein (of Galen) joins the straight sinus at the junction with the inferior sagittal sinus.

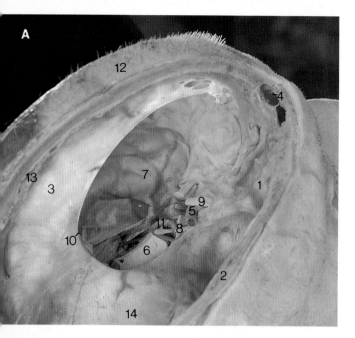

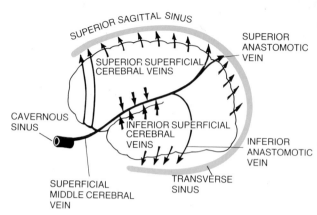

Venous drainage of the superior and lateral surfaces of the cerebrum.

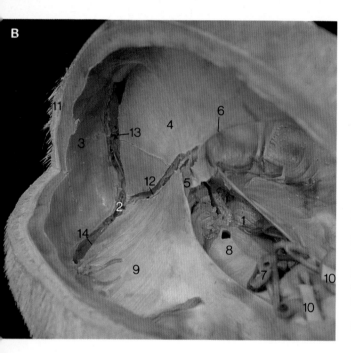

A The superior and inferior sagittal sinuses. x.59

1 Anterior cranial fossa
2 Diploë
3 Falx cerebri
4 Frontal sinus
5 Internal carotid artery
6 Midbrain
7 Middle cranial fossa
8 Oculomotor nerve
9 Optic nerve
10 Position of inferior sagittal sinus
11 Posterior cerebral artery
12 Scalp
13 Superior sagittal sinus
14 Tentorium cerebelli

B The dural venous sinuses. x.6

1 Cerebellum
2 Confluence of the sinuses
3 Dura mater
4 Falx cerebri
5 Great cerebral vein (of Galen)
6 Inferior sagittal sinus (position of)
7 Internal carotid artery
8 Midbrain
9 Tentorium cerebelli
10 Optic nerve
11 Scalp
12 Straight sinus
13 Superior sagittal sinus
14 Transverse sinus

• *Claudius Galen (A.D. 130-200) was a Roman physician to the gladiators, who became the accepted authority on human anatomy until the Renaissance.*

• *The direction of blood flow can vary in valveless veins.*

• *Blood seeping from a ruptured vein may collect between the dura and arachnoid mater to form a subdural haematoma. Elderly individuals have fragile veins. A slight blow to the head may lead to a subdural haematoma.*

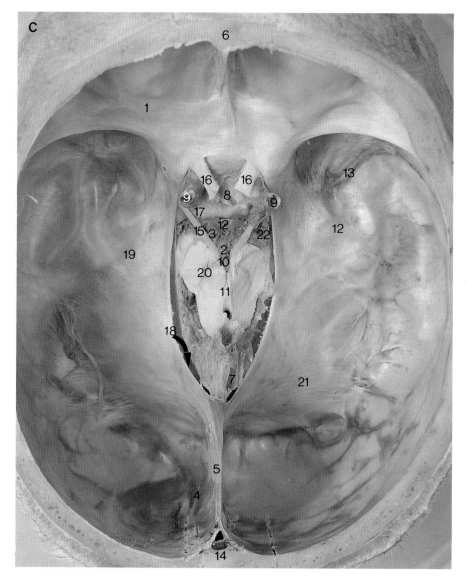

C A view from above of the floor of the cranial cavity to demonstrate the relationships of the cavernous sinus. x.86

1 Anterior cranial fossa
2 Basilar venous plexus
3 Cavernous sinus
4 Confluence of the sinuses
5 Falx cerebri
6 Frontal bone
7 Great cerebral vein
8 Hypophyseal fossa
9 Internal carotid artery
10 Interpeduncular fossa
11 Midbrain
12 Middle cranial fossa
13 Middle meningeal vessels
14 Occipital bone
15 Oculomotor nerve
16 Optic nerve
17 Posterior clinoid process
18 Posterior cranial fossa
19 Superior petrosal sinus
20 Substantia nigra
21 Tentorium cerebelli
22 Wall of cavernous sinus (cut edge)

A diagram to show the structures running in the walls of the cavernous sinus.

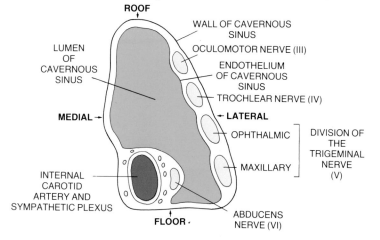

- *The posterior inter-cavernous sinus communicates between the left and right cavernous sinuses behind the hypophysis but cannot be seen in this specimen.*

- *If the internal carotid artery is ruptured in the cavernous sinus, arteriovenous communication results.*

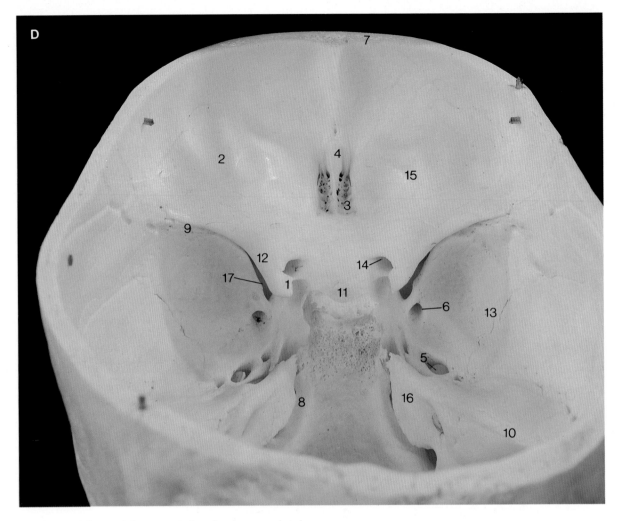

D The positions of the petrosal and sphenoparietal sinuses. The floor of the cranial cavity viewed from behind. The cranial vault has been removed. x1.3

1 Anterior clinoid process
2 Anterior cranial fossa
3 Cribriform plate of ethmoid bone
4 Crista galli
5 Foramen ovale
6 Foramen rotundum
7 Frontal bone
8 Groove for inferior petrosal sinus
9 Groove for sphenoparietal sinus
10 Groove for superior petrosal sinus
11 Hypophyseal fossa
12 Lesser wing of sphenoid
13 Middle cranial fossa
14 Optic canal
15 Orbital part of frontal bone
16 Petrous temporal bone
17 Superior orbital fissure

● *Note the thin parts of the squamous temporal, greater wing of sphenoid and frontal and parietal bones. This position is called the pterion. The* branches of the middle meningeal artery can easily be injured at this site.

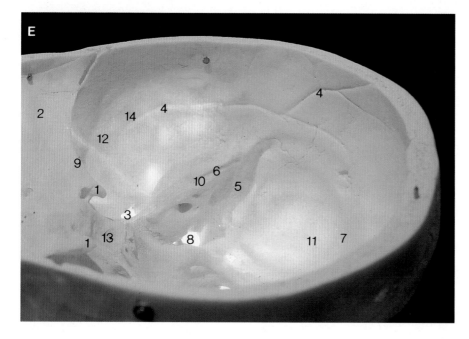

E The middle cranial fossa and the groove for the sigmoid sinus viewed from the side. The cranial vault has been removed. x.8

1 Anterior clinoid process
2 Anterior cranial fossa
3 Foramen ovale
4 Groove for middle meningeal artery
5 Groove for sigmoid sinus
6 Groove for superior petrosal sinus
7 Groove for transverse sinus
8 Jugular foramen
9 Lesser wing of sphenoid bone
10 Petrous part of temporal bone
11 Posterior cranial fossa
12 Pterion
13 Sella turcica (hypophyseal fossa)
14 Squamous part of temporal bone

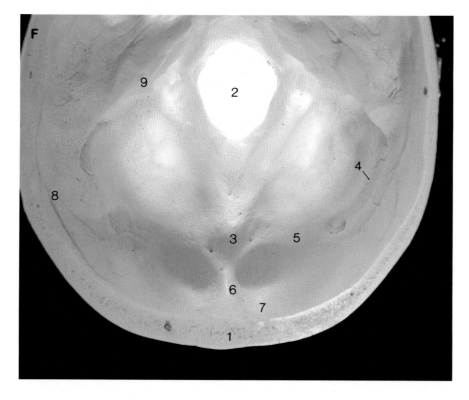

F The posterior cranial fossa and the grooves for its associated sinuses viewed from above. The vault has been removed. Note the density of the occipital bone. x.8

1 Diploë of the skull
2 Foramen magnum
3 Groove for confluence of the sinuses
4 Groove for sigmoid sinus
5 Groove for transverse sinus
6 Internal occipital protuberance
7 Occipital bone
8 Parietal bone
9 Petrous part of temporal bone

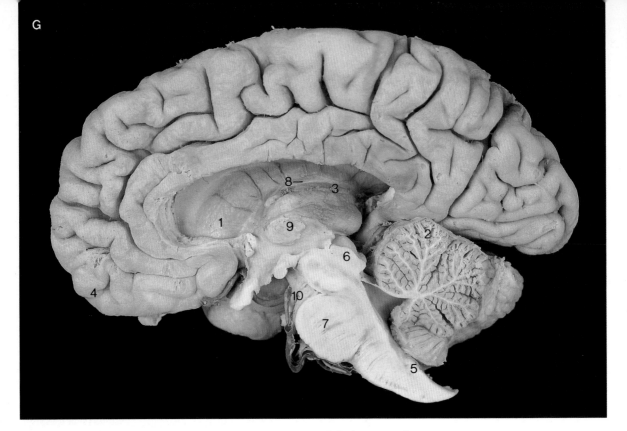

G The deep venous drainage of the caudate nucleus and thalamus. x.9

1 Caudate nucleus
2 Cerebellum
3 Choroid plexus of lateral ventricle
4 Frontal pole
5 Medulla oblongata
6 Midbrain
7 Pons
8 Thalamostriate vein (drains into the internal cerebral vein)
9 Thalamus
10 Vessels on surface of brainstem

• *The two internal cerebral veins join together to form the great cerebral vein (of Galen).*

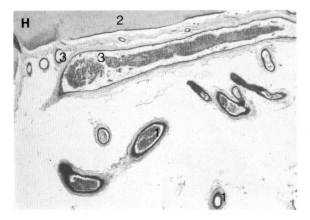

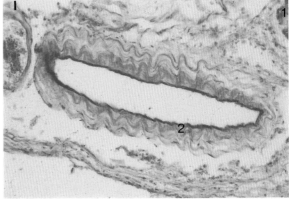

H Vessels on the surface of the medulla oblongata form a plexus with veins lying deep to the arteries. Van Gieson stain. x33

1 Artery
2 Medulla oblongata (surface)
3 Vein

Mr D. Adams

I A transverse section adjacent to the medulla oblongata to demonstrate the lack of muscle in the vein wall. Van Gieson stain. x167

1 Medulla oblongata
2 Vein

Blood-Brain and Blood-CSF Barriers

Neuronal function requires a micro-environment which is precisely controlled. Several mechanisms exist in the nervous system to isolate the brain and spinal cord from changes elsewhere in the body that might have an adverse effect. Collectively these mechanisms constitute the blood-brain barrier and the blood-CSF barrier. These barriers have five major functions:

a) Large molecules, for example plasma proteins, present in the blood are excluded from the CSF and nervous tissue.

b) The ionic composition and glucose concentration of the extracellular fluid in the nervous system is controlled at levels appropriate for neuronal function but not necessarily the same as those elsewhere in the body.

c) The brain and spinal cord are protected from the effect of neurotransmitters in the blood, for example, epinephrine from the adrenal gland.

d) Neurotransmitters produced in the CNS are prevented from leaking into the general circulation.

e) Toxins are excluded either because of their molecular size or because of their solubility. Only substances soluble in water and cell-membrane lipids can pass these barriers.

Anatomically the blood-brain barrier resides in the endothelium of capillaries in the nervous tissue. These have restricted permeability. The cells are attached to each other by tight (occluding) junctions which prevent large molecules, for example proteins, passing between the cells, effectively sealing off the lumen of the vessel from the extracellular space outside it. In addition, the endothelium shows few of the vesicles found in other capillary endothelia which are responsible for the transport of macromolecules across the cell.

The blood-CSF barrier exists in the choroid plexuses and in the arachnoid mater. Choroid plexus capillaries are fenestrated and highly permeable. However, the epithelial cells are attached to each other by tight junctions so that substances cannot pass between the epithelial cells into the CSF in the ventricles but have to be transported by the cells. Choroid plexus epithelial cells have active transport mechanisms for ions, glucose and amino acids but large molecules are unable to pass.

The subarachnoid space is sealed against free exchange of substances between the CSF in the space and blood in the vessels passing in or beside the space. A layer of flat, interdigitating cells, attached to each other by tight junctions, covers the outside of the arachnoid and the vessels crossing the subarachnoid space have endothelia with occluding tight junctions between the cells, sealing the lumen.

No barrier exists between the CSF in the ventricles or subarachnoid space and the nervous tissue because neither the astrocytes at the glia limitans nor the ependymal cells at the ventricular lumen have tight junctions. Water and electrolytes produced by metabolism pass freely between the brain and the CSF and are removed when the CSF is recirculated back to the blood via the arachnoid granulations. The CSF is performing the same function here that lymphatics do for other tissues. The CNS is devoid of lymphatic capillaries.

● *The pineal gland and the median eminence of the hypothalamus have fenestrated capillaries. In the hypothalamus these allow hypothalamic neurosecretions to enter the circulation (see Diencephalon, page 112).*

● *The blood-brain barrier is not fully developed at birth and albumin is present in the CSF.*

● *The subfornical organ (under the fornix), the area postrema (in the roof of the fourth ventricle) and the organum vasculosum of the lamina terminalis are areas with no blood-brain barrier. They are chemoreceptors—specific sense organs for blood-borne substances.*

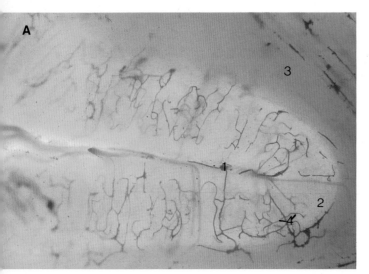

A A low power photomicrograph to show blood vessels entering the cerebellum as an example of the small blood vessels supplying the brain tissue. Golgi-Cox stain. x68
1 Blood vessel on surface
2 Cerebellar cortex
3 Cerebellar white matter
4 Penetrating vessels

B An histological section to show a capillary in the brainstem surrounded by multipolar neurons and nerve fibres. Cresyl violet stain. x669
1 Capillary
2 Cell body of neuron
3 Neuroglial cell nuclei
4 Neuronal processes or nerve fibres
5 Nucleus of neuron

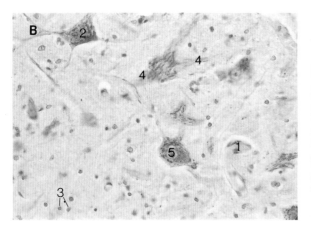

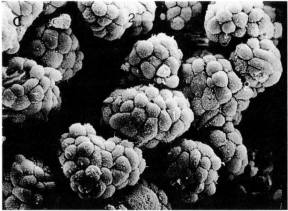

A blood-CSF barrier exists in the choroid plexus, where the epithelial cells are attached to one another by tight junctions, and in the arachnoid mater between the outermost arachnoid cells (arachnoid barrier layer).

C Scanning electron micrograph to show the epithelium of the choroid plexus which would be in contact with the cerebrospinal fluid. x405
1 Epithelial cell
2 Villi

D An histological section to show the arachnoid mater and the subarachnoid space. Solochrome cyanin and light green stain. x3.5
1 Arachnoid mater
2 Blood vessels in subarachnoid space
3 Grey matter of cerebral cortex
4 Subarachnoid space
5 Surface of arachnoid mater (arrow)

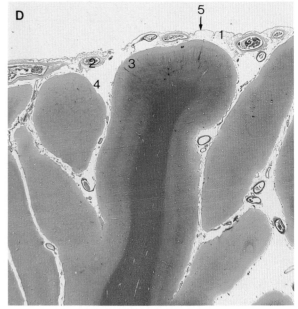

VENTRICLES

Deep inside the forebrain, midbrain and hindbrain is a series of connecting chambers (ventricles) lined with an epithelium called the ependyma. There are two large lateral ventricles inside the cerebral hemispheres (forebrain), each of which connects in the midline through the interventricular foramen (of Monro) which leads into the midline third ventricle. This connects through the narrow cerebral aqueduct (of Sylvius) in the midbrain to the midline fourth ventricle in the pons and medulla oblongata (hindbrain).

Projecting into each ventricle is a structure called the choroid plexus which produces cerebrospinal fluid (CSF). It consists of tufts of capillaries covered by an epithelium, the ependyma. As CSF is constantly produced it percolates through and fills all of the ventricles. It leaves the system by flowing out of three openings. In the hindbrain roof above the fourth ventricle is a midline median aperture (foramen of Magendie) and two lateral apertures (foramina of Luschka) which open from the sides of the fourth ventricle. CSF flows into and completely fills the subarachnoid space around the brain and spinal cord. Areas where the arachnoid and pia mater are widely separated are referred to as cisterns or cisternae.

Finally CSF then leaves the ventricular system through small openings in the superior sagittal sinus. These openings, found in the dura mater, have small projections of arachnoid bulging through them (arachnoid granulations). The CSF passes through the granulations and is carried away in the dural venous blood.

A A cast of the ventricles of the adult brain superimposed on the base of a brain to illustrate their position internally. x.65

1 Cerebral aqueduct
2 Anterior horn
3 Body
4 Posterior horn ⎬ Lateral ventricle
5 Inferior horn
6 Third ventricle
7 Fourth ventricle

RCS

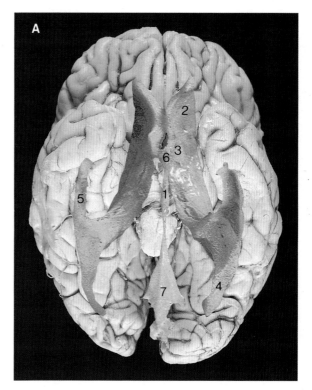

• *CSF cushions the brain and spinal cord by absorbing shocks.*

• *A lumbar puncture or spinal tap is made to measure the pressure of the intracranial CSF, to take a sample of spinal fluid, to introduce dyes, radio-opaque contrast media for diagnostic purposes and to administer anaesthetics and other drugs.*

• *CSF is a clear fluid similar to lymph and does not normally contain blood, pus or bacteria. In a spinal tap the levels of sugar, chloride and protein are measured. Any cells are counted and identified.*

• *One cause of hydrocephalus in newborn infants is an accumulation of CSF caused by an obstruction in the ventricular system. CSF is unable to flow out and accumulates in the ventricles.*

B The ventricles viewed from the medial aspect of a sagittal section. (Septum pellucidum has been removed). x.6

1 Anterior horn of lateral ventricle
2 Body of lateral ventricle
3 Choroid plexus
4 Corpus callosum
5 Diencephalon
6 Frontal lobe
7 Inferior horn of lateral ventricle
8 Occipital lobe
9 Parietal lobe
10 Posterior horn of lateral ventricle
11 Temporal lobe

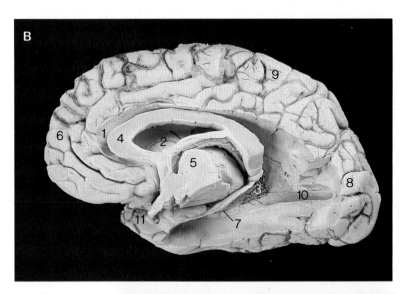

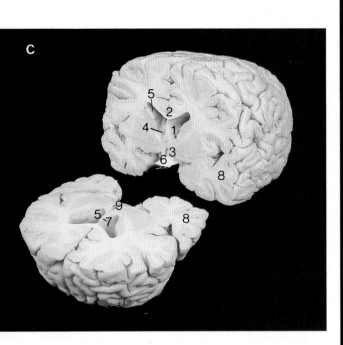

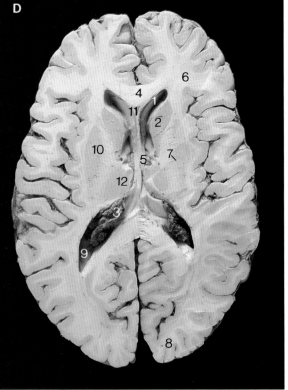

C A coronal section through the cerebral hemispheres and diencephalon to illustrate the position of the interventricular foramen between the lateral and third ventricles. x.5

1 Choroid plexus	6 Optic chiasma
2 Corpus callosum	7 Septum pellucidum
3 Hypothalamus	8 Temporal lobe
4 Interventricular foramen	9 Third ventricle
5 Lateral ventricle	

D An horizontal section through the brain to show the anterior and posterior horns of the lateral ventricles. x.6

1 Anterior horn of lateral ventricle	7 Globus pallidus
2 Caudate nucleus	8 Occipital lobe
3 Choroid plexus	9 Posterior horn of lateral ventricle
4 Corpus callosum	
5 Fornix	10 Putamen
6 Frontal lobe	11 Septum pellucidum
	12 Thalamus

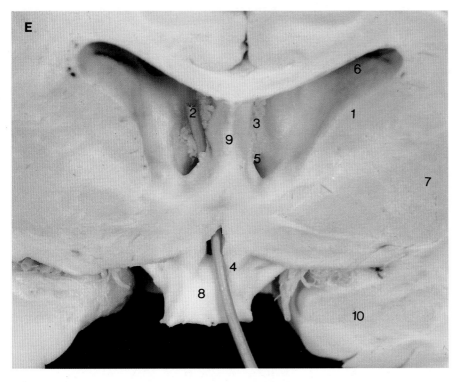

E A coronal section through the diencephalon to illustrate the relationship between the interventricular foramen and the third ventricle. x1.9

1 Caudate nucleus
2 Connection between lateral and third ventricle (shown by the position of a red wire)
3 Choroid plexus
4 Hypothalamus
5 Interventricular foramen
6 Lateral ventricle
7 Lentiform nucleus
8 Optic chiasma
9 Septum pellucidum
10 Temporal lobe

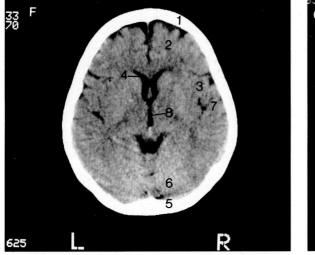

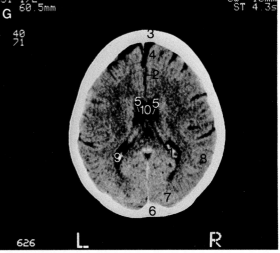

F Computerized axial tomography (CAT) scan image to show the third and lateral ventricles.

1 Frontal bone	5 Occipital bone
2 Frontal lobe	6 Occipital lobe
3 Insula	7 Temporal lobe
4 Lateral ventricle	8 Third ventricle

Elscint Ltd

G CAT scan image to show posterior horn of the lateral ventricle.

1 Choroid plexus (shows calcification in this instance)	5 Lateral ventricle
	6 Occipital bone
	7 Occipital lobe
2 Falx cerebri	8 Parietal lobe
3 Frontal bone	9 Posterior horn of ventricle
4 Frontal lobe	10 Septum pellucidum

Elscint Ltd

• *In chronic alcoholism there is atrophy of the cerebral cortex and an apparent increase in the size of the ventricles.*

H The choroid plexus of the lateral ventricle viewed *in situ* from the lateral surface. x.7

1 Choroid plexus
2 Frontal lobe
3 Insula
4 Lateral ventricle
5 Parietal lobe
6 Occipital lobe
7 Temporal lobe

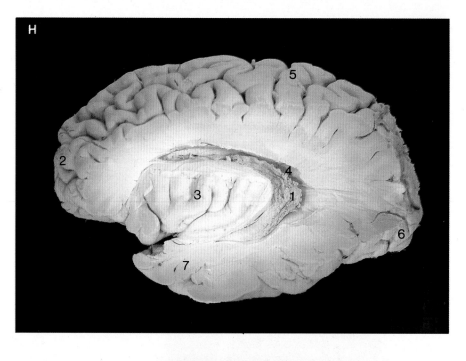

I An histological section to show the choroid plexus of the lateral ventricle, stained with phosphotungstic acid and haematoxylin. x4.8

1 Caudate nucleus
2 Choroid plexus
3 Corpus callosum
4 Lateral ventricle
5 Thalamus

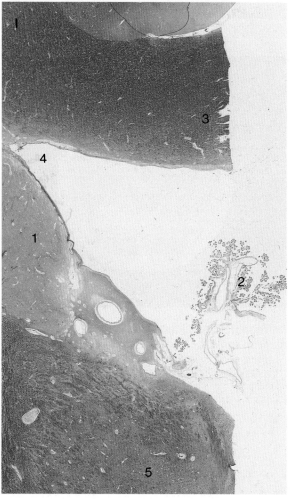

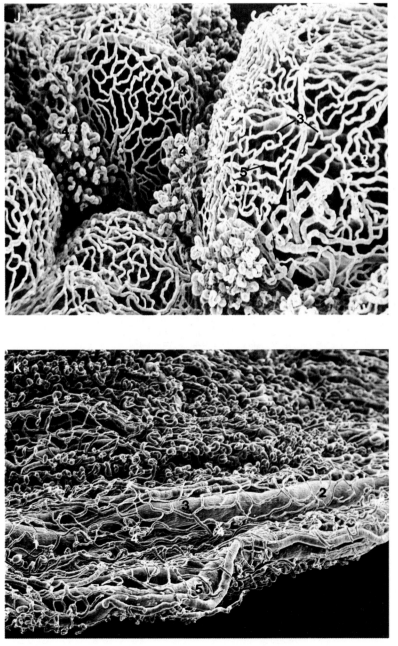

J-K Capillaries of the choroid plexus form either dichotomous or glomerular formations.

J Scanning electron micrograph of a cast of the capillary network in the choroid plexus. x99

Dr E. Motti

1 Artery
2 Capillary
3 Dichotomous branching
4 Glomerular formation
5 Vein

K A cast of an artery and a vein surrounded by capillary meshes. x111

Dr E. Motti

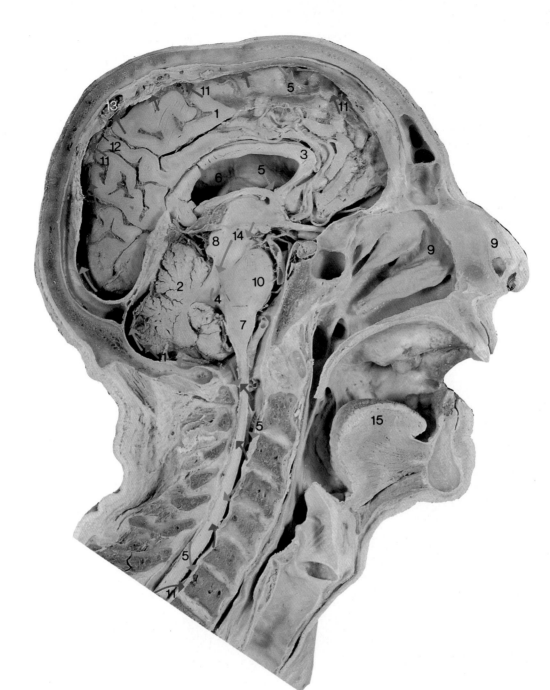

L Sagittal section of a head to illustrate the circulation of cerebrospinal fluid through the ventricles and subarachnoid space and its return to the blood circulation. x.64

1 Cerebral hemisphere
2 Cerebellum
3 Corpus callosum
4 Fourth ventricle
5 Green arrows (circulation of CSF)
6 Lateral ventricle
7 Medulla oblongata
8 Midbrain

9 Nose
10 Pons
11 Red arrows (return of CSF to blood circulation)
12 Subarachnoid space
13 Superior sagittal sinus
14 Third ventricle
15 Tongue

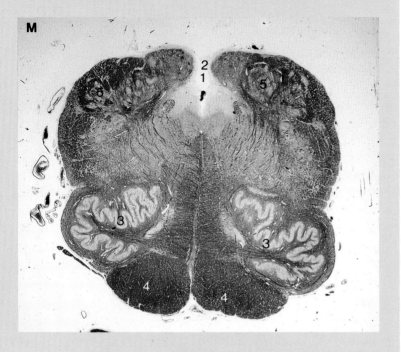

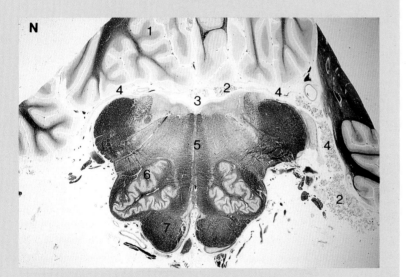

Foramina of the fourth
ventricle.

M Transverse section of medulla
oblongata passing through the
median aperture of the fourth
ventricle. Myelin stain. x5.1
1 Fourth ventricle
2 Median aperture
  (foramen of Magendie)
3 Olive
4 Pyramid
5 Posterior (dorsal) column nuclei

MHMS

N Transverse histological section
of medulla and cerebellum passing through the lateral apertures
of the fourth ventricle. Weigert
stain. x2.6
1 Cerebellum
2 Choroid plexus of fourth ventricle
3 Fourth ventricle
4 Lateral aperture
  (foramen of Luschka)
5 Medulla oblongata
6 Olive
7 Pyramid

MHMS

● *The lateral aperture is not a
well-defined opening, but a gap
between the cerebellum and
medulla. The choroid plexus
protrudes through it.*

O-Q The subarachnoid space.

O The subarachnoid space on the parietal lobe (opened by removing the arachnoid mater). x5.7
1 Arachnoid granulations
2 Arachnoid mater
3 Gyri
4 Frontal lobe
5 Longitudinal fissure
6 Occipital lobe
7 Parietal lobe
8 Subarachnoid space (arrow: space between pia mater investing the brain and the arachnoid mater)

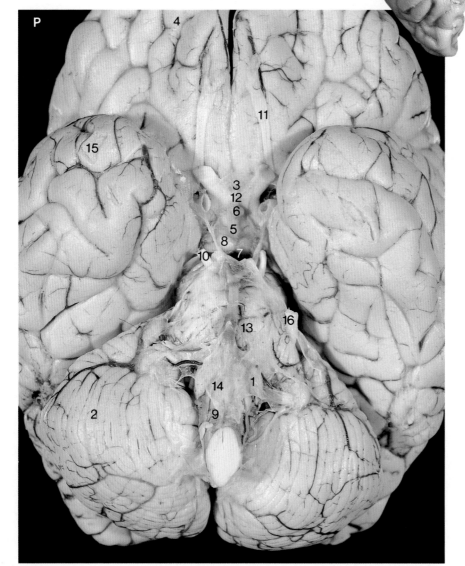

P The base of the brain with the arachnoid mater *in situ* to show the major cisternae associated with the ventral aspect of the brainstem. The interpeduncular cisterna has been partly opened to reveal the hypothalamus. x17.8
1 Arachnoid mater
2 Cerebellum
3 Cisterna of the optic chiasma
4 Frontal lobe
5 Hypothalamus
6 Infundibulum
7 Interpeduncular cisterna
8 Mamillary body
9 Medulla oblongata
10 Oculomotor nerve
11 Olfactory tract
12 Optic chiasma
13 Pons
14 Pontine cisterna
15 Temporal lobe
16 Trigeminal nerve

Q

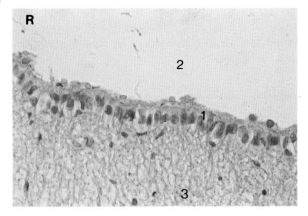

Q A sagittal section of the head to illustrate the cisternae. x.56

  1 Cerebello-medullary cisterna
  2 Cerebellum
  3 Cisterna of the great cerebral vein (of Galen)
     (or cisterna ambiens)
  4 Falx cerebri
  5 Frontal lobe
  6 Interpeduncular cisterna
  7 Lateral ventricle
  8 Medulla oblongata
  9 Midbrain
10 Mouth
11 Nose
12 Pontine cisterna
13 Pons
14 Spinal cord

● *All the ventricles are lined by an epithelium called the ependyma.*

R An histological section of the ependyma lining the fourth ventricle. Haematoxylin and eosin stain. x557

1 Ependyma
2 Fourth ventricle
3 Nervous tissue

CEREBRAL HEMISPHERES

The two cerebral hemispheres are the largest part of the brain and cover many other structures. The right and left cerebral hemispheres are connected to one another inferiorly by a band of transversely running white fibres called the corpus callosum. Each hemisphere has four lobes named after their position in the skull, i.e. frontal, parietal, temporal and occipital. Inside, each cerebral hemisphere has a C-shaped lateral ventricle. In the floor and medial walls of the hemispheres are collections of grey matter, (basal ganglia or nuclei) and nerve fibres.

Many functions have been localized to specific regions of the brain. For example, the frontal lobe is generally concerned with personality and higher centres for voluntary motor activities. The temporal lobe deals with sensations of smell, taste and hearing; the parietal lobe is concerned with the peripheral sensations and the occipital lobe with vision. Speech is associated with the frontal and temporal lobes in the major or dominant hemisphere i.e. the left hemisphere in right-handed individuals.

The surface of each hemisphere is covered by broad folds of grey matter (gyri) and spaces or furrows (sulci) between the gyri. Many of the gyri and sulci are variable in position but a small number are constant due to their development and are important functionally.

Buried immediately below the lateral sulcus is an island of cerebral cortex called the insula. This was buried during embryonic development when adjoining cortical areas overgrew this region.

The grey matter (cortex) covering the surface of the hemispheres is composed of neuronal cell bodies, their proximal neurites, blood vessels and supporting neuroglial cells. The neurons are of various types and some areas contain a concentration of certain types of multipolar neurons. Predominantly sensory (afferent) areas (postcentral gyrus) contain more stellate neurons while motor (efferent) areas (precentral gyrus) contain a greater proportion of the larger type of pyramidal cells. In the phylogenetically older areas of cortex in the temporal lobe (areas with a longer evolutionary history), three layers are distinguishable; while in the newer areas (neocortex), which include most of the cerebral cortex, there are six layers.

The white matter consists of myelinated nerve fibres (axons) embedded in neuroglia. The nerve fibres in the white matter form nerve tracts which connect different areas of the same hemisphere (short and long association fibres) or connect one hemisphere with the other hemisphere (commissural fibres) or are afferent and efferent fibres (projection fibres) which pass from and to the brain stem or spinal cord, sometimes via masses of grey matter (basal nuclei) buried inside the cerebral hemisphere.

The two cerebral hemispheres, however, are not identical. Left/right asymmetries appear in fetal development and persist into childhood and adulthood. They may lead to hand preference and cerebral dominance for language.

The lateral ventricle is larger on the left and the left lateral sulcus is longer and straighter than the right. In many right handers the right frontal lobe is larger than the left and the left temporal and occipital lobes are larger than the right. The corpus callosum is larger in left-handed and ambidextrous people, reflecting a greater interconnectedness of the two hemispheres.

• *Lesions involving the frontal lobe produce motor and autonomic disturbances and alteration in character and behaviour are apparent. Certain types of pain are no longer perceivable.*

• *Lesions involving the temporal lobe may produce disturbances in hearing, memory and in emotional behaviour.*

• *Lesions in the parietal lobe produce a disturbance or loss of function in perception of shape, size and texture (agnosia), and are associated with difficulties in writing and talking (sensory aphasia) and memory.*

• *Destruction of the cortical visual areas of the occipital lobes produces blindness, although the pupillary reactions to light persist.*

• *Specific speech areas are located in the frontal, parietal and temporal lobes. Lesions in these areas affect the use of language.*

Gyri and Sulci

Maps of the brain are based on the positions of constant gyri (folds) and sulci (furrows). Some of the gyri have specific functions. Areas of cortex adjacent to these are called association areas if they are related in function. Often they are concerned with interpretation which is called gnosis (to know). The entire brain surface is further subdivided into numbered areas which can be referred to for position of functions. Several different systems exist; Brodmann's is useful for localizing function, while von Economo's is based on wider cellular differences between the layers and von Bonin's is based on the distribution of fibres spreading out from the thalamus into the cortex.

If certain areas are damaged on the dominant side of the brain, normal functioning is impaired.

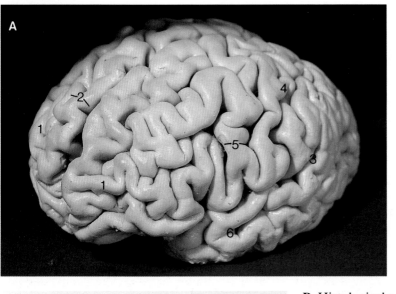

A Gyri and sulci on a lateral view of the brain. (The dura mater and arachnoid mater have been removed.) x.52
1 Frontal lobe
2 Gyri
3 Occipital lobe
4 Parietal lobe
5 Sulci
6 Temporal lobe

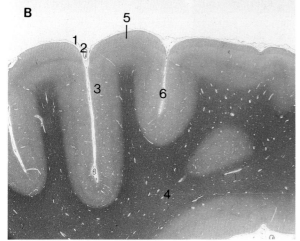

B Histological section to show gyri and sulci of the temporal lobe, stained with solochrome cyanin and nuclear fast red. x2.9
1 Arachnoid mater
2 Blood vessel
3 Cerebral cortex (grey matter)
4 Cerebral white matter
5 Gyrus
6 Sulcus

● *Aphasia is the inability to understand or express language in symbols. Damage to Brodmann's area 39 (angular gyrus) produces a sensory (receptor) aphasia called alexia or visual aphasia 'word blindness'. The printed word is meaningless. Damage to area 22 (sensory) produces auditory aphasia or word deafness. Damage to areas 44 and 45 (Broca's area) produces a motor aphasia in which the patient cannot convert thoughts into speech sounds. For areas see page 88.*

● *Agraphia is the loss of the ability to write.*

● *Apraxia is the inability to carry out learned voluntary acts.*

C-E Gyri and sulci which have relatively constant locations on every brain.

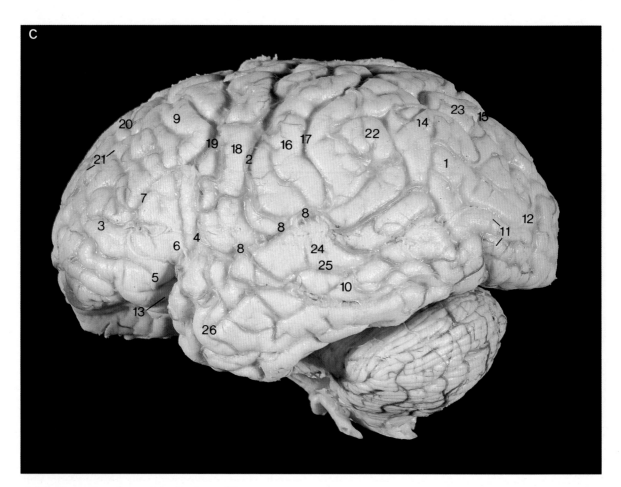

C The lateral surface of the brain. x.95

1 Angular gyrus
2 Central sulcus
3 Frontal lobe
4 Pars opercularis ⎫
5 Pars orbitalis ⎬ Inferior frontal gyrus
6 Pars triangularis ⎭
7 Inferior frontal sulcus
8 Lateral fissure (Sylvian fissure)
9 Middle frontal gyrus
10 Middle temporal gyrus
11 Occipital gyri
12 Occipital lobe
13 Orbital gyri

14 Parietal lobe
15 Parieto-occipital sulcus
16 Postcentral gyrus
17 Postcentral sulcus
18 Precentral gyrus
19 Precentral sulcus
20 Superior frontal gyrus
21 Superior frontal sulcus
22 Supramarginal gyrus
23 Superior parietal lobule
24 Superior temporal gyrus
25 Superior temporal sulcus
26 Temporal lobe

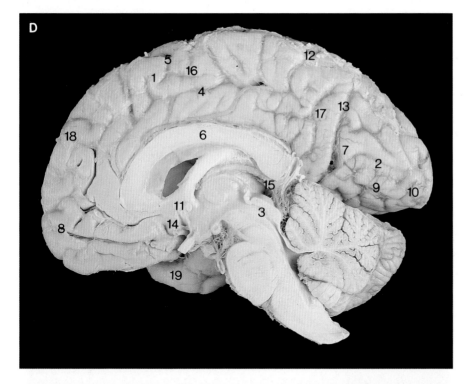

D The medial surface of the brain. x.78

1 Anterior paracentral lobule
2 Calcarine sulcus
3 Cerebral aqueduct
4 Cingulate sulcus
5 Central sulcus
6 Corpus callosum
7 Cuneate gyrus
8 Frontal lobe
9 Lingual gyrus
10 Occipital lobe
11 Paraterminal gyri
12 Parietal lobe
13 Parieto-occipital sulcus
14 Paraolfactory gyri
15 Pineal gland (body)
16 Posterior paracentral lobule
17 Precuneate gyrus
18 Superior frontal gyrus
19 Temporal lobe

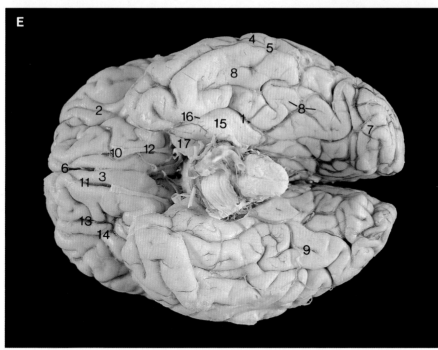

E The base of the hemi-spheres. x.63

1 Collateral sulcus
2 Frontal lobe
3 Gyrus rectus
4 Inferior temporal gyrus
5 Inferior temporal sulcus
6 Longitudinal fissure
7 Occipital lobe
8 Occipitotemporal gyri
9 Occipitotemporal sulcus
10 Olfactory bulb
11 Olfactory sulcus
12 Olfactory tract
13 Orbital gyri
14 Orbital sulcus
15 Parahippocampal gyrus
16 Rhinal sulcus
17 Uncus

F-N Brodmann's areas related to function.

Pioneering studies by Brodmann (1904) originally described 47 areas with distinct boundaries in the six-layered neocortex of the brain. These areas were based on minute histological variations. Many of these have since been ascribed functions and are designated below as motor, sensory, (including touch, taste and sight), speech and hearing, and the limbic system (including mood, behaviour and smell). The remaining numbered areas are indeterminate functionally and appear on page **89**.

This method of describing the brain was once thought to be outdated, but recent work in cellular neuroanatomy and neurophysiology has re-emphasised the importance of a detailed knowledge of cellular arrangements (cytoarchitectonics) for an understanding of cortical function. These studies have confirmed the validity of Brodmann's original concept.

F Brodmann's areas with motor functions. (Lateral view). x.68

4 Precentral gyrus (general movement control)

6
8 } 'Pre-motor' (some general movement, connections to basal ganglia, and controls eye movements)
9

44
45 } Broca's area (parts of these areas control speech movements; also see Hearing and Language below)

G Brodmann's areas with motor functions. (Medial view) x.68

4 Precentral gyrus (leg and foot movements)

6
8 } 'Pre-motor' (some general movement, connections to basal ganglia)
9

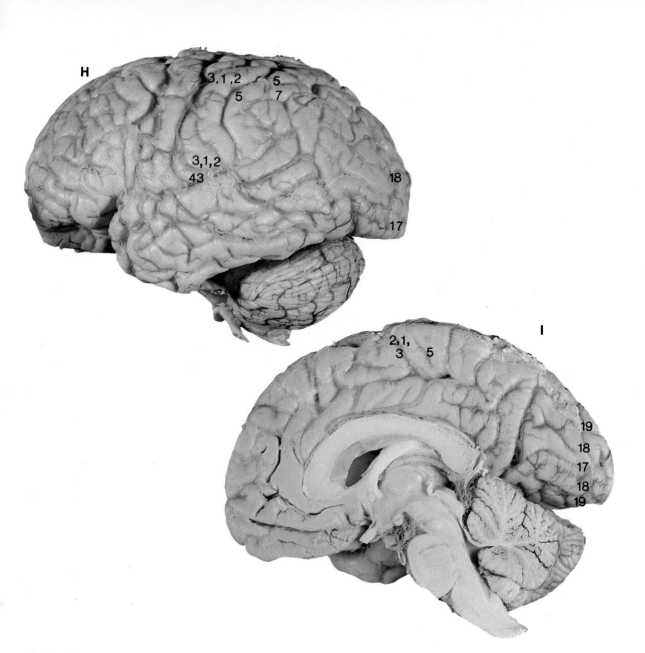

H Brodmann's areas with sensory functions (touch, taste, sight). (Lateral view) x.68

1 ⎫
2 ⎬ Postcentral gyrus (touch, pain, temperature,
3 ⎭ conscious proprioception)

5 ⎫ Parietal lobe (sensory association cortex:
7 ⎬ interpretation of senses perceived
   ⎭ in areas 1, 2 and 3).
43 Adjacent to the most inferior part of post
     central gyrus, 1, 2 and 3 (taste)
17 Lips of the calcarine sulcus (vision)
18 Remainder of occipital lobe (visual association for
     interpretation of visual information).

I Brodmann's areas with sensory functions (touch and sight). Medial view x.68

1 ⎫
2 ⎬ Postcentral gyrus (touch, pain, temperature,
3 ⎭ conscious proprioception)

5 Parietal lobe (sensory association cortex:
    interpretation of senses perceived in areas **1, 2** and
    3).

17 Lips of calcarine sulcus (vision)

18 ⎫ Remainder of occipital lobe (visual
19 ⎬ association for interpretation of visual
    ⎭ information).

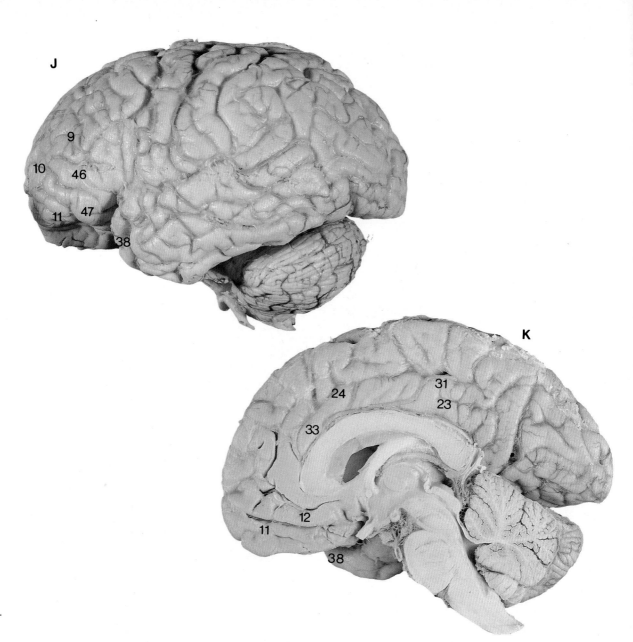

J Brodmann's areas concerned with emotion, mood and behaviour, including the limbic system. (Lateral view) x.68

9	(Upper part)	
10		Superior, middle and inferior
11	(Anterior	gyri of frontal lobe. 'Higher'
46	part)	intellectual functions
47		
38	Anterior pole of temporal lobe	Complex memory and imaging processes

K Brodmann's areas concerned with emotion, mood and behaviour, including the limbic system. (Medial view) x.68

23		
24	Cingulate gyrus	May add emotional 'Tone'
31	(see limbic system)	to sensory experience
33		including pain
11	Orbital region of	May have an inhibitory
12	frontal lobe	effect on expression of emotions
38	Anterior pole of temporal lobe	Complex memory and imaging processes

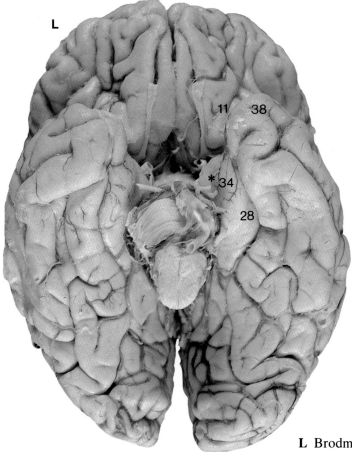

L Brodmann's areas concerned with olfactory functions and those concerned with emotion, mood, and behaviour, including the limbic system. (Basal view) x.77

	*Uncus	Olfactory
28	Parahippocampal gyrus (anterior part)	Olfactory
34	Adjacent to uncus	Olfactory
11	Posterior end of orbital gyri of frontal lobe	Olfactory
28	Parahippocampal gyrus	Memory
38	Anterior pole of temporal lobe	Complex memory and imaging processes

The uncus is not included in Brodmann's map because it is not formed of six-layered neocortex. It is the primary olfactory cortex; the other numbered areas are probably association cortex.

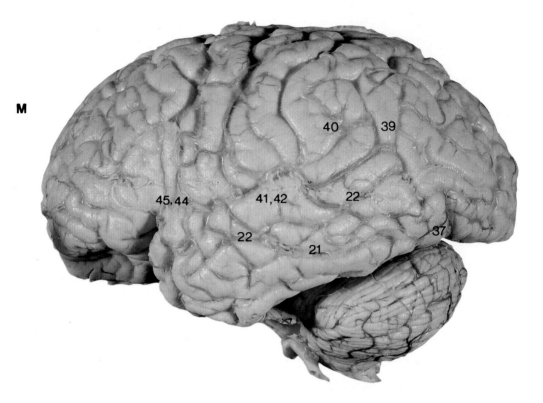

M

M Brodmann's areas concerned with hearing and language. (Lateral view) x.92

41 **42**	Middle of superior temporal gyrus	Primary auditory cortex Perception of sound
22	Superior temporal gyrus and part of the middle temporal gyrus	Auditory association cortex for interpretation of sound including speech (see **22*** below)
44 **45**	Part of pars triangularis and pars opercularis of inferior frontal gyrus	Broca's area for control of speech movements

22 *	Posterior end of the superior temporal gyrus	Wernicke's area or sensory speech area. Comprehension of speech and formulation of speech content
39	Angular gyrus	Important in reading
40	Supramarginal gyrus	Comprehension and ability to repeat speech
21	Middle temporal gyrus	Auditory memory
37	On border between temporal and occipital lobes	Mainly visual memory (possibly including written language)

* The uncus is not included in Brodmann's map because it is not formed of six-layered neocortex. It is the primary olfactory cortex; the other numbered areas are probably association cortex.

● *Language involves listening, comprehension and speech. In most people the left hemisphere is dominant in language functions, although the right is important for the emotional 'tone' and expression of spoken words.*

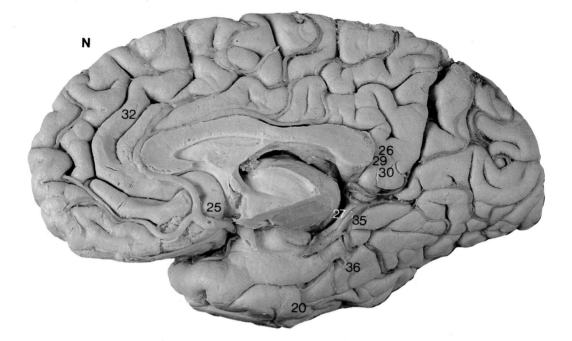

N Brodmann's areas which have no clearly determined function (indeterminate). (Medial view) x.79

25   Adjacent to olfactory tract in frontal lobe

26 ⎫
27 ⎪
29 ⎬ Behind the splenium of the corpus callosum.
30 ⎪ Connect cingulate and parahippocampal gyri
35 ⎭

36   Occipitotemporal gyrus

20   Inferior temporal gyrus
32   Medial side of frontal lobe above cingulate
      gyrus

13 ⎫
14 ⎪ Areas ascribed to the insula on the grounds of
15 ⎬ comparative anatomy
16 ⎭

Alternatives to Brodmann's methods for anatomical mapping of the cerebral cortex place less emphasis on small local variations in histology (cytoarchitecture).

The von Economo system recognizes five types of six-layered neocortex based on variation in the relative thickness of the cellular layers. The Bailey and von Bonin system divides the cortex into nine sections according to their afferent connections with the thalamus.

● *The existence of gender differences in the pattern of cortical gyri and sulci is controversial. Individual differences between persons of the same sex may be greater than any overall differences between males and females. However, in structures connected with reproductive functions distinct sexual dimorphism has been demonstrated in laboratory mammals and there is reason to believe that differences also exist in Man.*

A Map of the Cerebral Cortex based on the Distribution of Fibres from the Thalamus, according to Bailey and von Bonin.

It is useful to compare this diagram with that of the thalamic peduncles (see page 116).

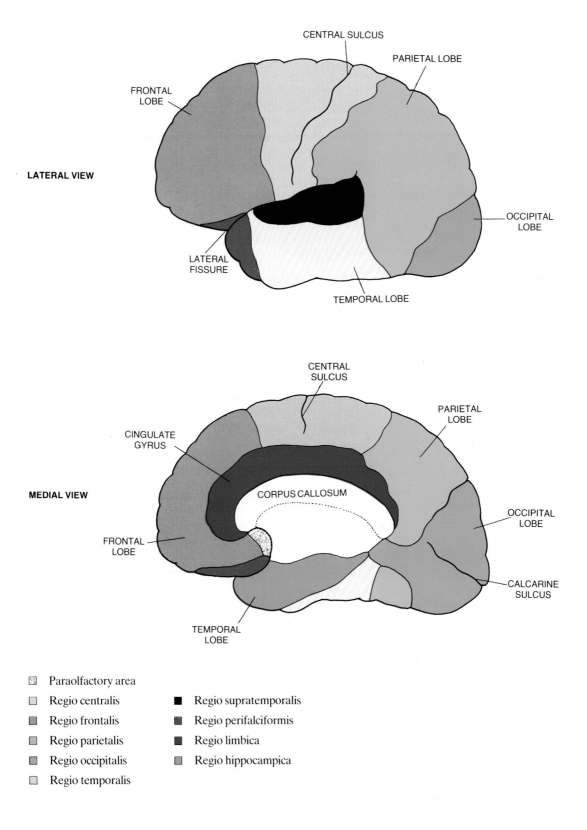

LATERAL VIEW

CENTRAL SULCUS

PARIETAL LOBE

FRONTAL LOBE

OCCIPITAL LOBE

LATERAL FISSURE

TEMPORAL LOBE

MEDIAL VIEW

CENTRAL SULCUS

PARIETAL LOBE

CINGULATE GYRUS

CORPUS CALLOSUM

OCCIPITAL LOBE

FRONTAL LOBE

CALCARINE SULCUS

TEMPORAL LOBE

Paraolfactory area

Regio centralis

Regio frontalis

Regio parietalis

Regio occipitalis

Regio temporalis

Regio supratemporalis

Regio perifalciformis

Regio limbica

Regio hippocampica

Histology of the Cerebral Cortex

Most parts of the cerebral hemisphere are covered by cortex comprising six layers of neurons. This type of cortex is known as neocortex or isocortex. Modified forms of cortex are found in cortical areas associated with the limbic. system; the cortex of the hippocampal formation, parahippocampal gyrus and uncus is three-layered (allocortex); that of the insula and cingulate gyrus has six indistinct layers (mesocortex). While the layers run parallel to the cortical surface, functionally the cells are associated in columns at right angles to the cortical surface, spanning all the layers. Cortical cells form synapses with each other. They also connect with association and projection fibres entering the cortex from the cerebral white matter and project fibres into the white matter.

Within the basic six-layer pattern different parts of the cortex show minor variations in their cellular arrangements (cytoarchitecture) and fibre distribution (myeloarchitecture). Some of these can be correlated with the localization of specific cortical functions (see Brodmann's areas).

Layer I contains some small cells but consists mainly of intracortical fibres.

Layer II contains small, mainly stellate cells connected in local circuits.

Layer III cells are predominantly pyramidal in shape and give rise to commissural and association fibres.

Layer IV is well-developed in cortical areas with a sensory function (for example, Brodmann's areas 1,2,3 (somatic sensory), 41 and 42 (hearing), and 17 (vision)) and poorly represented in motor cortex (for example, area 4). Its cells are granular in form and it receives many projection fibres from thalamic nuclei which are components of specific sensory pathways.

Layer V cells are mostly pyramidal and give off projection fibres to the basal ganglia, brainstem and spinal cord. This layer predominates in motor cortex.

Layer VI cells are variable in shape and send fibres to the thalamus.

Some pyramidal cells are present in all layers except layer I.

Using specific cytochemical techniques a variety of neurotransmitters can be identified in the cortical cells and fibres. Pyramidal cells are excitatory in function and contain glutamate. Non-pyramidal cells predominantly use gamma-amino-butyric acid (GABA). Some cells contain neuro-peptide transmitters either alone or co-localized with GABA. These are not confined to any one layer. Fibres entering the cortex from subcortical structures may be noradrenergic (transmitter noradrenaline); serotonergic (transmitter serotonin); dopaminergic (transmitter dopamine) or cholinergic (transmitter acetylcholine). In addition, there are corticopetal fibres (from the thalamus and the basal ganglia) for which the transmitters are unknown.

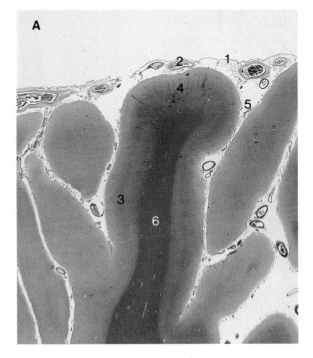

A A low power view of part of an histological section of cerebral hemisphere to differentiate the grey matter of the cortex on its surface from the white matter inside. Solochrome cyanin and light green stain. x3.5

1 Arachnoid mater
2 Blood vessel
3 Cortex
4 Gyrus
5 Sulcus
6 White matter

● *In Alzheimer's disease there is a loss of cholinergic axons to the cortex from the basal forebrain, particularly the nucleus of Meynert (see page 93).*

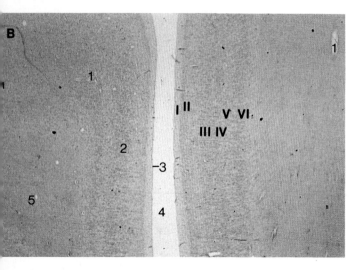

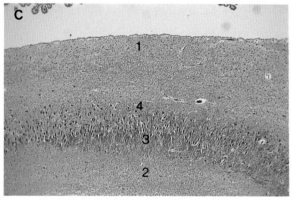

C An histological section to show the three layers of cells in the cortex of Ammon's horn, part of the hippocampus. Cresyl violet stain. x56
1 Alveus (fibres)
2 Molecular layer (stratum radiatum)
3 Pyramidal cell layer
4 Stratum oriens or polymorphic cell layer

CAM

B Section through the cortex of the frontal lobe to show the six-layered structure of neocortex. Cresyl violet stain. x7
1 Blood vessel
2 Cerebral cortex (the layers are numbered I-VI)
3 Pia mater
4 Sulcus
5 White matter

OXF

D A paraffin wax section through layers I to IV of the primary visual cortex of the occipital lobe to show neurons and fibres. Myelin stain. x55
1 Blood vessel
2 Intracortical fibres of layer I
3 Layer I
4 Layer II
5 Layer III
6 Layer IV
7 Neuronal cell body
8 Outer band of Baillarger
9 Projection fibres

CAM

● *The outer band of Baillarger is formed by thalamic afferent fibres entering layer IV. It is therefore well developed in sensory areas of cortex. In the visual cortex it is especially prominent and known as the stria of Gennari.*

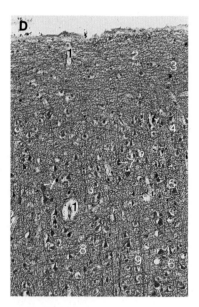

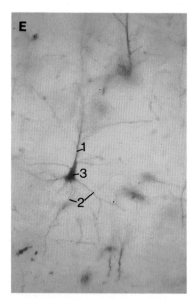

E A pyramidal cell from layer V of the temporal lobe cortex. Golgi-Cox stain. x223
1 Apical dendrite
2 Basal processes
3 Cell body

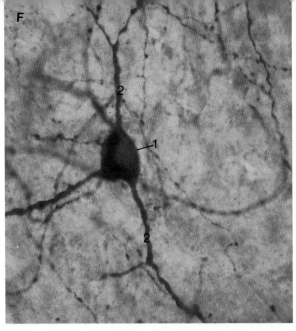

F-H Examples of the use of specific immunocyto-chemical staining methods to demonstrate the presence of neuropeptides in neurons of the cerebral neocortex. Neuropeptides, of which neuropeptide Y and somatostatin are examples, are a group of substances which may act as modulators of the sensitivity of neurons to other transmitters rather than as transmitters in their own right. They may coexist in the same cell with other transmitter substances.

F A neuropeptide Y containing neuron in the normal temporal neocortex, from a surgical specimen. The dark staining demonstrates the presence of neuropeptide Y in this cell. x1100
1 Cell body
2 Cell processes

Dr Victoria Chan-Palay

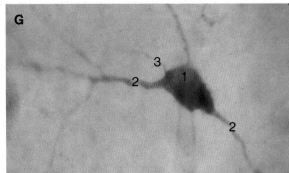

G Somatostatin-immunoreactive non-pyramidal neuron from layer V of the frontal cortex. x733
1 Cell body
2 Cell processes
3 Thin axon-like process

Dr Eva Braak

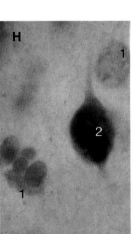

H Somatostatin-immuno-reactive non-pyramidal neuron from layer VI of the frontal neocortex. Surrounding non-reactive cells are demonstrated by gallocyanin-chromalum counterstain. x648
1 Non-reactive cells
2 Somatostatin-immuno-reactive cell

Dr Eva Braak

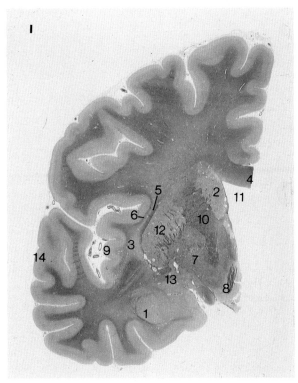

I A coronal section of one cerebral hemisphere to show the position of the substriatal grey matter, in which the nucleus of Meynert is situated. Phosphotungstic acid and haematoxylin stain. x1.1

1 Amygdaloid nucleus	8	Hypothalamus
2 Caudate nucleus	9	Insula
3 Claustrum	10	Internal capsule
4 Corpus callosum	11	Lateral ventricle
5 External capsule	12	Putamen
6 Extreme capsule	13	Substriatal grey matter
7 Globus pallidus	14	Temporal lobe

Short and Long Association Fibres

Association fibres connect different areas in the same hemisphere. They are divided into short and long groups. The short fibres connect adjacent gyri and dip below the floor of the intervening sulcus. The long fibres connect different lobes. There are four main deep bundles of long fibres; the uncinate fasciculus, the superior longitudinal fasciculus (including the arcuate fasciculus) the inferior longitudinal fasciculus, and the cingulum. The first two are placed laterally in the brain.

The uncinate fasciculus connects parts of the orbital, middle and inferior frontal gyri with anterior portions of the temporal lobe. A deeply placed part also connects the frontal and occipital lobes. The inferior longitudinal fasciculus connects the occipital lobe to the temporal lobe.

The superior longitudinal fasciculus connects the frontal to the occipital temporal and parietal lobes. The fronto-occipital fasciculus connects the frontal lobe to the occipital and temporal lobes. The arcuate fasciculus, sometimes described as part of this fasciculus, connects the middle frontal gyri to parts of the temporal lobe.

The cingulum is the principal medially placed long association bundle. It connects regions of the frontal and parietal lobes with the parahippocampal area and adjacent temporal region.

Short Association Fibres

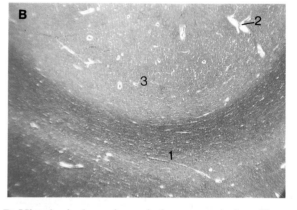

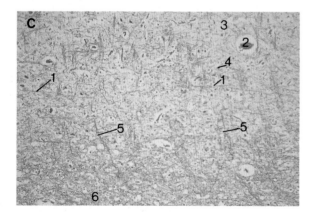

A Short association fibres between gyri in the frontal lobe. x1.5

1 Grey matter
2 Gyri
3 Short association fibres
4 Sulci
5 White matter

B Histological section of short association fibres between gyri of the frontal lobe. Solochrome cyanin and nuclear fast red stain. x22

1 Association fibres
2 Blood vessel
3 Cortex

C Higher magnification view of an histological section through the transition between the grey matter of the cerebral cortex and the white matter. Projection fibres (see page **97**) which enter and leave the cortex run at right angles to the cortical surface, while the association fibres run parallel to it. Luxol fast blue and cresyl violet stain. x356

1 Association fibres
2 Blood vessel
3 Grey matter
4 Neuronal cell body
5 Projection fibres
6 White matter

Long Association Fibres

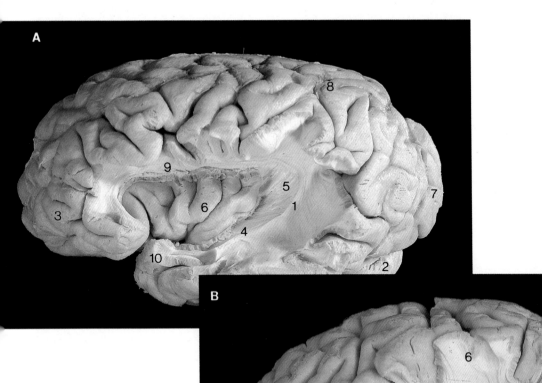

A The bundle of long association fibres called the superior longitudinal fasciculus lies immediately deep to the gyri and sulci laterally. x.77

  1 Arcuate fasciculus
  2 Cerebellum
  3 Frontal lobe
  4 Inferior longitudinal fasciculus
  5 Inferior occipitofrontal fasciculus
  6 Insula
  7 Occipital lobe
  8 Parietal lobe
  9 Superior longitudinal fasciculus
10 Temporal lobe

B Association fibres located immediately deep to the gyri and sulci on the lateral surface (including those of the insula).* x.75

  1 Arcuate fasciculus
  2 Extreme capsule
  3 Frontal pole
  4 Occipital pole
  5 Inferior longitudinal fasciculus
  6 Short association fibres
  7 Superior longitudinal fasciculus
  8 Temporal pole
  9 Uncinate fasciculus

* The freezing and thawing technique used to prepare this specimen causes a colour change. Brains may become yellow.

C The long association fibres in the cingulate and hippocampal gyri are known as the cingulum. Medial aspect of the brain with the cortex of the cingulate gyrus removed to reveal the cingulum. x.92

1 Cerebral aqueduct	**6** Frontal lobe	**11** Optic nerve	**16** Tectum of midbrain
2 Cingulum	**7** Genu (of corpus callosum)	**12** Parahippocampal gyrus	**17** Temporal lobe
3 Corpus callosum	**8** Hypothalamus	**13** Parietal lobe	**18** Thalamus
4 Crus cerebri	**9** Mamillary body	**14** Septum pellucidum	
5 Diencephalon	**10** Occipital lobe	**15** Splenium (of corpus callosum)	

Projection Fibres

Projection fibres which are both afferent and efferent, connect the spinal cord, brainstem, diencephalon and deep telencephalic nuclei with the cerebral cortex. Within the cerebral hemisphere the projection fibres are 'fan-shaped', the internal capsule forming the handle of the 'fan', as the fibres pass between the grey nuclear masses (the basal ganglia) lying in the floor of each cerebral hemisphere (see page **102**). Immediately above the nuclear masses, the fibres radiate vertically to the cerebral cortex, forming the 'fan' itself, the corona radiata. Most of these fibres lie deep to the association fibres and intersect the commissural fibres. They include all the major ascending (sensory) and descending (motor) pathways. The internal capsule is supplied by central branches of the middle and anterior cerebral arteries.

As the internal capsule passes between the nuclear masses it conforms to the shapes of their outlines and is divided into an anterior and a posterior limb which are joined at the genu.

The anterior limb contains the frontopontine and thalamocortical fibres. The genu contains corticonuclear fibres. The anterior one-half to two-thirds of the posterior limb contains thalamocortical fibres (general somatic sensory pathway) and corticospinal fibres.

The most posterior of the internal capsule fibres are 'retrolentiform' as they lie posterior to one of the nuclear masses (the lentiform nucleus). The retrolentiform region contains fibres of the auditory and of the optic radiations. Lesions in the internal capsule cause widespread neurological defects due to interruptions of a variety of nervous pathways.

The external capsule lies superficial to the basal ganglia. It also contains projection fibres. Its composition is incompletely known but it contains corticostriate fibres ending in the putamen and corticoreticular connections to the reticular formation. These also run in the internal capsule.

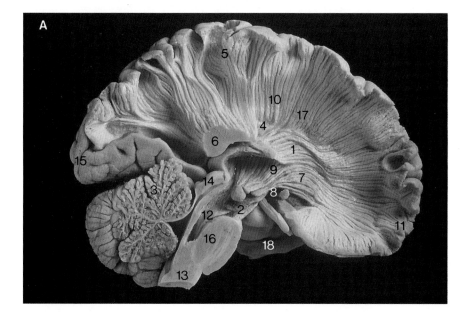

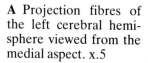

A Projection fibres of the left cerebral hemisphere viewed from the medial aspect. x.5

1 Anterior thalamic peduncle (or radiation)
2 Basis pedunculi
3 Cerebellum
4 Caudate nucleus
5 Corona radiata
6 Corpus callosum
7 Corticohypothalamic fibres in the internal capsule
8 Corticonigral tract
9 Corticorubral tract
10 Corticostriate fibres
11 Frontal lobe
12 Medial lemniscus
13 Medulla
14 Midbrain
15 Occipital lobe
16 Pons
17 Superior thalamic peduncle (or radiation)
18 Temporal lobe

Prof. N. Gluhbegovic

● *Corticohypothalamic, corticonigral, corticorubral and corticostriate fibres are descending pathways. The thalamic peduncles are ascending pathways.*

B Horizontal section of brain showing the relationship between internal, external and extreme capsules, the thalamus and the basal ganglia. Mulligan stain. x.70

1 Anterior limb of internal capsule
2 Caudate nucleus
3 Cerebellum
4 Claustrum
5 Corpus callosum
6 External capsule
7 Extreme capsule
8 Fornix
9 Frontal lobe
10 Genu of internal capsule
11 Insula
12 Lateral ventricle
13 Lentiform nucleus
14 Posterior limb of internal capsule (lenticulothalamic portion)
15 Retrolentiform part of posterior limb of the internal capsule
16 Thalamus
17 Third ventricle

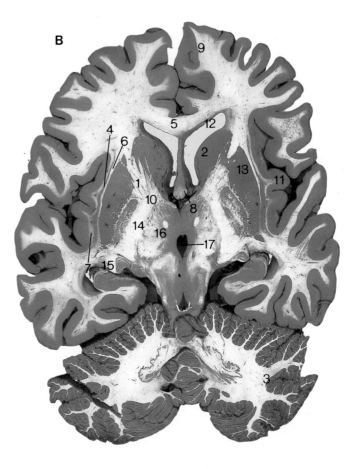

C Thick coronal slice of brain to show the passage of the projection fibres between the brainstem through the internal capsule into the cerebral hemisphere. Mulligan stain. x.74

1 Cerebral white matter
2 Corpus callosum
3 Crus cerebri (cerebral peduncle)
4 Fornix
5 Frontal lobe
6 Hippocampal formation
7 Internal capsule (posterior limb)
8 Lateral ventricle
9 Midbrain
10 Pons
11 Substantia nigra
12 Temporal lobe
13 Thalamus

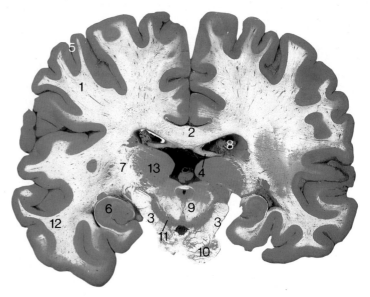

D A paraffin wax coronal section passing through one cerebral hemisphere, the caudal end of the diencephalon, the midbrain and the pons, showing the sublenticular portion of the posterior limb of the internal capsule. Solochrome cyanin and nuclear fast red stain. x1.6

1 Caudate nucleus
2 Cerebral aqueduct
3 Cerebral peduncle
4 Cingulate gyrus
5 Claustrum
6 Corona radiata
7 Corpus callosum
8 Decussation of the superior cerebellar peduncle
9 External capsule
10 Extreme capsule
11 Fornix
12 Habenular nuclei and stria medullaris thalami
13 Hippocampus
14 Insula
15 Internal capsule (posterior limb)
16 Internal capsule (sublenticular portion)
17 Lateral geniculate body
18 Lateral posterior nucleus of thalamus
19 Lateral ventricle
20 Midbrain
21 Pons
22 Putamen
23 Temporal lobe
24 Ventral posterior thalamic nuclei
25 Visual (optic) radiation

D

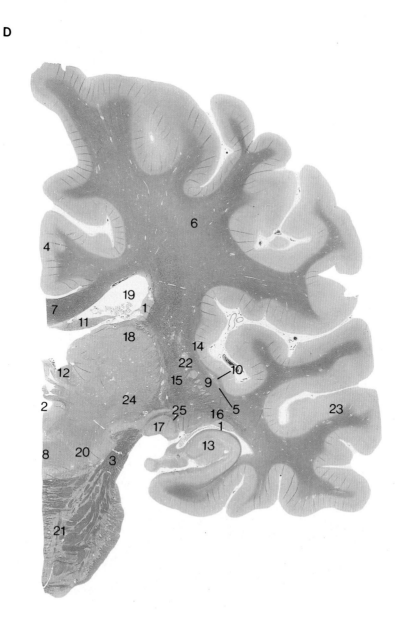

Insula

The insula is an area of cerebral cortex buried deep to the lateral sulcus. It is not visible unless the two gyri adjacent to the lateral sulcus are separated.

Histologically the anterior part of the insula is granular and the posterior part is agranular. The insula is believed to be associated with visceral functions such as autonomic and emotional responses to external stimuli. Though many of its fibre connections are unknown, it is recognized that the anterior part of the insula is connected to the olfactory and taste areas of the cerebral cortex. The posterior part is connected to the auditory cortex and to a somatic sensory area of the parietal operculum known as SII because it is secondary to the main somatic sensory area.

Immediately deep (medial) to the insula are the external capsule and the lentiform nucleus.

A-B Position of the insula.

A A lateral view of the brain with a coloured overlay to indicate the position of the insula buried below the surface. x.57
1 Cerebellum
2 Frontal lobe
3 Insula (coloured overlay)
4 Lateral sulcus
5 Occipital lobe
6 Parietal lobe
7 Temporal lobe

B Cerebral hemisphere dissected from the lateral side to reveal the insula. x.61
1 Frontal lobe
2 Frontal operculum (cut)
3 Insula
4 Occipital lobe
5 Parietal lobe
6 Parietal operculum (cut)
7 Temporal lobe
8 Temporal operculum (cut)

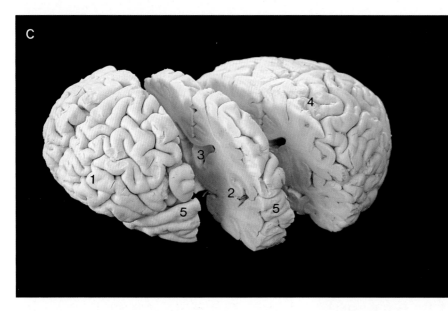

C A coronal section through the insula. x.51
1 Frontal lobe
2 Insula
3 Lateral ventricle
4 Parietal lobe
5 Temporal lobe

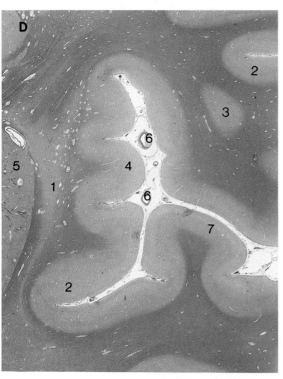

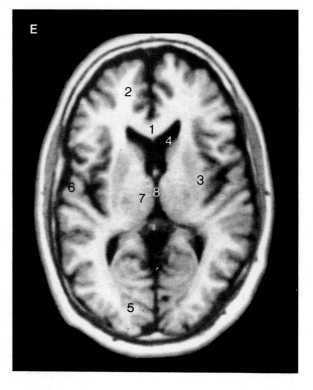

D Histological section to show the insula and the middle cerebral vessels. Section stained with solochrome cyanin and nuclear fast red. x2.5
1 Claustrum
2 Cortex
3 Frontal operculum
4 Insula
5 Lentiform nucleus
6 Middle cerebral artery
7 Temporal operculum

E Transverse image of the normal adult brain as seen by the nuclear magnetic resonance (NMR) technique.
1 Corpus callosum
2 Frontal lobe
3 Insula
4 Lateral ventricle
5 Occipital lobe
6 Temporal lobe
7 Thalamus
8 Third ventricle

Dr G. Bydder

Basal Ganglia or Basal Nuclei

The basal nuclei are well-defined masses of grey matter which are grouped together, embedded in the subcortical white matter of the telencephalon around the lateral ventricle. They can only be seen when the brain has been sectioned or dissected. The basal ganglia are the corpus striatum, amygdaloid nucleus and claustrum. The corpus striatum, substantia nigra and subthalamic nucleus are all areas concerned with motor functions.

The corpus striatum is divided into two parts (the caudate and lentiform nuclei) by a band of white matter called the internal capsule.

From a functional viewpoint, the substantia nigra and subthalamic nucleus may also be considered as parts of the basal ganglia, but the amygdaloid nucleus is not (see Limbic System).

The caudate nucleus forms a 'C' shape closely applied to the contours of the lateral ventricle (along the floor of the anterior horn and body, and the roof of the inferior horn). It ends anteriorly in apparent continuity with the amygdaloid nucleus (or 'amygdala').

The lentiform (lens-shaped) nucleus lies deep to the insula, and is divided by a vertical sheet of white matter into a dark, large lateral portion (putamen) and an inner, paler portion (globus pallidus).

The amygdaloid nucleus is concerned with olfactory reflexes and is part of the limbic system, concerned with aggressive and sexual behaviour.

The claustrum is a thin sheet of grey matter whose function is unknown.

There are afferent and efferent connections between the corpus striatum and the cerebral cortex, thalamus, subthalamus and brainstem (see Movement Control on page **253-255**).

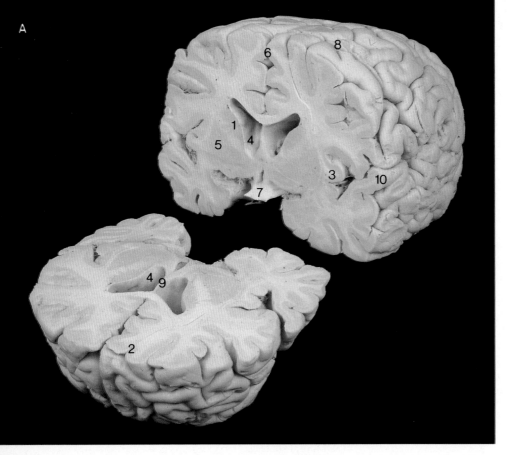

A Coronal section through the cerebral hemispheres and the diencephalon to illustrate the position of the caudate and lentiform nuclei. x.75

1 Caudate nucleus
2 Frontal lobe
3 Insula
4 Lateral ventricle
5 Lentiform nucleus
6 Longitudinal fissure
7 Optic chiasma
8 Parietal lobe
9 Septum pellucidum
10 Temporal lobe

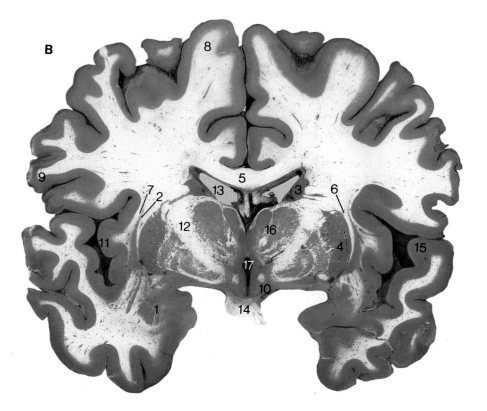

B Thick stained coronal slice through both cerebral hemispheres at the level of the optic chiasma to show the caudate, lentiform and amygdaloid nuclei. Mulligan stain. x.88

1 Amygdaloid nucleus (amygdala)
2 Claustrum
3 Caudate nucleus ⎫
4 Lentiform nucleus ⎬ Corpus striatum
5 Corpus callosum
6 External capsule

7 Extreme capsule
8 Frontal lobe
9 Frontal operculum
10 Hypothalamus
11 Insula
12 Internal capsule

13 Lateral ventricle
14 Optic chiasma
15 Temporal lobe
16 Thalamus
17 Third ventricle

C-H If the brain is dissected from the lateral side the caudate and lentiform nuclei and associated white matter are revealed in sequence.

C The extreme capsule lies immediately deep to the gyri and sulci of the insula. x.66
1 Corona radiata
2 Extreme capsule
3 Frontal lobe
4 Occipital lobe
5 Parietal lobe

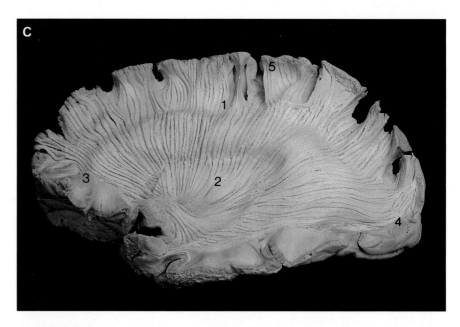

D The brain dissected from the lateral surface to show the claustrum. x.64
1 Claustrum
2 Corona radiata
3 External capsule
4 Frontal lobe
5 Inferior longitudinal fasciculus
6 Occipital lobe
7 Parietal lobe
8 Temporal lobe
9 Uncinate fasciculus

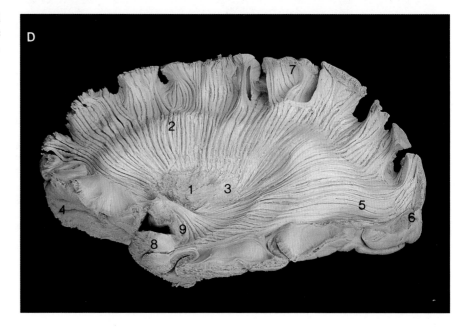

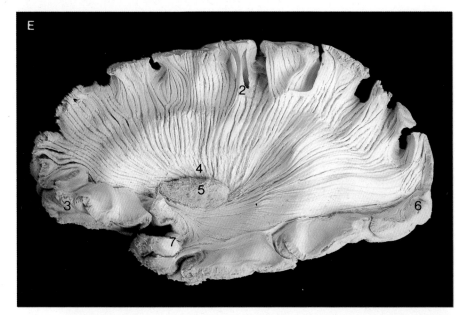

1 Cerebellum
2 Corona radiata
3 Frontal lobe
4 Internal capsule
5 Lentiform nucleus
6 Occipital lobe
7 Temporal lobe

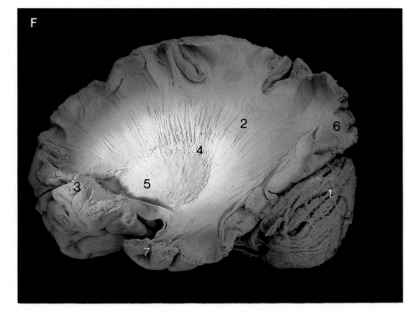

F Deeper dissection from the lateral side to show the lentiform nucleus. x.57

G The lentiform and caudate nuclei as viewed from the lateral surface. x.65

1 Caudate nucleus
2 Cerebellum
3 Choroid plexus
4 Corpus callosum
5 Frontal lobe
6 Lateral ventricle
7 Lentiform nucleus
8 Occipital lobe
9 Parietal lobe
10 Temporal lobe

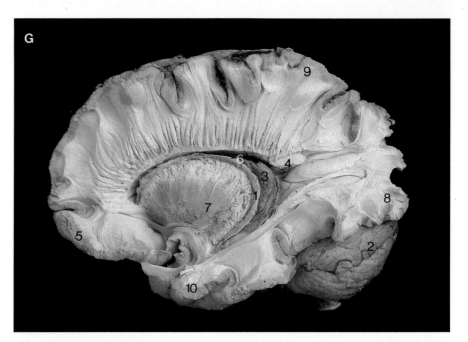

H Caudate nucleus and diencephalon in a dissection of the medial side of the brain. x.62

1 Caudate nucleus
2 Cerebellum
3 Fornix
4 Frontal lobe
5 Internal capsule
6 Mamillary body
7 Mamillothalamic tract
8 Midbrain
9 Occipital lobe
10 Optic chiasma
11 Pons
12 Stria terminalis
13 Thalamic nuclei

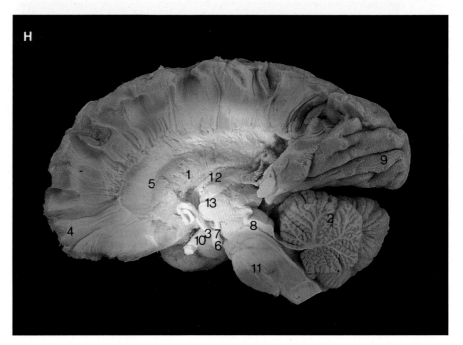

I-J Sections to demonstrate connections between the rostral part (head) of the caudate nucleus and the lentiform nucleus across the internal capsule.

The striped or striated appearance caused by these connections gives rise to the name 'corpus striatum'.

I Thick coronal section through both cerebral hemispheres. Mulligan stain. x.69

1 Caudate nucleus	**7** Frontal lobe
2 Claustrum	**8** Insula
3 Connections between the caudate nucleus and the lentiform nucleus	**9** Internal capsule
	10 Lateral ventricle
	11 Lentiform nucleus
4 Corpus callosum	**12** Longitudinal fissure
5 External capsule	**13** Septum pellucidum
6 Extreme capsule	**14** Temporal lobe

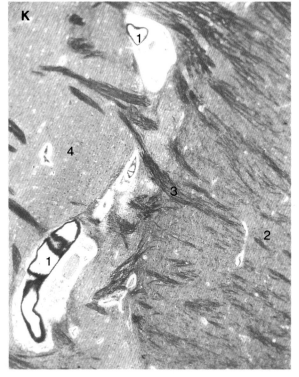

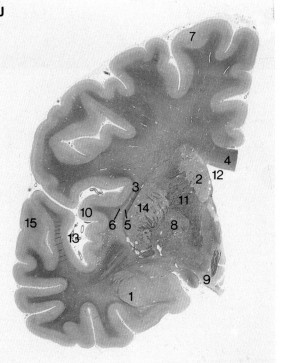

J An histological section through a cerebral hemisphere to show the structure of the corpus striatum. The relationship between the caudate, lentiform and amygdaloid nuclei is also illustrated. Phosphotungstic acid and haematoxylin stain. x1.05

1 Amygdaloid nucleus	**9** Hypothalamus
2 Caudate nucleus	**10** Insula
3 Claustrum	**11** Internal capsule
4 Corpus callosum	**12** Lateral ventricle
5 External capsule	**13** Middle cerebral artery
6 Extreme capsule	**14** Putamen
7 Frontal lobe	**15** Temporal lobe
8 Globus pallidus	

K Histological section to show nerve fibres passing between the putamen and the globus pallidus. A higher magnification of Figure **J**. Phosphotungstic acid and haematoxylin stain. x27

1 Blood vessel
2 Globus pallidus
3 Nerve fibres
4 Putamen

● *The term 'pallidus', i.e. pale, describes the appearance of this structure in unstained sections or in sections stained to demonstrate grey matter, for example with Mulligan stain.*

L-P Dissections and histological preparations to show the relationships of the basal ganglia.

L-O The dissections in **L, N** and **O** are the same specimen to show the relationship between the corpus striatum and thalamus.

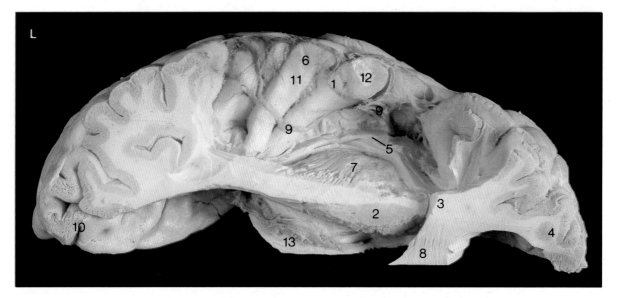

L A cerebral hemisphere dissected from above to show the medial to lateral relationships of the thalamus, caudate nucleus and lentiform nucleus. x.95

1 Auditory cortex	**6** Lateral aspect	**11** Superior temporal gyrus
2 Caudate nucleus	**7** Lentiform nucleus	**12** Temporal lobe
3 Corpus callosum	**8** Medial aspect	**13** Thalamus
4 Frontal lobe	**9** Middle cerebral artery (branches)	
5 Insula	**10** Occipital lobe	

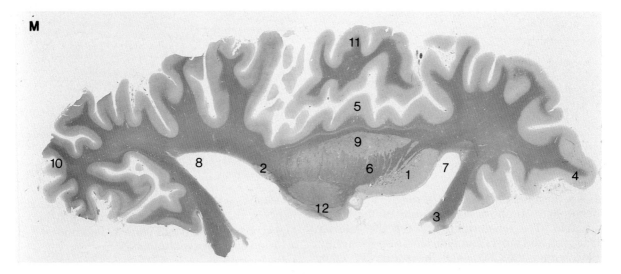

M Horizontal histological section through one cerebral hemisphere to illustrate the relationships of the caudate and lentiform nuclei to the thalamus. Solochrome cyanin and nuclear fast red stain. x.90

1 Caudate nucleus (head)	**5** Insula	**9** Lentiform nucleus
2 Caudate nucleus (tail)	**6** Internal capsule	**10** Occipital lobe
3 Corpus callosum	**7** Lateral ventricle (anterior horn)	**11** Temporal lobe
4 Frontal lobe	**8** Lateral ventricle (posterior horn)	**12** Thalamus

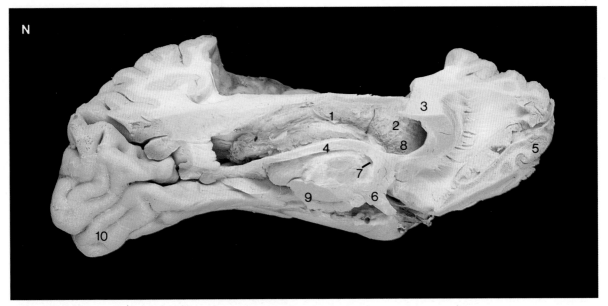

N A cerebral hemisphere dissected from the medial side to show the superior to inferior relationships of the thalamus and caudate nucleus. The septum pellucidum has been removed. x.87

1 Caudate nucleus (body)
2 Caudate nucleus (head)
3 Corpus callosum
4 Fornix

5 Frontal lobe
6 Hypothalamus
7 Interventricular foramen
8 Lateral ventricle

9 Midbrain
10 Occipital lobe

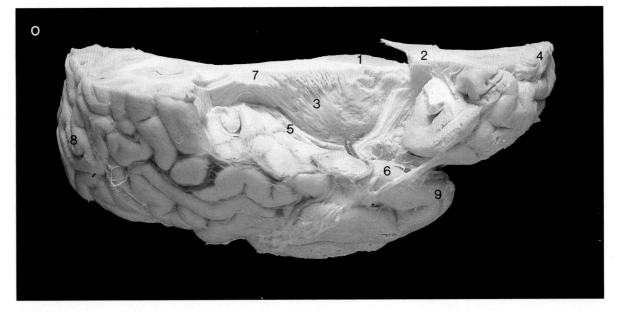

O A cerebral hemisphere dissected from the lateral surface to illustrate the relationships between the external capsule and lentiform nucleus. x.87

1 Caudate nucleus
2 Corpus callosum
3 External capsule

4 Frontal lobe
5 Inferior longitudinal fasciculus
6 Lateral aspect

7 Medial aspect
8 Occipital lobe
9 Temporal lobe

P Coronal histological section through part of one cerebral hemisphere showing the caudate and lentiform nuclei, thalamus and subthalamus. Solochrome cyanin and light green stain. x2.45

1 Caudate nucleus (body)	11 Lentiform nucleus
2 Caudate nucleus (tail)	12 Subthalamus
3 Corpus callosum	13 Thalamus
4 External capsule	
5 Extreme capsule	
6 Fornix	
7 Insular cortex	
8 Internal capsule	
9 Lateral ventricle (body)	
10 Lateral ventricle (inferior horn)	

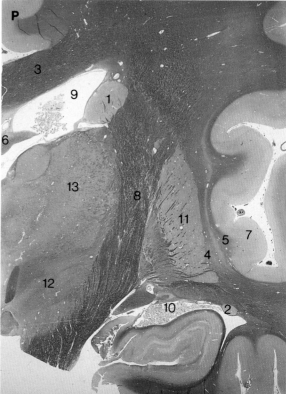

Q-S Sections to illustrate the position and structure of the substantia nigra.

Q An half brain dissected from the medial side to demonstrate the position and relationships of the substantia nigra and red nucleus. x.66

1 Anterior commissure	10 Mamillothalamic tract
2 Caudate nucleus	11 Medulla
3 Cerebellum	12 Midbrain
4 Cerebral aqueduct	13 Pons
5 Cerebral hemisphere	14 Red nucleus
6 Cerebral peduncle	15 Substantia nigra
7 Inferior colliculus	16 Superior colliculus
8 Fourth ventricle	17 Thalamus
9 Mamillary body	

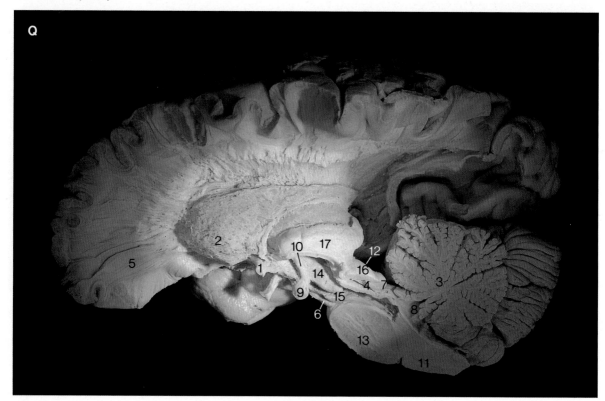

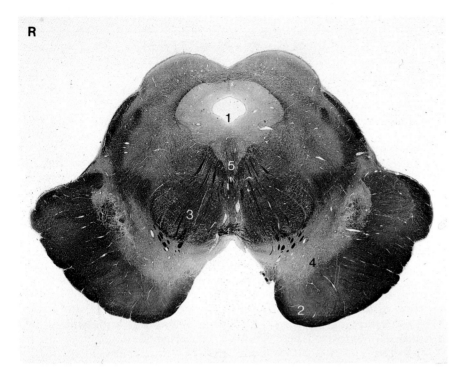

R A transverse histological section of the midbrain to show the position of the substantia nigra. Weigert-Pal stain. x4.9

1 Cerebral aqueduct
3 Red nucleus
5 Tegmentum
2 Cerebral peduncle
4 Substantia nigra

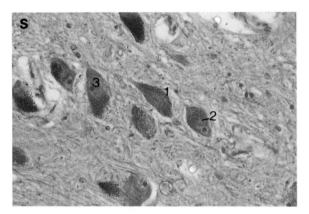

S Cells of the substantia nigra showing their brown neuromelanin pigmentation. Solochrome cyanin and nuclear fast red stain. x446
1 Cell body
2 Neuromelanin
3 Nucleus

DIENCEPHALON

The name 'diencephalon' means 'between brain', and refers to the part lying between the brainstem and the cerebral hemispheres. The diencephalon surrounds the third ventricle and is subdivided into four parts—the thalamus, the subthalamus, the hypothalamus and the epithalamus.

The thalamus is a paired structure, with right and left thalami forming the upper part of the lateral walls of the third ventricle. Each is an oval mass of grey matter divided into medial, lateral and anterior parts by a Y-shaped band of white matter, the internal medullary lamina. Several nuclei, each with different connections (see diagrams on page **116**) may be found within the divisions.

The thalamus is linked to the sensory systems, basal ganglia, cerebellum, brainstem and cerebral cortex. These connections enable the thalamus to act as an intermediary between subcortical structures and the cerebral cortex. Most cortical connections are grouped in bundles, the thalamic peduncles or radiations. Thalamic nuclei connected to localized areas of cerebral cortex are often called 'specific nuclei' and those not so connected have 'nonspecific' connections. Some nuclei fall into both categories. The medial and lateral geniculate bodies lie slightly separated from the main mass of the thalamus. They are part of the auditory and visual pathways respectively.

The subthalamus lies below and caudal to the thalamus. It contains the subthalamic nucleus, a prominent nucleus, which is part of the system for movement coordination in the basal ganglia.

The hypothalamus lies below the rostral end of the thalamus, forming the floor and lower part of the lateral walls of the third ventricle. It contains several nuclei and has a variety of important functions. Through its connections with the autonomic nervous system, it is involved in the regulation of body temperature and the circulation. It also controls food and water intake. As a part of the endocrine system it regulates the activity of the anterior lobe of the hypophysis by producing hormones known as releasing and inhibitory factors. These hormones are released into blood vessels in the median eminence and are carried by a system of portal vessels to the capillary plexus of the adenohypophysis. Antidiuretic hormone and oxytocin, which are stored in the posterior lobe of the hypophysis, are produced in large neurosecretory cells in the supraoptic and paraventricular nuclei. The hypothalamus is also a component of the limbic system involved in emotional behaviour.

The hypothalamus is anatomically and physiologically linked to the hypophysis or pituitary gland. The hypophysis consists of two parts, the adenohypophysis or anterior lobe and the neurohypophysis or posterior lobe. The adenohypophysis has no neural connections with the hypothalamus but is linked to it via its blood supply, the portal system. It is composed of endocrine cells of epithelial origin from the roof of the stomodeum. The neurohypophysis is in direct neural continuity with the hypothalamus. It develops as an outgrowth from the diencephalon in the embryo. The hypophyseal stalk contains tracts connecting it to the adult hypothalamus. Neurosecretory neurons in the hypothalamus secrete hormones, the releasing factors, into capillaries of the portal system in the hypothalamus. These substances are transported via portal veins in the hypophyseal stalk to a second capillary bed in the adenohypophysis which supplies the endocrine cells. These cells respond to the releasing factors by producing hormones which regulate the activity of other endocrine glands throughout the body. A textbook of endocrinology should be consulted for further information on the structure and functions of the hypophysis.

The main tracts of the hypothalamus are the fornix, medial forebrain bundle, mamillothalamic tract and dorsal longitudinal fasciculus.

The epithalamus lies above the thalamus. It consists of the habenular nuclei and their associated tracts, and the pineal gland. The habenular nuclei and their tracts are part of the limbic system. The pineal gland is an endocrine gland and its cells, the pinealocytes, produce a hormone melatonin, which is associated with reproductive behaviour and the regulation of physiological and behavioural rhythms, for example the sleep/wake cycle. Melatonin secretion shows a diurnal rhythm related to light and darkness.

The pineal gland is believed to have evolved from a median third eye in extinct lower vertebrates. In modern vertebrates it is no longer photosensitive itself, but receives information about light levels indirectly via a complex neural pathway from the retina (see diagram).

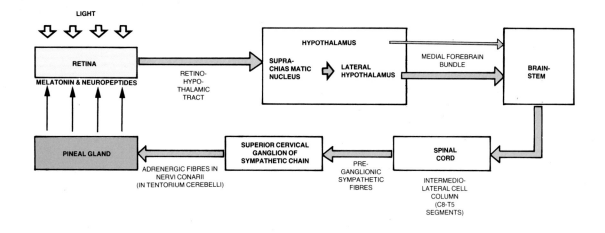

- *In the thalamic syndrome, pain perception is distorted or exaggerated on the side opposite the lesion.*

- *Rudimentary awareness of sensations, especially pain, exists at thalamic level.*

- *The rhythmic pattern of melatonin secretion is disturbed by 'jet lag'.*

A series of diagrams to illustrate the afferent and efferent connections of the thalamus.

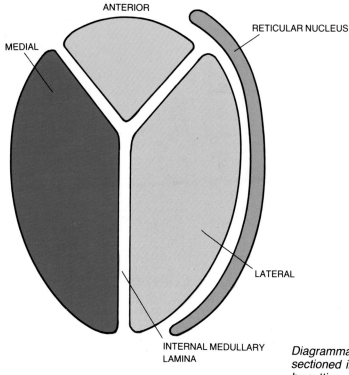

Diagrammatic view of the thalamus from above, as if sectioned into anterior, medial and lateral subdivisions by cutting along the internal medullary lamina.

The thalamus viewed from the lateral side as if cut into dorsal and ventral tiers of lateral thalamic nuclei.

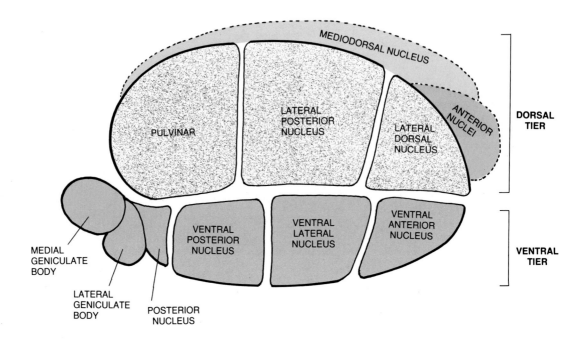

Diagrammatic view of the thalamus sectioned to show the mediodorsal nucleus and the intralaminar nuclei.

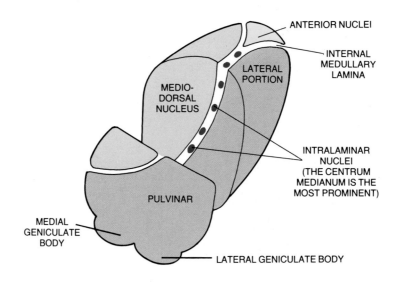

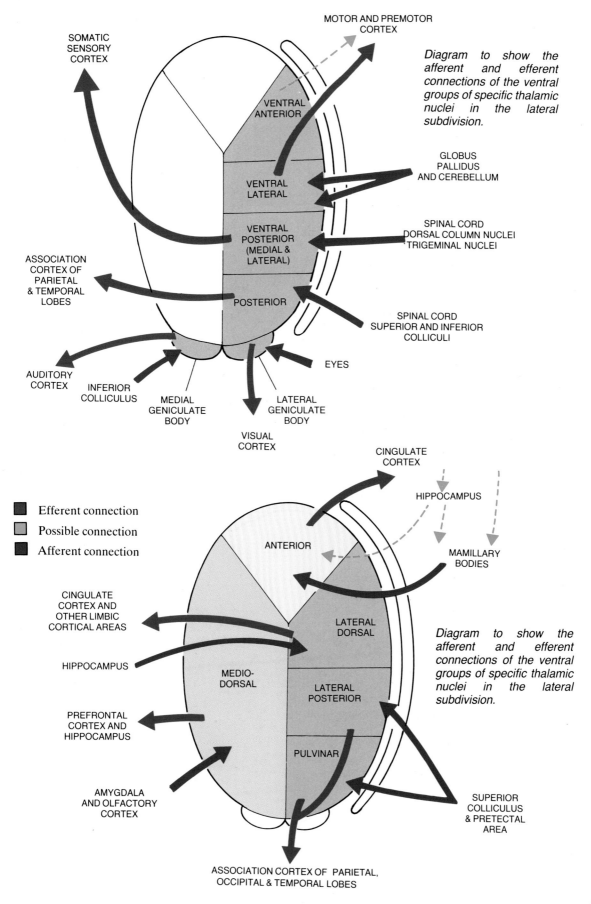

MOTOR AND PREMOTOR CORTEX

SOMATIC SENSORY CORTEX

Diagram to show the afferent and efferent connections of the ventral groups of specific thalamic nuclei in the lateral subdivision.

VENTRAL ANTERIOR

VENTRAL LATERAL

GLOBUS PALLIDUS AND CEREBELLUM

VENTRAL POSTERIOR (MEDIAL & LATERAL)

SPINAL CORD DORSAL COLUMN NUCLEI TRIGEMINAL NUCLEI

ASSOCIATION CORTEX OF PARIETAL & TEMPORAL LOBES

POSTERIOR

SPINAL CORD SUPERIOR AND INFERIOR COLLICULI

EYES

AUDITORY CORTEX

INFERIOR COLLICULUS

MEDIAL GENICULATE BODY

LATERAL GENICULATE BODY

VISUAL CORTEX

CINGULATE CORTEX

HIPPOCAMPUS

■ Efferent connection

■ Possible connection

■ Afferent connection

ANTERIOR

MAMILLARY BODIES

CINGULATE CORTEX AND OTHER LIMBIC CORTICAL AREAS

LATERAL DORSAL

Diagram to show the afferent and efferent connections of the ventral groups of specific thalamic nuclei in the lateral subdivision.

HIPPOCAMPUS

MEDIO-DORSAL

LATERAL POSTERIOR

PREFRONTAL CORTEX AND HIPPOCAMPUS

PULVINAR

AMYGDALA AND OLFACTORY CORTEX

SUPERIOR COLLICULUS & PRETECTAL AREA

ASSOCIATION CORTEX OF PARIETAL, OCCIPITAL & TEMPORAL LOBES

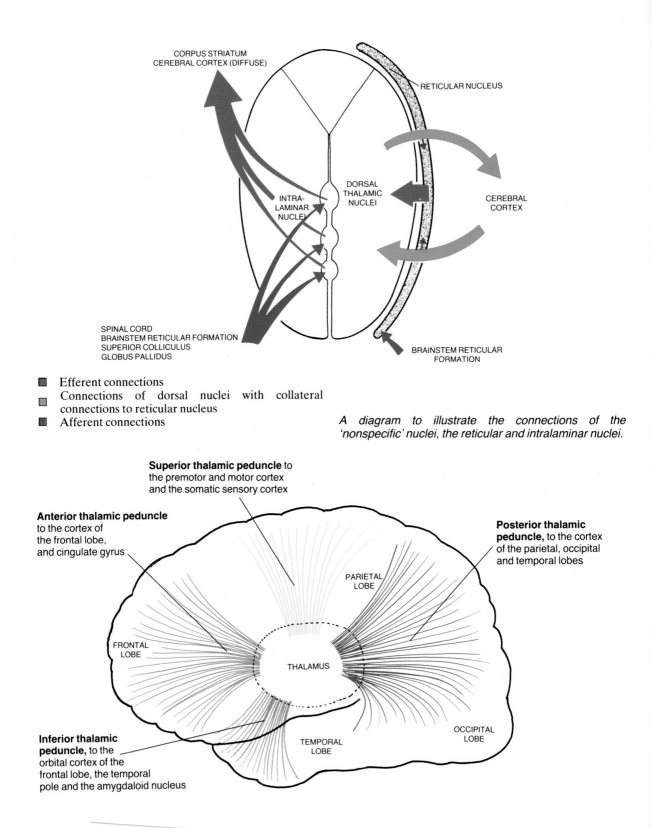

CORPUS STRIATUM
CEREBRAL CORTEX (DIFFUSE)

RETICULAR NUCLEUS

DORSAL
THALAMIC
NUCLEI

INTRA-
LAMINAR
NUCLEI

CEREBRAL
CORTEX

SPINAL CORD
BRAINSTEM RETICULAR FORMATION
SUPERIOR COLLICULUS
GLOBUS PALLIDUS

BRAINSTEM RETICULAR
FORMATION

■ Efferent connections

■ Connections of dorsal nuclei with collateral connections to reticular nucleus

■ Afferent connections

A diagram to illustrate the connections of the 'nonspecific' nuclei, the reticular and intralaminar nuclei.

Superior thalamic peduncle to the premotor and motor cortex and the somatic sensory cortex

Anterior thalamic peduncle to the cortex of the frontal lobe, and cingulate gyrus

Posterior thalamic peduncle, to the cortex of the parietal, occipital and temporal lobes

PARIETAL
LOBE

FRONTAL
LOBE

THALAMUS

Inferior thalamic peduncle, to the orbital cortex of the frontal lobe, the temporal pole and the amygdaloid nucleus

TEMPORAL
LOBE

OCCIPITAL
LOBE

Diagram to show the thalamic peduncles (radiations) projected onto the brain surface, lateral view.

A-E Dissections and histological preparations showing the anatomy of the diencephalon as a whole.

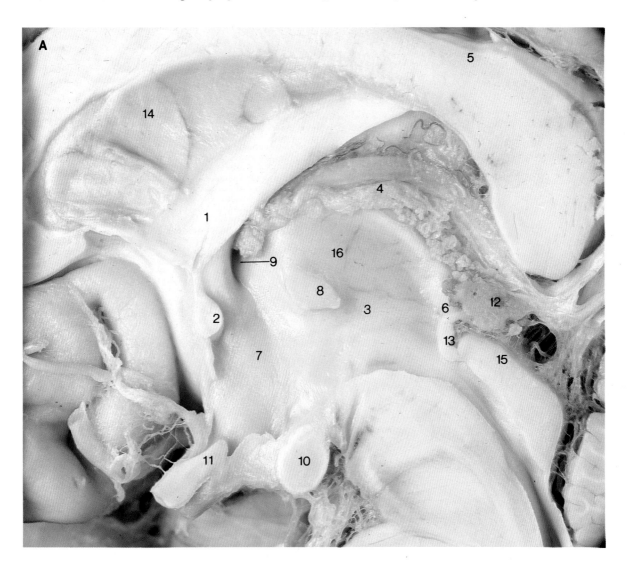

A Sagittal section of the brain to show the positions of the thalamus, hypothalamus and epithalamus. x2.2

1 Anterior column of fornix	**7** Hypothalamus	**13** Posterior commissure
2 Anterior commissure	**8** Interthalamic connection or adhesion	**14** Septum pellucidum
3 Cavity of third ventricle	**9** Interventricular foramen	**15** Superior colliculus
4 Choroid plexus of third ventricle	**10** Mamillary body	**16** Thalamus
5 Corpus callosum	**11** Optic chiasma	
6 Epithalamus	**12** Pineal body (gland) (part of epithalamus)	

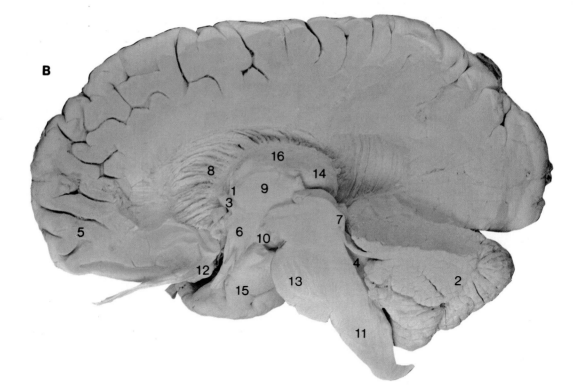

B A sagittal section of brain dissected on the medial side to show the shapes and relationships of the thalamus and hypothalamus. Part of the cerebellum has been removed. x1

1 Anterior portion of thalamus
2 Cerebellum
3 Fornix
4 Fourth ventricle
5 Frontal lobe
6 Hypothalamus
7 Inferior colliculus
8 Internal capsule
9 Interthalamic adhesion
10 Mamillary body
11 Medulla oblongata
12 Optic chiasma
13 Pons
14 Pulvinar of thalamus
15 Temporal lobe
16 Thalamus

OXF

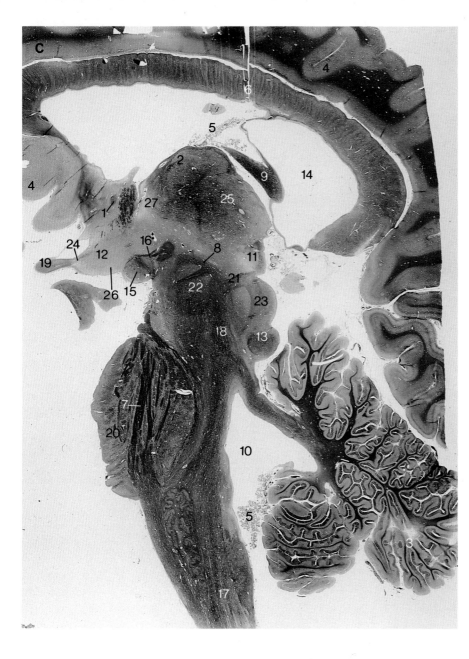

C A sagittal histological section of the brainstem and part of the forebrain to illustrate the nuclei and tracts of the diencephalon. Myelin stain. x2.4

1 Anterior commissure
2 Anterior thalamic nuclei
3 Cerebellum
4 Cerebral cortex
5 Choroid plexus
6 Corpus callosum
7 Corticospinal tract
8 Fasciculus retroflexus (or habenulointerpeduncular tract)
9 Fornix
10 Fourth ventricle
11 Habenular area (trigone)
12 Hypothalamus
13 Inferior colliculus
14 Lateral ventricle
15 Mamillary body of hypothalamus
16 Mamillothalamic tract
17 Medulla oblongata
18 Midbrain
19 Optic chiasma
20 Pons
21 Pretectal area
22 Red nucleus
23 Superior colliculus
24 Supraoptic region of hypothalamus
25 Thalamus
26 Tuberal region of hypothalamus
27 Ventral thalamic nuclei

CAM

119

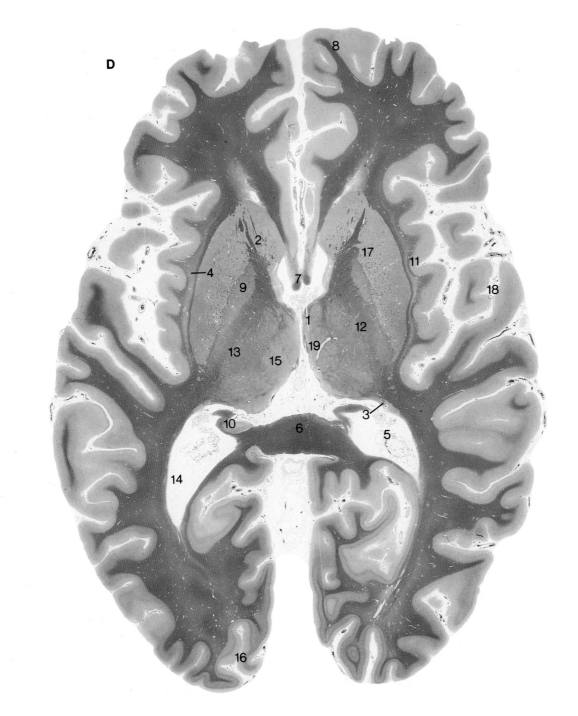

D Horizontal section through the brain showing the division of the thalamus into medial, lateral and anterior nuclear groups and the relationship between the thalamus and the basal ganglia. Solochrome cyanin and nuclear fast red stain. x1.1

1 Anterior thalamic nuclei
2 Caudate nucleus (head)
3 Caudate nucleus (tail)
4 Claustrum
5 Choroid plexus
6 Corpus callosum
7 Fornix

8 Frontal lobe of cerebral hemisphere
9 Globus pallidus
10 Hippocampus
11 Insula
12 Internal capsule
13 Lateral thalamic nuclei

14 Lateral ventricle
15 Medial thalamic nuclei
16 Occipital lobe
17 Putamen
18 Temporal lobe
19 Thalamus

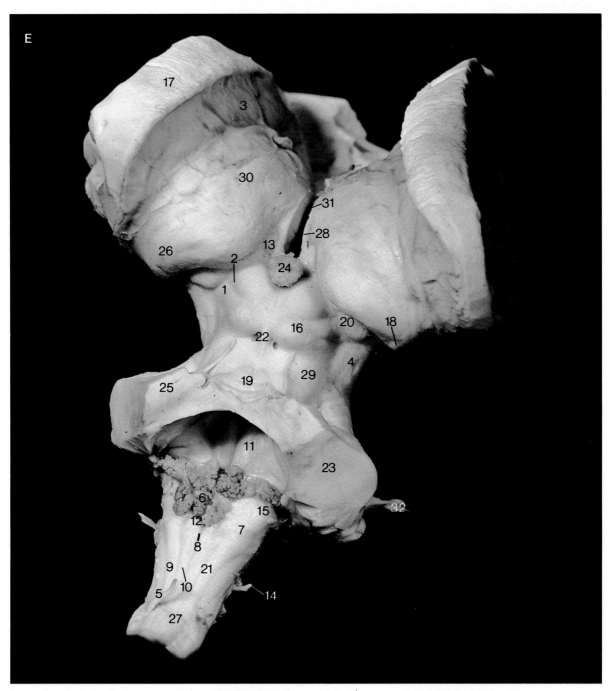

E A dissection of the diencephalon and brainstem viewed from the dorsal surface. x1.65

1 Brachium of inferior colliculus	**12** Gracile tubercle	**23** Middle cerebellar peduncle
2 Brachium of superior colliculus	**13** Habenula	**24** Pineal gland
3 Caudate nucleus	**14** Hypoglossal nerve rootlets	**25** Pons
4 Cerebral peduncle	**15** Inferior cerebellar peduncle	**26** Pulvinar of thalamus
5 Cervical dorsal root	**16** Inferior colliculus	**27** Spinal cord
6 Choroid plexus	**17** Internal capsule	**28** Stria medullaris thalami
7 Cuneate tubercle	**18** Lateral geniculate body	**29** Superior cerebellar peduncle
8 Dorsal median sulcus	**19** Lingula of cerebellum	**30** Thalamus
9 Fasciculus cuneatus	**20** Medial geniculate body	**31** Third ventricle
10 Fasciculus gracilis	**21** Medulla oblongata	**32** Trigeminal nerve
11 Fourth ventricle	**22** Midbrain	

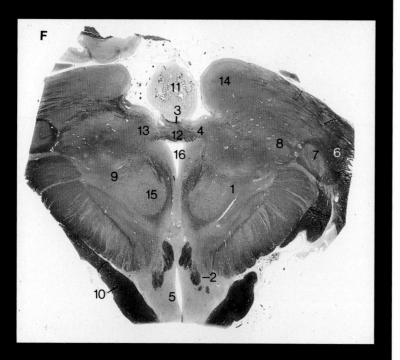

F-J Sections through the diencephalon at various levels to demonstrate the nuclei of the thalamus, and the structure of the subthalamus and epithalamus.

F A section passing through the transition between the midbrain and diencephalon. Myelin stain and counterstain. x1.9
1 Dentatorubrothalamic fibres
2 Fornix
3 Habenular commissure
4 Habenular nucleus
5 Hypothalamus
6 Internal capsule
7 Lateral geniculate body
8 Medial geniculate body
9 Medial lemniscus, spinothalamic and trigeminothalamic tracts
10 Optic tract
11 Pineal gland
12 Posterior commissure
13 Pretectal nuclei
14 Pulvinar of thalamus
15 Red nucleus
16 Third ventricle becoming cerebral aqueduct

MHMS

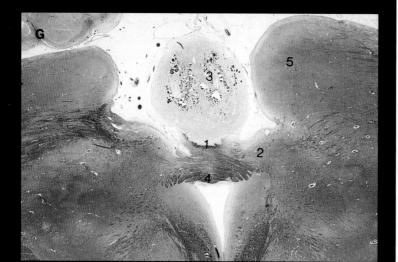

G An higher magnification view of the epithalamus to demonstrate the habenular nuclei and the habenular commissure. Myelin stain and counterstain. x3.4
1 Habenular commissure
2 Habenular nucleus
3 Pineal gland
4 Posterior commissure
5 Pulvinar of thalamus

MHMS

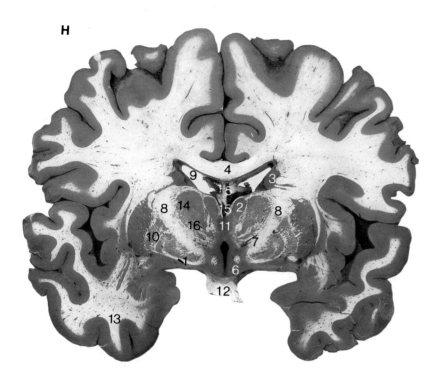

H A coronal thick slice through the forebrain at the rostral end of the diencephalon to show the anterior part of the thalamus, the hypothalamus and their relationships. Mulligan stain. x.86

1 Ansa lenticularis
2 Anterior thalamic nucleus
3 Caudate nucleus
4 Corpus callosum
5 Fornix
6 Hypothalamus
7 Inferior thalamic peduncle (radiation)
8 Internal capsule
9 Lateral ventricle
10 Lentiform nucleus
11 Midline thalamic nuclei
12 Optic chiasma
13 Temporal lobe
14 Thalamus
15 Third ventricle
16 Ventral anterior thalamic nucleus

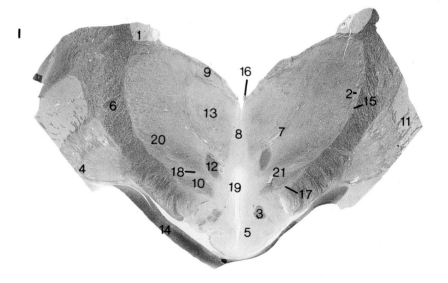

I An histological section passing through the middle of the thalamus, with adjacent portions of the subthalamus and hypothalamus. Myelin stain. x2.3

1 Caudate nucleus
2 External medullary lamina
3 Fornix
4 Globus pallidus
5 Hypothalamus
6 Internal capsule
7 Internal medullary lamina

8 Interthalamic adhesion and midline thalamic nuclei
9 Lateral dorsal thalamic nucleus
10 Lenticular fasciculus
11 Lentiform nucleus
12 Mamillothalamic tract

13 Medial (or mediodorsal) thalamic nucleus
14 Optic tract
15 Reticular thalamic nucleus
16 Stria medullaris thalami

17 Subthalamic nucleus
18 Thalamic fasciculus
19 Third ventricle
20 Ventral lateral thalamic nucleus
21 Zona incerta

CXWMS

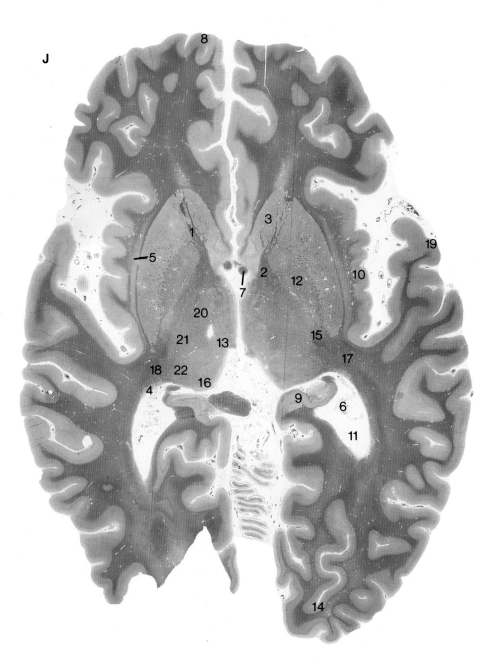

J An horizontal section through both cerebral hemispheres and diencephalon to show the medial and ventral thalamic nuclei and the anterior and somatic sensory thalamic radiations. Solochrome cyanin and nuclear fast red stain. x1.1

1 Anterior limb of internal capsule
2 Anterior thalamic peduncle (radiation)
3 Caudate nucleus (head)
4 Caudate nucleus (tail)
5 Claustrum
6 Choroid plexus
7 Fornix
8 Frontal lobe
9 Hippocampus
10 Insula
11 Lateral ventricle
12 Lentiform nucleus
13 Medial thalamic nuclei
14 Occipital lobe
15 Posterior limb of internal capsule
16 Pulvinar of thalamus
17 Retrolentiform part of internal capsule
18 Somatic sensory thalamic peduncle (radiation)
19 Temporal lobe
20 Ventral anterior thalamic nucleus
21 Ventral lateral thalamic nucleus
22 Ventral posterior thalamic nucleus

K-S Dissections and histological preparations to demonstrate the anatomy and relationships of the hypothalamus.

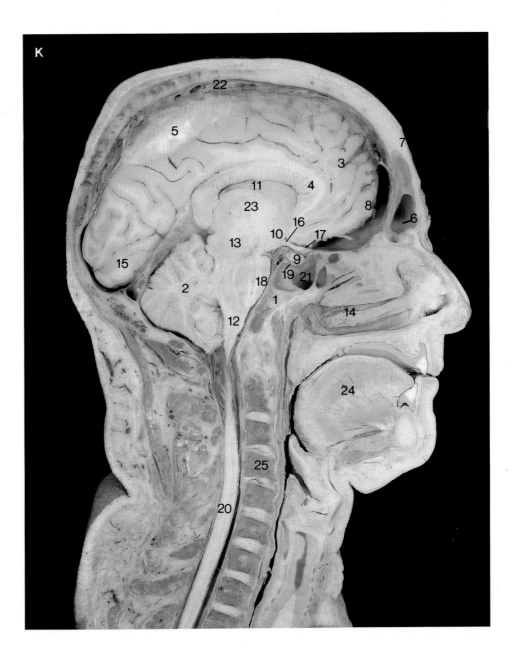

K A sagittal section of the head to show the relationships of the hypothalamus *in situ*. x.54

1 Body of sphenoid bone	**10** Hypothalamus	**19** Sella turcica (hypophyseal fossa)
2 Cerebellum	**11** Lateral ventricle	**20** Spinal cord
3 Cerebral hemisphere	**12** Medulla oblongata	**21** Sphenoidal air sinus
4 Corpus callosum	**13** Midbrain	**22** Superior sagittal sinus
5 Falx cerebri	**14** Nasal cavity	**23** Thalamus
6 Frontal air sinus	**15** Occipital lobe	**24** Tongue
7 Frontal bone	**16** Optic chiasma	**25** Vertebral column
8 Frontal lobe	**17** Optic nerve	
9 Hypophysis	**18** Pons	

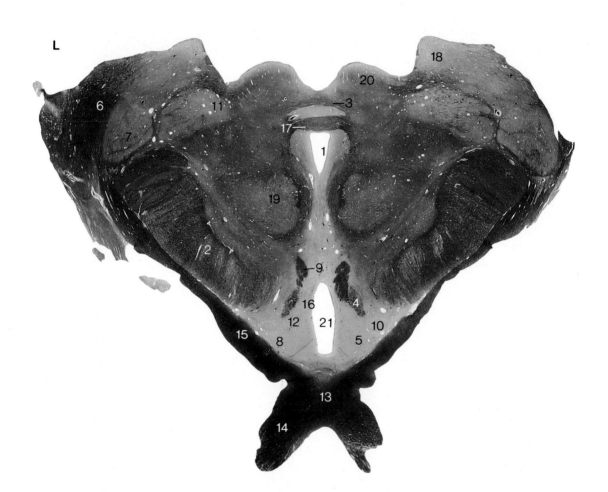

L A section through the transition between the midbrain and diencephalon orientated to pass through the optic chiasma. Weigert stain. x3

1 Cerebral aqueduct
2 Crus cerebri
3 Commissure of the superior colliculus
4 Fornix
5 Hypothalamus
6 Internal capsule
7 Lateral geniculate body

8 Lateral area of hypothalamus
9 Mamillothalamic tract
10 Medial forebrain bundle
11 Medial geniculate body
12 Medial hypothalamic area
13 Optic chiasma
14 Optic nerve

15 Optic tract
16 Periventricular hypothalamic area
17 Posterior commissure
18 Pulvinar of thalamus
19 Red nucleus
20 Superior colliculus
21 Third ventricle

M-P Sections to illustrate the structure of the neuroendocrine nuclei of the chiasmatic region of the hypothalamus.

M-N Sections to show the position and structure of the supraoptic nucleus. Weigert stain.

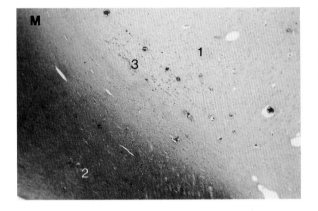

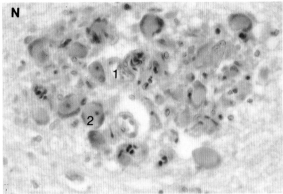

M A low power view showing the supraoptic nucleus and the optic tract. x22
1 Grey matter of hypothalamus
2 Optic tract
3 Supraoptic nucleus

N An high magnification view of the specialised neurosecretory cells and profuse blood supply of the supraoptic nucleus. x558
1 Capillary
2 Neurosecretory cell

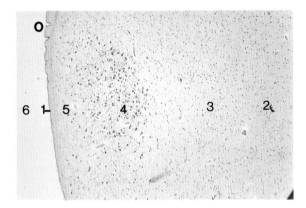

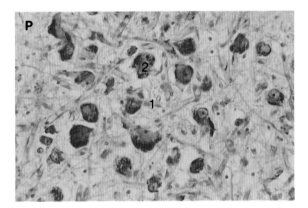

O A section to illustrate the position and structure of the paraventricular nucleus. Cresyl violet stain. x33
1 Ependyma
2 Lateral hypothalamic area
3 Medial hypothalamic area
4 Paraventricular nucleus
5 Periventricular hypothalamic area
6 Third ventricle

P High magnification view of the paraventricular nucleus showing its neurosecretory cells and profuse blood supply. Cresyl violet stain. x446
1 Capillary
2 Neurosecretory cell

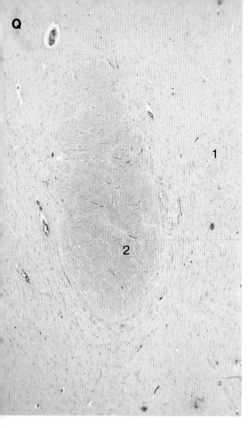

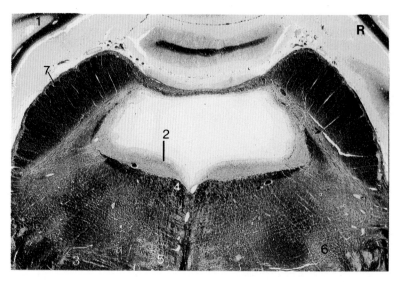

R A transverse paraffin wax section of the pons to show the dorsal longitudinal fasciculus, a connection between the hypothalamus and brainstem parasympathetic nuclei. Weigert stain. x7
1 Cerebellum
2 Dorsal longitudinal fasciculus
3 Medial lemniscus
4 Medial longitudinal fasciculus
5 Pons
6 Reticular formation
7 Superior cerebellar peduncle

Q A section showing the lateral area of the hypothalamus with the medial forebrain bundle. Weigert stain. x28
1 Grey matter of lateral hypothalamus
2 Medial forebrain bundle

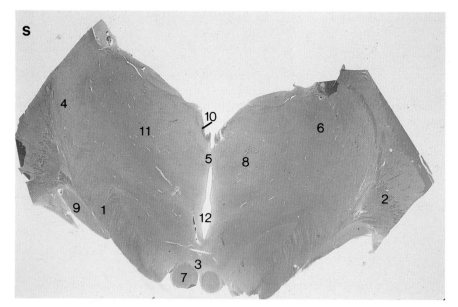

S A coronal section through the caudal end of the diencephalon to demonstrate the position of the mamillary bodies in relation to other diencephalic structures. Luxol fast blue stain. x2.3
1 Crus cerebri
2 Globus pallidus
3 Hypothalamus
4 Internal capsule
5 Interthalamic adhesion
6 Lateral thalamic nuclei
7 Mamillary body
8 Medial thalamic nuclei
9 Optic tract
10 Stria medullaris thalami
11 Thalamus
12 Third ventricle

COMMISSURAL FIBRES

Commissures pass from one side of the brain to the other carrying impulses in both directions. There are several bundles of commissural fibres; the corpus callosum, anterior commissure, posterior commissure, hippocampal commissure (commissure of the fornix) and habenular commissure.

The corpus callosum connects broad regions of the cortex in all the lobes with the corresponding regions in the other hemisphere. It is divided into four regions; the rostrum, genu, body and splenium. The rostrum and genu connect anterior parts of the frontal lobe and their radiating fibres form the forceps minor (frontal forceps). The body connects the remainder of the frontal lobe and the parietal lobe. The splenium connects regions of the temporal and occipital lobes and their radiating fibres form the forceps major. A group of fibres in the splenium (tapetum) sweeps inferiorly over the ventricle and optic radiation and connects with the temporal lobe.

The anterior commissure is a small bundle of fibres shaped like bicycle-handlebars straddling the midline. It is divided into two parts: fibres lying rostrally in the commissure connecting the olfactory structures and fibres lying caudally connecting the middle and inferior temporal gyri.

The posterior commissure lies in the lower part of the pineal stalk. Its composition is poorly understood but one important component consists of fibres crossing the midline from the pretectal area to the contralateral Edinger-Westphal nucleus from which the constrictor muscle of the pupil is supplied (see Brainstem Cranial Nerve Nuclei on page **152**). These are part of the pathway for the pupillary light reflex. Both pupils constrict when a light is shone into one because of this commissural connection. This is known as the consensual light reflex.

The fornix is the main tract of the limbic system connecting the hippocampus with the hypothalamus. Most of its fibres are ipsilateral but some cross, forming the hippocampal commissure.

Small commissures also link the colliculi of the midbrain. The habenular commissure lies in the upper part of the pineal stalk and connects the two habenular nuclei to the contralateral olfactory areas. The habenular nuclei are part of the limbic system.

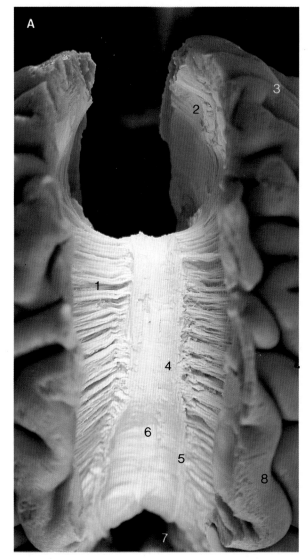

A The corpus callosum connecting the two hemispheres as viewed from above. x1.5

1 Corpus callosum (commissural fibres)
2 Frontal forceps
3 Frontal lobe
4 Indusium griseum
5 Lateral longitudinal stria
6 Medial longitudinal stria
7 Occipital lobe
8 Parietal lobe

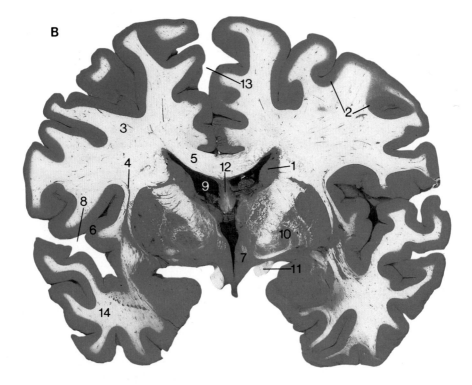

B Thick coronal slice of the cerebral hemispheres to show the corpus callosum. Mulligan stain. x.73

1 Caudate nucleus
2 Cerebral cortex (grey matter)
3 Cerebral white matter
4 Claustrum
5 Corpus callosum
6 Insula
7 Hypothalamus
8 Lateral sulcus
9 Lateral ventricle
10 Lentiform nucleus
11 Optic tract
12 Septum pellucidum
13 Superior longitudinal fissure
14 Temporal lobe

C Paraffin wax histological section of the corpus callosum showing the indusium griseum. Cresyl violet stain. x167

1 Corpus callosum
2 Indusium griseum

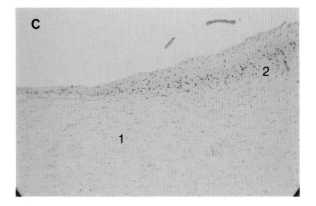

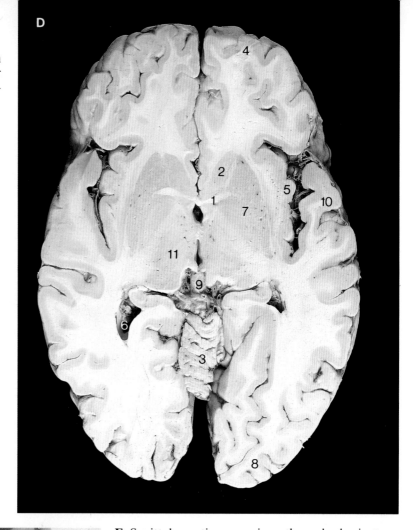

D Horizontal section through the brain showing the anterior commissure. Note its 'bicycle-handlebar' shape. x.68

1 Anterior commissure
2 Caudate nucleus
3 Cerebellum
4 Frontal lobe
5 Insula
6 Lateral ventricle
7 Lentiform nucleus
8 Occipital lobe
9 Pineal gland
10 Temporal lobe
11 Thalamus

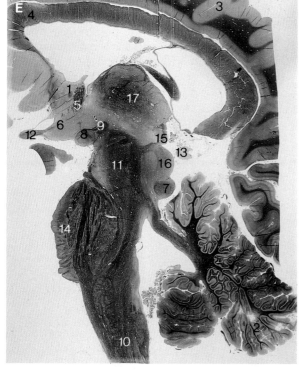

E Sagittal section passing through brainstem, cerebellum, diencephalon and part of cerebral hemisphere showing the anterior and posterior commissures and the corpus callosum. Myelin stain. x1.5

1 Anterior commissure
2 Cerebellum
3 Cerebral hemisphere
4 Corpus callosum
5 Fornix
6 Hypothalamus
7 Inferior colliculus
8 Mamillary body
9 Mamillothalamic tract
10 Medulla oblongata
11 Midbrain
12 Optic chiasma
13 Pineal gland
14 Pons
15 Posterior commissure
16 Superior colliculus
17 Thalamus

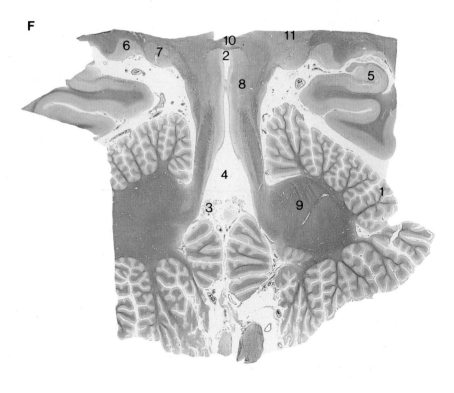

F Longitudinal section of brainstem showing the posterior commissure. Solochrome cyanin and nuclear fast red stain. x1.2

1 Cerebellum
2 Cerebral aqueduct
3 Choroid plexus
4 Fourth ventricle
5 Hippocampal formation
6 Lateral geniculate body
7 Medial geniculate body
8 Midbrain
9 Middle cerebellar peduncle
10 Posterior commissure
11 Thalamus

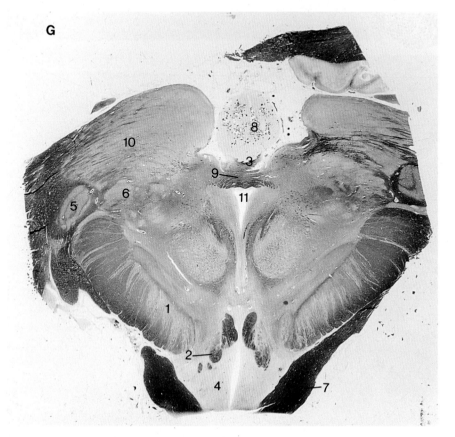

G Histological section through the transition between the midbrain and diencephalon orientated to pass through the posterior and habenular commissures. Weigert-Pal stain. x2.3

1 Cerebral peduncle
2 Fornix
3 Habenular commissure
4 Hypothalamus
5 Lateral geniculate body
6 Medial geniculate body
7 Optic tract
8 Pineal gland
9 Posterior commissure
10 Thalamus
11 Third ventricle

MHMS

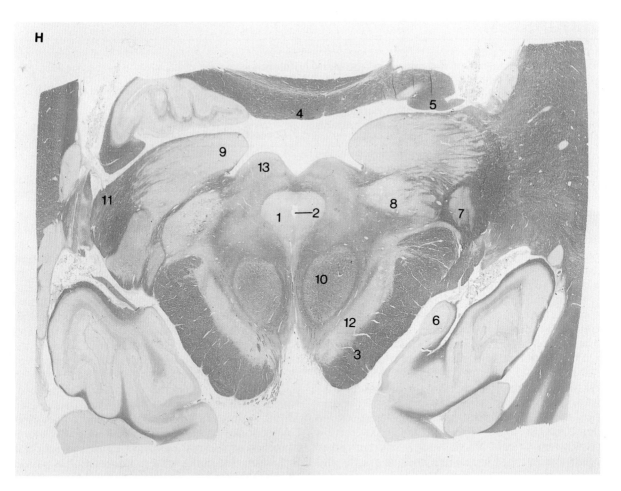

H Paraffin wax histological section through the brainstem at the junction of midbrain and diencephalon, to demonstrate the hippocampal commissure (commissure of the fornix). Luxol fast blue stain. x2.4

  1 Central grey matter of midbrain
  2 Cerebral aqueduct
  3 Cerebral peduncle
  4 Commissure of fornix
  5 Crus of fornix
  6 Hippocampal formation
  7 Lateral geniculate body
  8 Medial geniculate body
  9 Pulvinar of thalamus
 10 Red nucleus
 11 Retrolentiform part of internal capsule
 12 Substantia nigra
 13 Superior colliculus

CAM

BRAINSTEM

The brainstem consists of the midbrain, the pons and the medulla. All of these are midline structures which are overgrown by the cerebral hemispheres during development. Therefore, most parts of the brainstem can only be seen when the brain is viewed from below or in section.

Rostrally the brainstem is continuous with the diencephalon. Caudally it blends with the first cervical segment of the spinal cord. Dorsally it is connected to the cerebellum by the superior, middle and inferior cerebellar peduncles.

The brainstem lies on the floor of the cranial cavity. The medulla rests on the basi-occiput, the pons on the sphenoid bone as far forward as the dorsum sellae. The midbrain passes through the tentorial notch of the tentorium cerebelli.

All of the cranial nerves except the first and second arise from the brainstem; the first (olfactory) nerve is composed of processes of bipolar neurons in the olfactory epithelium and the second (optic) nerve is a drawn-out brain pathway rather than a true peripheral nerve. Cranial nerves III to XII which originate from the brainstem arise from or terminate in aggregations of grey matter (i.e. nerve cells) which form nuclei. These will be described in more detail in the next section (Brainstem Cranial Nerve Nuclei). Certain other brainstem nuclei, for example nucleus gracilis and nucleus cuneatus, are not associated with cranial nerves, but form part of sensory or motor functional systems. The most important of these will be covered in the section on sensory and motor pathways (see page **182-183**).

The white matter of the brainstem is arranged in bundles or tracts. These may be local connections within the brainstem itself or projection fibres linking brainstem structures to other parts of the central nervous system, often as parts of functional systems.

The most important tracts clearly visible in brainstem sections are listed below.

1 Sensory pathways or ascending tracts
Medial lemniscus: touch, pressure, conscious proprioception
Spinothalamic tracts: touch, pain, temperature
Spinocerebellar tracts: unconscious proprioception
Lateral lemniscus: auditory
Spinal tract and nucleus of the trigeminal nerve: touch, pain, temperature from head
Solitary tract: taste

2 Motor pathways for movement control
Corticospinal tract ⎫
Corticobulbar tracts ⎬ Pyramidal tracts

Rubrospinal tract ⎫
Tectospinal tract ⎪
Vestibulospinal tract ⎬ Extrapyramidal tracts
Reticulospinal tract ⎭

3 Connections with the cerebellum
Inferior, middle and superior cerebellar peduncles

4 Connecting brainstem nuclei to each other
Medial longitudinal fasciculus

The connections and functions of these tracts are described more fully on pages **182-196** and **231-242**.

Between the well-defined nuclei and tracts, the brainstem consists of more diffusely arranged nervous tissue, the reticular formation. This forms a longitudinally orientated core to the brainstem, within which there are cell groupings (reticular nuclei), which have a number of important functions. The medullary and pontine reticular formations contain the 'vital centres', controlling respiration and the circulation. The medial part of the reticular formation from mid-pons to mid-medulla is called the magnocellular nucleus, which gives rise to the reticulospinal tracts (see Motor Pathways). The lateral reticular nucleus has connections with the cerebellum. Collateral branches of sensory pathways enter the reticular formation. Incoming sensory information is passed to the thalamus, then to wide areas of the cerebral cortex. It forms the reticular activating system, which controls the sleep-wake cycle and maintains cortical activity. The midline raphe nucleus gives rise to the raphespinal pathways to the spinal trigeminal nucleus and the posterior horn of the spinal cord. The transmitter for this pathway is 5-HT. It is an inhibitory pathway for pain impulses, part of the 'gate' mechanism for preventing painful sensations from reaching consciousness.

● *An alternative definition of the brainstem includes the diencephalon.*

● *Brainstem injuries may be fatal by directly damaging reticular formation centres for control of vital functions.*

● *Uncal tumours of the temporal lobe may cause the temporal lobe to herniate into the tentorial notch, compressing the midbrain. Herniation (coning) can also occur in a patient with a raised intracranial pressure if a lumbar puncture is performed, due to sudden decompression when CSF is withdrawn.*

A-E The anatomy and relationships of the brainstem *in situ*.

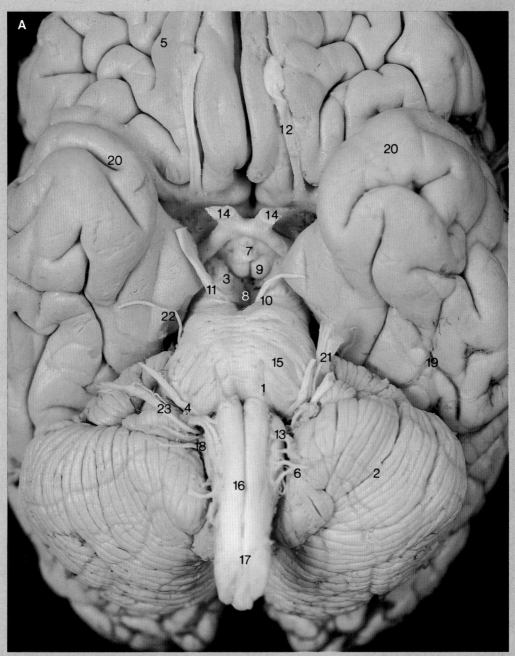

A The brain viewed from the basal aspect to show the brainstem and associated structures including the blood vessels and cranial nerves. The meninges have been removed. x1.2

  1 Abducens nerve (VI)
  2 Cerebellum
  3 Cerebral peduncle
  4 Facial nerve and nervus
     intermedius (VII)
  5 Frontal lobe
  6 Hypoglossal nerve (XII) roots
  7 Hypothalamus
  8 Interpeduncular fossa

  9 Mamillary body
 10 Midbrain
 11 Oculomotor nerve (III)
 12 Olfactory tract
 13 Olive
 14 Optic nerve (II)
 15 Pons
 16 Pyramid
 17 Pyramidal decussation

 18 Roots of glossopharyngeal (IX),
     vagus (X), and accessory
     (XI) nerves
 19 Surface blood vessels
 20 Temporal lobe
 21 Trigeminal nerve (V)
 22 Trochlear nerve (IV)
 23 Vestibulocochlear nerve (VIII)

B-C A dissection and an NMR (nuclear magnetic resonance) image to demonstrate the relationships of the brainstem in the cranial cavity.

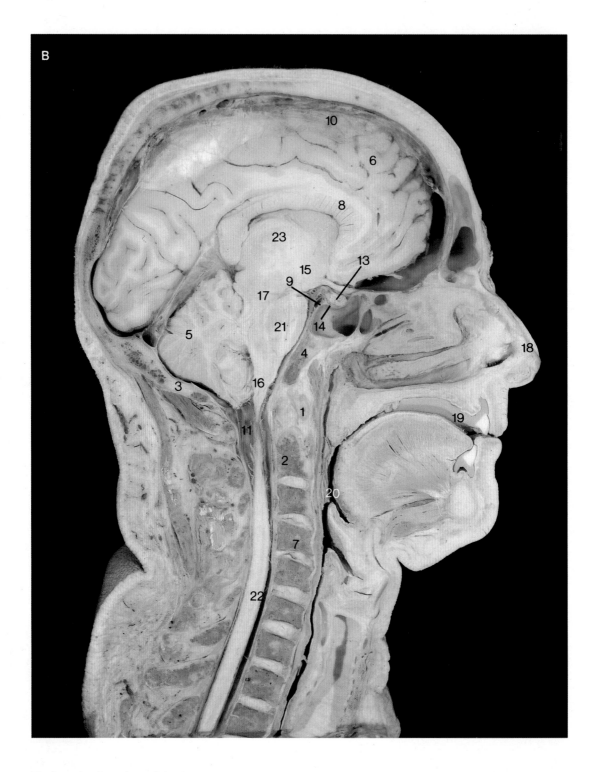

B A sagittal section of the head. x.6

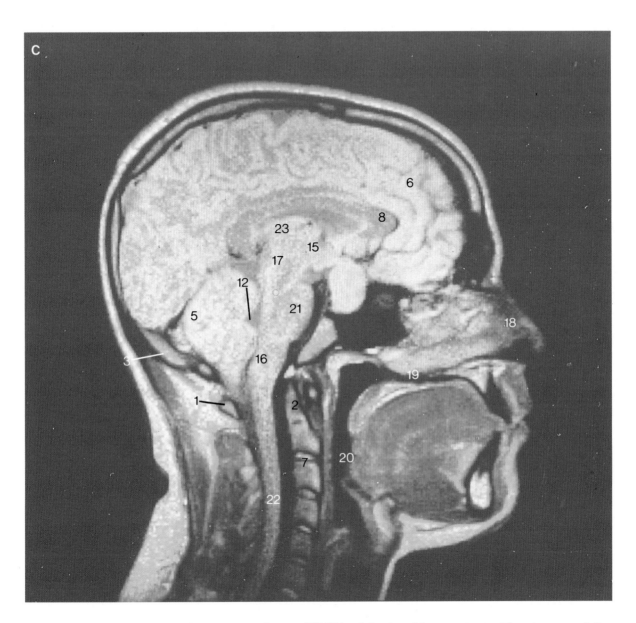

C A sagittal nuclear magnetic resonance image (NMR) of the head in a patient with a tumour of the hypophysis. Three different black-and-white images were superimposed to form this colour composite by displaying the first as red, second as green, and third as shades of blue. This allows simultaneous viewing of all three original images and can simplify their interpretation.

1 Atlas	9 Dorsum sellae	17 Midbrain
2 Axis	10 Falx cerebri	18 Nose
3 Basi occiput	11 Foramen magnum	19 Oral cavity
4 Body of sphenoid	12 Fourth ventricle	20 Pharynx
5 Cerebellum	13 Hypophysis	21 Pons
6 Cerebral hemisphere	14 Hypophyseal fossa	22 Spinal cord
7 Cervical vertebra	15 Hypothalamus	23 Thalamus
8 Corpus callosum	16 Medulla oblongata	

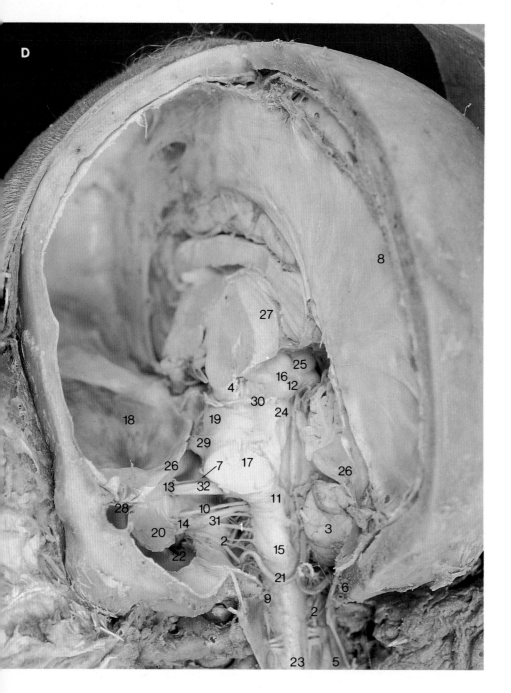

D Oblique posterior view of a dissection to display some cranial nerves leaving the brainstem through their foramina in the skull. Almost all of the cerebellum, the right cerebral hemisphere and the right side of the tentorium cerebelli have been removed. x.67

 1 Accessory nerve (cranial root) (XI)
 2 Accessory nerve (spinal root) (XI)
 3 Cerebellum
 4 Cerebral peduncle
 5 Dura mater
 6 Edge of foramen magnum
 7 Facial nerve (VII)
 8 Falx cerebri
 9 First cervical nerve root (C1)
10 Glossopharyngeal nerve (IX)
11 Inferior cerebellar peduncle
12 Inferior colliculus
13 Internal auditory meatus
14 Jugular foramen
15 Medulla
16 Midbrain
17 Middle cerebellar peduncle
18 Middle cranial fossa
19 Pons
20 Posterior cranial fossa
21 Posterior inferior cerebellar artery
22 Sigmoid sinus
23 Spinal cord
24 Superior cerebellar peduncle
25 Superior colliculus
26 Tentorium cerebelli
27 Thalamus
28 Transverse sinus
29 Trigeminal nerve (V)
30 Trochlear nerve (IV)
31 Vagus nerve (X)
32 Vestibulocochlear nerve (VIII)

OXF

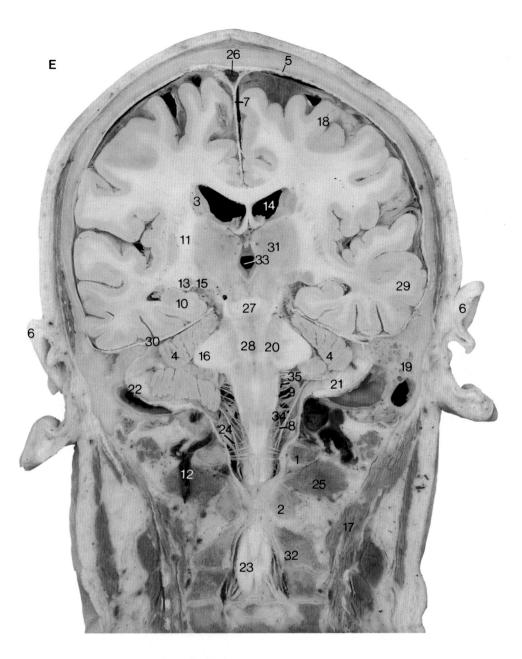

E A coronal section of the head and neck viewed from behind. The specimen shows the relationships of the brainstem *in situ* and its continuity with the spinal cord and diencephalon (thalamus). x.7

1	Atlas	**13**	Lateral geniculate body	**25** Subcapital muscles
2	Axis	**14**	Lateral ventricle	**26** Superior sagittal sinus
3	Caudate nucleus	**15**	Medial geniculate body	**27** Tegmentum of midbrain
4	Cerebellum	**16**	Middle cerebellar peduncle	**28** Tegmentum of pons
5	Dura mater	**17**	Muscles of posterior triangle of	**29** Temporal lobe
6	Ear		the neck	**30** Tentorium cerebelli
7	Falx cerebri	**18**	Parietal lobe	**31** Thalamus
8	First cervical nerve root (C1)	**19**	Petrous temporal bone	**32** Third cervical vertebra
9	Glossopharyngeal and vagus	**20**	Pons	**33** Third ventricle
	nerve roots	**21**	Posterior cranial fossa	**34** Vertebral artery
10	Hippocampus	**22**	Sigmoid sinus	**35** Vestibulocochlear nerve (VIII)
11	Internal capsule	**23**	Spinal cord	
12	Internal jugular vein	**24**	Spinal root of accessory nerve (XI)	

UN

139

F-I Dissections and histological preparations to demonstrate the anatomy of the isolated brainstem.

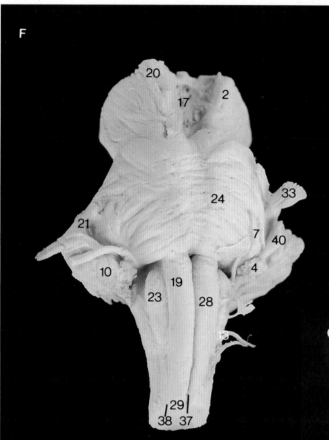

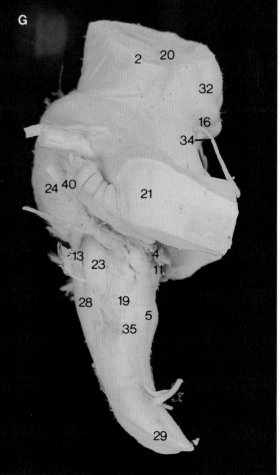

F The brainstem viewed from the ventral aspect. x1.3

G The same brainstem viewed from the left side. x1.3

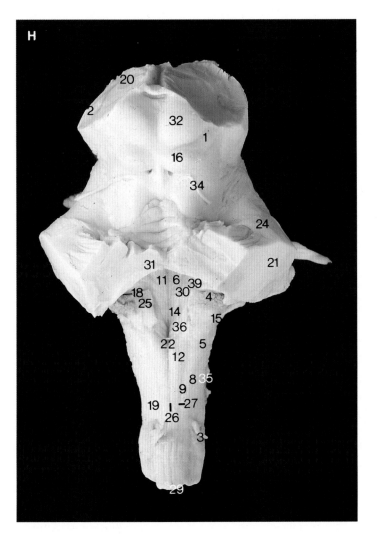

H A dorsal view of the brainstem in **F**. x1.4

1 Brachium of inferior colliculus	**15** Inferior cerebellar peduncle	**29** Spinal cord
2 Cerebral peduncle	**16** Inferior colliculus	**30** Stria medullaris
3 Cervical (C1) dorsal roots	**17** Interpeduncular fossa	**31** Superior cerebellar peduncle
4 Choroid plexus of fourth ventricle	**18** Lateral recess of fourth ventricle	**32** Superior colliculus
5 Cuneate tubercle	**19** Medulla oblongata	**33** Trigeminal nerve (V)
6 Facial colliculus	**20** Midbrain	**34** Trochlear nerve (IV)
7 Facial nerve (VII)	**21** Middle cerebellar peduncle	**35** Tuberculum cinereum
8 Fasciculus cuneatus	**22** Obex	**36** Vagal trigone
9 Fasciculus gracilis	**23** Olive	**37** Ventral (anterior) median fissure
10 Flocculus of cerebellum	**24** Pons	**38** Ventrolateral (anterolateral) sulcus
11 Fourth ventricle	**25** Posterior inferior cerebellar artery	**39** Vestibular area
12 Gracile tubercle	**26** Posterior (dorsal) median sulcus	**40** Vestibulocochlear nerve
13 Hypoglossal nerve (XII)	**27** Posterolateral (dorsolateral) sulcus	
14 Hypoglossal trigone	**28** Pyramid	

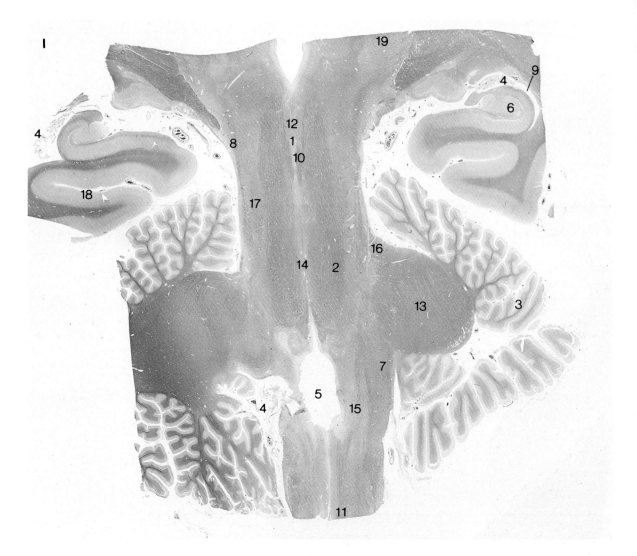

I A longitudinal histological section through the brainstem with part of the cerebellum and thalamus. This section shows tracts passing through the brainstem and connecting it to adjacent structures. Solochrome cyanin and nuclear fast red stain. x2.1

 1 Central grey matter
 2 Central tegmental tract
 3 Cerebellum
 4 Choroid plexus
 5 Fourth ventricle
 6 Hippocampal formation
 7 Inferior cerebellar peduncle

 8 Lateral lemniscus
 9 Lateral ventricle
10 Medial longitudinal fasciculus
11 Medulla oblongata
12 Midbrain
13 Middle cerebellar peduncle
14 Pons

15 Solitary tract
16 Spinocerebellar tract
17 Superior cerebellar peduncle
18 Temporal lobe cortex
19 Thalamus

Midbrain

The midbrain can be divided into three zones visible in transverse sections. The roof or tectum comprises mainly the superior and inferior colliculi and lies dorsal to the cerebral aqueduct (of Sylvius). Below this is the tegmentum which contains a variety of nuclei and tracts. The base of the midbrain consists of the two crura cerebri. These are made up of descending motor pathways, the corticospinal, corticobulbar and corticopontine tracts. One crus cerebri plus one half of the tegmentum constitutes a cerebral peduncle.

J A dissection of the midbrain *in situ* demonstrating its anatomy and relationships. x.91

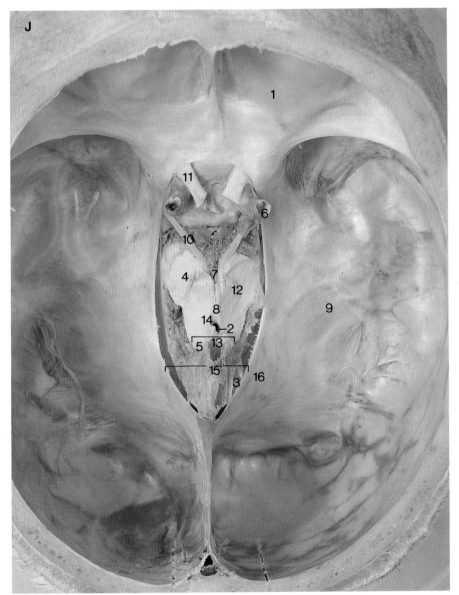

1 Anterior cranial fossa
2 Cerebral aqueduct
3 Cerebellum
4 Crus cerebri
5 Inferior colliculus
6 Internal carotid artery
7 Interpeduncular fossa
8 Midbrain
9 Middle cranial fossa
10 Oculomotor nerve
11 Optic nerve
12 Substantia nigra
13 Tectum
14 Tegmentum
15 Tentorial notch
16 Tentorium cerebelli

Pons

The pons consists of a large basal or basilar portion and a small dorsal or tegmental portion in the floor of the fourth ventricle. Corticospinal and corticobulbar fibres run longitudinally through the basilar portion. Transverse pontine fibres which are axons of the neurons comprising the pontine nuclei cross it to enter the cerebellum in the middle cerebellar peduncle. The tegmental portion contains cranial nerve nuclei and a variety of ascending and descending tracts.

K-O Dissections and histological preparations to demonstrate the anatomy of the pons.

K The pons viewed from the ventral aspect to show its general anatomy and relationships. The cerebellum has been removed. x1.8

1 Basilar portion of pons
2 Crus cerebri of midbrain
3 Facial nerve (VII)
4 Hypoglossal nerve (XII)
5 Interpeduncular fossa
6 Occipital lobe
7 Oculomotor nerve (III)
8 Olive
9 Posterior cerebral artery
10 Posterior communicating artery
11 Pyramid of medulla oblongata
12 Temporal lobe
13 Transverse pontine fibres
14 Trigeminal nerve (V)
15 Vestibulocochlear nerve (VIII)

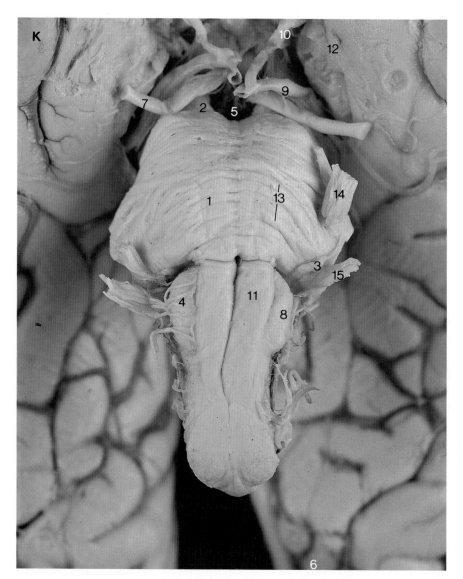

• *The name 'pons' means 'bridge' and refers to the bridge-like appearance created by the transverse pontine fibres forming the middle cerebellar peduncles.*

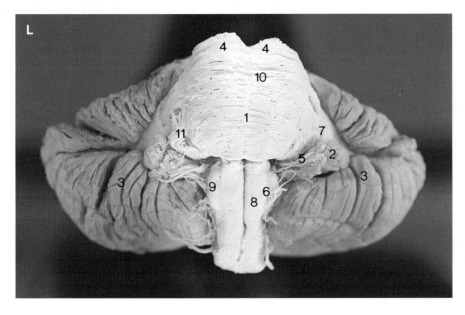

L A superficial dissection of the brainstem and cerebellum showing transverse pontine fibres crossing the basilar portion of the pons and entering the middle cerebellar peduncle. x.1

1 Basilar portion of pons
2 Cerebellar flocculus
3 Cerebellar hemisphere
4 Crus cerebri
5 Facial nerve (VII)
6 Hypoglossal nerve (XII)
7 Middle cerebellar peduncle
8 Pyramid of medulla oblongata
9 Olive
10 Transverse pontine fibres
11 Vestibulocochlear nerve (VIII)

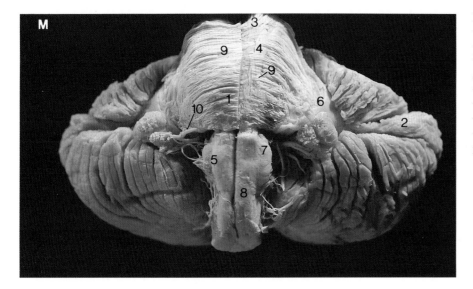

M A deep dissection of the left-hand side of the pons. This demonstrates the corticospinal fibres coursing longitudinally through the basilar portion of the pons, interweaving with the transverse pontine fibres. x1.3

1 Basilar portion of pons
2 Cerebellum
3 Crus cerebri of midbrain
4 Corticospinal fibres
5 Medulla oblongata
6 Middle cerebellar peduncle
7 Olive
8 Pyramid
9 Transverse pontine fibres
10 Vestibulocochlear and facial nerves (VIII and VII)

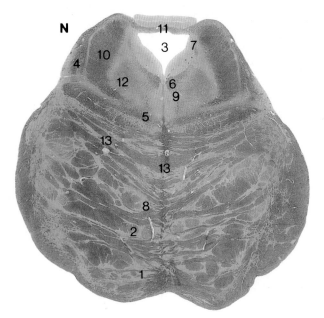

N A transverse section of the pons rostral to the middle cerebellar peduncle. Weigert stain. x4

  1 Basilar portion of pons
  2 Corticospinal/corticobulbar fibres
  3 Fourth ventricle
  4 Lateral lemniscus
  5 Medial lemniscus
  6 Medial longitudinal fasciculus
  7 Mesencephalic nucleus and tract of trigeminal nerve
  8 Pontine nuclei
  9 Reticular formation
10 Superior cerebellar peduncle
11 Superior medullary velum
12 Tegmental portion of pons
13 Transverse pontine fibres

O A transverse section through the pons and the middle cerebellar peduncle. Luxol fast blue stain. x44

  1 Basilar portion of pons
  2 Corticospinal tract
  3 Facial nerve (VII)
  4 Fourth ventricle
  5 Medial lemniscus
  6 Middle cerebellar peduncle
  7 Reticular formation
  8 Spinothalamic tracts
  9 Tegmental portion of pons
10 Trapezoid body
11 Trigeminal nerve fibres
12 Vestibular nuclei

CAM

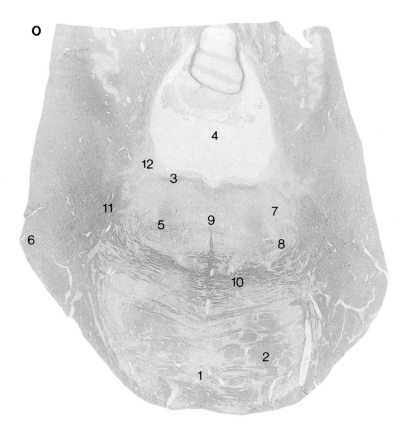

Medulla Oblongata

The medulla oblongata is the hindmost portion of the brainstem. At its caudal end its structure shows a gradual transition to that of the first cervical segment of the spinal cord. Rostrally it is continuous with the pons. Tracts ascending and descending between the spinal cord and higher brain centres all pass through the medulla. It also contains several cranial nerve nuclei and other nuclei associated with functional systems.

P-R Sections showing the structure and relationships of the medulla oblongata.

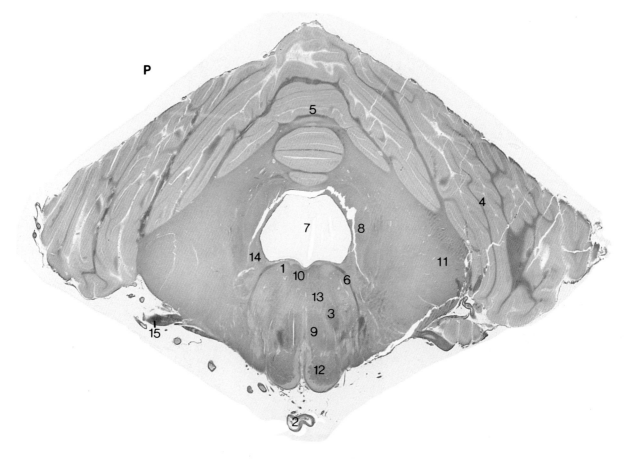

P A coronal section through the brainstem at the junction between the pons and the medulla oblongata, with the cerebellum attached. Weigert-Pal stain, celloidin-embedded section cut by Mr P.A. Runnicles. x1.7

1 Abducens nucleus	**6** Facial nerve (VII)	**11** Middle cerebellar peduncle
2 Basilar artery	**7** Fourth ventricle	**12** Pyramid
3 Central tegmental tract	**8** Inferior cerebellar peduncle	**13** Reticular formation
4 Cerebellar hemisphere	**9** Medial lemniscus	**14** Vestibular nuclei
5 Cerebellar vermis	**10** Medial longitudinal fasciculus	**15** Vestibulocochlear nerve (VIII)

MHMS

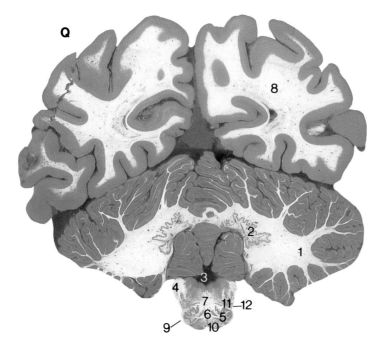

Q Thick coronal slice through the brain showing the anatomy and relationships of the medulla oblongata at the level of the olive. Mulligan stain. x.89

1 Cerebellum
2 Dentate nucleus
3 Fourth ventricle
4 Inferior cerebellar peduncle
5 Inferior olivary nucleus
6 Medial lemniscus
7 Medulla oblongata
8 Occipital lobe
9 Olive
10 Pyramid
11 Spinal trigeminal nucleus and tract
12 Tuberculum cinereum

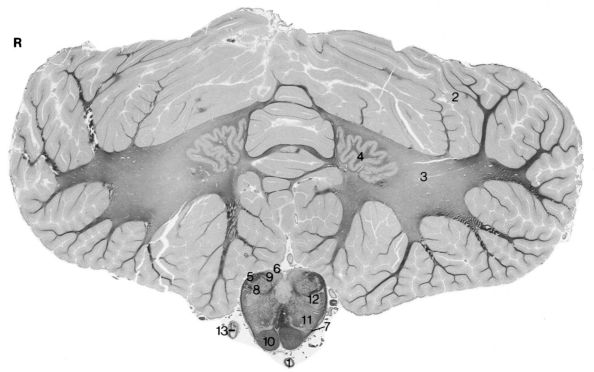

R Coronal section through the brainstem and cerebellum showing the anatomy and relationships of the medulla oblongata caudal to the olive. Weigert-Pal stain and celloidin embedded section cut by Mr P.A. Runnicles. x1.6

1 Anterior spinal artery	6 Fasciculus gracilis	11 Reticular formation
2 Cerebellar cortex	7 Medulla oblongata	12 Spinal trigeminal nucleus and tract
3 Cerebellar white matter	8 Nucleus cuneatus	13 Vertebral artery
4 Dentate nucleus	9 Nucleus gracilis	
5 Fasciculus cuneatus	10 Pyramid	

MHMS

S-T Transverse sections through the junction between the lower medulla oblongata and the first cervical segment of the spinal cord. In this transitional zone the arrangement of grey matter changes from the discrete nuclei typical of the brainstem to the central butterfly-shaped mass of spinal cord grey matter. The most prominent feature of the white matter is the pyramidal decussation. The pyramidal or corticospinal tract is the major nervous pathway for the control of voluntary movement. It connects the motor cortex of the cerebral hemisphere with the contralateral side of the spinal cord. Approximately 80 per cent of its fibres decussate at the transition from brainstem to spinal cord. The resulting concentration of decussating fibres is known as the pyramidal decussation.

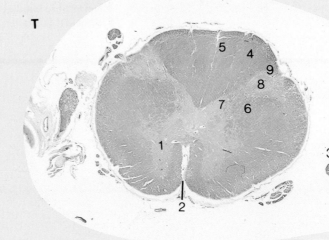

S A section of medulla oblongata passing through the pyramidal decussation.
Thionin stain. x7.3

1 Accessory nerve nucleus
2 Anterior horn
3 Arachnoid mater
4 Central grey matter
5 Fasciculus cuneatus
6 Fasciculus gracilis
7 Nucleus cuneatus
8 Nucleus gracilis
9 Pyramidal decussation
10 Spinal trigeminal nucleus
11 Spinal trigeminal tract
12 Vertebral artery

T A section through the first cervical segment (C1) of the spinal cord.
Myelin stain. x5.1

1 Anterior (ventral) horn
2 Anterior (ventral) median sulcus
3 Cervical nerve roots
4 Fasciculus cuneatus
5 Fasciculus gracilis
6 Lateral corticospinal tract
7 Posterior (dorsal) horn
8 Spinal trigeminal nucleus
9 Spinal trigeminal tract
10 Vertebral artery

U-Y Sections to illustrate the position and histology of the reticular formation.

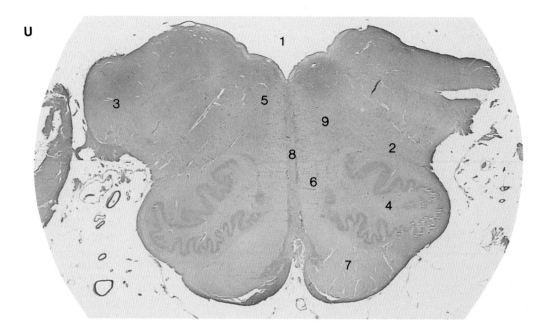

U A transverse section of the upper medulla oblongata showing the most important reticular nuclei. Thionin stain. x6.8

1 Fourth ventricle
2 Lateral reticular nucleus
3 Inferior cerebellar peduncle
4 Inferior olivary nucleus
5 Magnocellular nucleus
6 Medial lemniscus
7 Pyramid
8 Raphe nucleus
9 Reticular formation

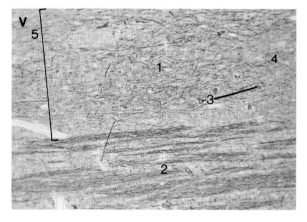

V Section to contrast the histology of the reticular formation in the medulla with that of a myelinated tract, the medial lemniscus. Palmgren stain. x55

1 Loosely arranged nerve fibres
2 Medial lemniscus
3 Nerve cell bodies
4 Nerve fibre bundles
5 Reticular formation

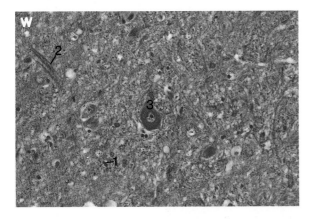

W High power view of the reticular formation in the pons to show widely scattered cells and fibres. Luxol fast blue and acid fuchsin stain. x356
1 Glial cell nucleus
2 Nerve fibres
3 Neuron

CXWMS

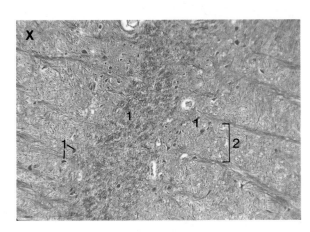

X A section of the medulla oblongata at the same level as section 'U' to demonstrate the relationship between the raphe nucleus and the medial lemniscus. Palmgren stain. x167
1 Cells of raphe nucleus
2 Fibres of medial lemniscus

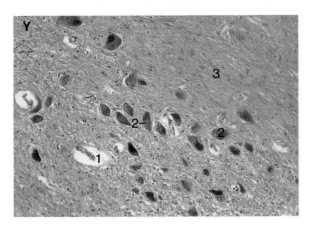

Y A section to show the pigmented cells of the locus coeruleus. Haematoxylin and eosin stain. x140
1 Blood vessel
2 Pigmented neurons
3 Unpigmented nervous tissue

Some groups of cells in the reticular formation are pigmented. The largest of these is the locus coeruleus in the floor of the fourth ventricle. The noradrenergic neurons of this nucleus have widespread connections throughout the brain.

● *General anaesthetics suppress transmission through the reticular activating system.*

● *Stimulation of reticular formation pathways inhibitory to pain transmission may explain acupuncture analgesia.*

● *Serotonin is a widespread inhibitory transmitter in the reticular formation. Tryptophane is a precursor of serotonin synthesis. It is present in milk. This may account for the effectiveness of milk based drinks relieving insomnia in many individuals.*

151

BRAINSTEM CRANIAL NERVE NUCLEI

Cranial nerves III to XII arise from the brainstem and appear in order from rostral to caudal. The oculomotor (III) and trochlear (IV) nerves emerge from the midbrain; the trigeminal (V), abducens (VI), facial (VII) and vestibulocochlear (VIII) nerves emerge from the pons and the junction between the pons and medulla oblongata; and the glossopharyngeal (IX), vagus (X), accessory (XI) and hypoglossal (XII) nerves emerge from the medulla oblongata.

● *Cranial nerves III-XII beyond their exit from the skull are considered as part of the peripheral nervous system and are not covered in this book.*

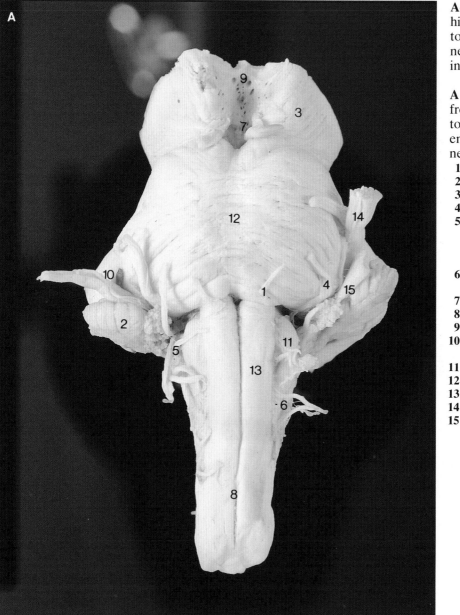

A-M Dissections and histological preparations to demonstrate cranial nerves and their nuclei in the brainstem.

A The brainstem viewed from below (anteriorly) to demonstrate the emergence of cranial nerves. x1.68

1 Abducens nerve (VI)
2 Cerebellar flocculus
3 Crus cerebri
4 Facial nerve (VII)
5 Glossopharyngeal (IX), vagus (X) and accessory (XI) nerve rootlets
6 Hypoglossal nerve rootlets (XII)
7 Interpeduncular fossa
8 Medulla oblongata
9 Midbrain
10 Middle cerebellar peduncle
11 Olive
12 Pons
13 Pyramid
14 Trigeminal nerve (V)
15 Vestibulocochlear nerve (VIII)

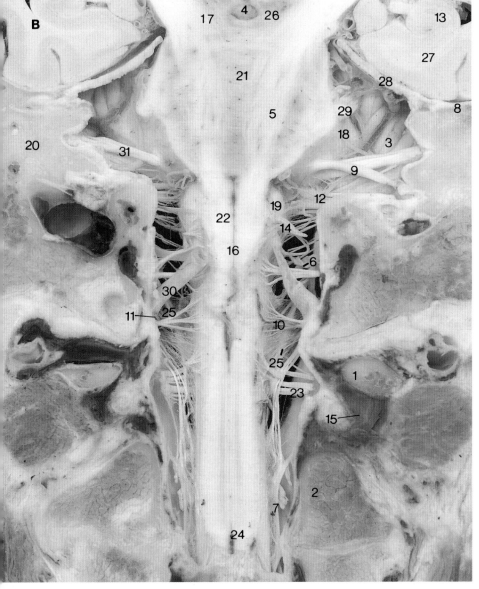

B An anterior view of a coronal section through the brainstem *in situ* to show cranial nerve roots and upper cervical spinal nerve roots in relation to the skull and vertebral column. x1.7

1 Atlas
2 Axis
3 Cerebellum
4 Cerebral aqueduct
5 Corticospinal tract
6 Cranial root of accessory nerve (XI)
7 Denticulate ligament
8 Dura mater
9 Facial nerve (VII)
10 First cervical nerve (C1) roots
11 Foramen magnum
12 Glossopharyngeal nerve (IX)
13 Hippocampal formation
14 Hypoglossal nerve (XII)
15 Internal jugular vein
16 Medulla oblongata
17 Midbrain
18 Middle cerebellar peduncle
19 Olive
20 Petrous temporal bone
21 Pons
22 Pyramid
23 Second cervical nerve (C2) roots
24 Spinal cord
25 Spinal root of accessory nerve (XI)
26 Tegmentum of midbrain
27 Temporal lobe
28 Tentorium cerebelli
29 Trigeminal nerve (V)
30 Vertebral artery
31 Vestibulocochlear nerve (VIII)

UN

- For the optic and olfactory nerves see *Special Senses on page 197 and page 224.*

- *Unlike spinal nerves which all contain both sensory and motor fibres, cranial nerves may be either mixed or purely motor, or sensory. The mixed cranial nerves contain fibres associated with both motor and sensory brainstem nuclei.*

- *Motor cranial nerve nuclei supplying extraocular and tongue muscles lie closer to the midline of the brainstem than autonomic or sensory nuclei.*

Nuclei of the Oculomotor and Trochlear Nerves

C-E Histological preparations to illustrate the anatomy of the oculomotor and trochlear nuclei and nerves.

The oculomotor nucleus contains an autonomic component, the Edinger-Westphal nucleus to supply the pupillary sphincter and ciliary muscle. Groups of somatic motor cells within the main nucleus supply the superior, medial and inferior rectus and the inferior oblique muscles of the eye, and the levator palpebrae superioris muscle of the upper eyelid.

C An oblique section through the midbrain, passing through the rostral end of one inferior colliculus and the caudal end of the contralateral superior colliculus, demonstrating the nucleus and fibres of the oculomotor nerve. Weigert stain. x4.1

1 Anterolateral system
2 Central tegmental tract
3 Cerebral aqueduct
4 Crus cerebri
5 Edinger-Westphal nucleus
6 Inferior colliculus
7 Interpeduncular fossa
8 Lateral lemniscus
9 Medial lemniscus
10 Medial longitudinal fasciculus
11 Oculomotor nerve fibres (III)
12 Oculomotor nucleus
13 Peri aqueductal grey matter
14 Substantia nigra
15 Superior cerebellar peduncle
16 Superior colliculus

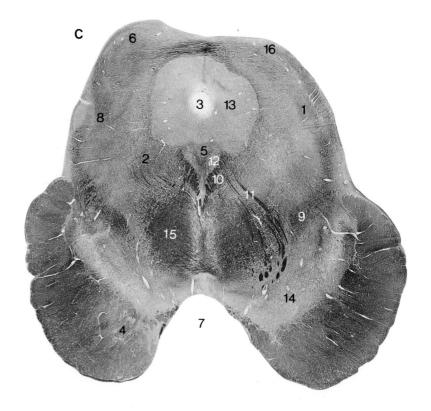

The trochlear nerve (IV) supplies only the superior oblique muscle of the eye. It is the only nerve which emerges from the dorsum of the brainstem. From the nucleus the nerve fibres pass caudally and decussate in the superior medullary velum over the fourth ventricle before leaving the brain.

D A transverse section of the tectum and tegmentum of the midbrain to show the position of the nucleus of the trochlear nerve. Weigert stain. x2.2

1 Cerebral aqueduct
2 Crus cerebri
3 Decussation of superior cerebellar peduncle
4 Inferior colliculus (tectum)
5 Lateral lemniscus
6 Medial lemniscus
7 Medial longitudinal fasciculus
8 Periaqueductal grey matter
9 Reticular formation
10 Tegmentum
11 Trochlear nucleus

MHMS

E A transverse section of the rostral end of the pons immediately behind the inferior colliculus, to demonstrate the decussation and emergence of the fibres of the trochlear nerve. Weigert stain. x3

1 Basilar portion of pons
2 Central tegmental tract
3 Corticospinal tract
4 Decussating fibres of trochlear nerve (IV)
5 Emerging fibres of trochlear nerve (IV)
6 Fourth ventricle
7 Lateral lemniscus
8 Medial lemniscus
9 Medial longitudinal fasciculus
10 Superior cerebellar peduncle
11 Superior medullary velum
12 Transverse pontine fibres

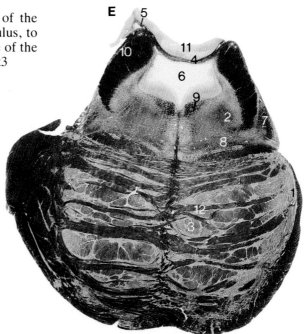

Nuclei of the Trigeminal Nerve

Four nuclei are associated with the trigeminal nerve. A chain of sensory nuclei receiving fibres from the nerve extends through the brainstem and down into the spinal cord as far as the third cervical segment. Of these the spinal nucleus (or nucleus of the descending tract of V) is concerned with touch, pain and temperature, the principal (or main) sensory nucleus with touch, and the mesencephalic nucleus with proprioception. The motor nucleus lies in the pons. Its fibres enter only the mandibular division of the trigeminal nerve and innervate muscles of mastication. Maxillary and ophthalmic divisions of the nerve are sensory.

● *The spinal nucleus of the trigeminal nerve receives afferent fibres from all three divisions of the trigeminal nerve. It also receives fibres from the facial, glossopharyngeal and vagus nerves and upper cervical segments of the spinal cord. It, therefore, receives a complete 'map' of sensory information from the head, beyond the territory of the trigeminal nerve itself.*

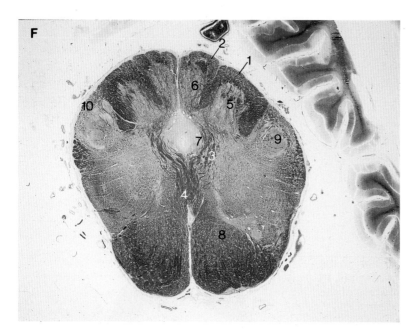

F A transverse section of the caudal end of the medulla oblongata showing the spinal nucleus and spinal tract of the trigeminal nerve. Weigert-Pal stain. x5.3

1 Fasciculus cuneatus
2 Fasciculus gracilis
3 Internal arcuate fibres
4 Medial lemniscus
5 Nucleus cuneatus
6 Nucleus gracilis
7 Position of X and XII nuclei
8 Pyramid
9 Spinal nucleus of the trigeminal nerve
10 Spinal tract of the trigeminal nerve

MHMS

G A transverse section through the pons to demonstrate the nuclei of the trigeminal nerve and some features of the abducens and facial nerves. Weigert stain. x3.3

1 Abducens nerve (VI)
2 Abducens nucleus
3 Corticospinal tract
4 Facial nerve (VII)
5 Fourth ventricle
6 Lateral lemniscus
7 Mesencephalic tract and nucleus of trigeminal nerve
8 Middle cerebellar peduncle
9 Motor nucleus of trigeminal nerve
10 Pontine genu of facial nerve
11 Principal sensory nucleus of trigeminal nerve
12 Spinal tract and nucleus of trigeminal nerve
13 Trigeminal nerve fibres (V)

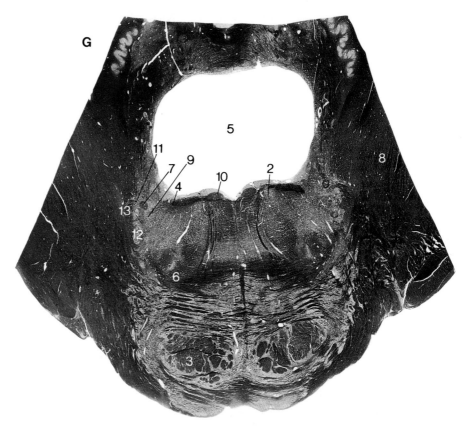

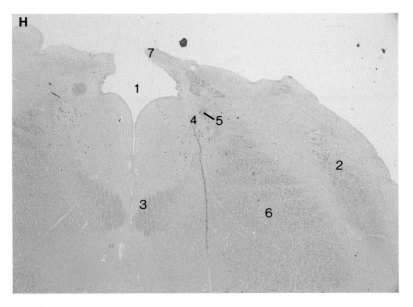

H A section of part of the floor of the fourth ventricle in the rostral third of the pons to show the mesencephalic tract and nucleus of the trigeminal nerve. The pink line on this section is a fold in the tissue (artefact). Luxol fast blue and acid fuchsin stain. x8.7

1 Fourth ventricle
2 Medial lemniscus
3 Medial longitudinal fasciculus
4 Mesencephalic nucleus of trigeminal nerve
5 Mesencephalic tract of trigeminal nerve
6 Superior cerebellar peduncle
7 Superior medullary velum

CXWMS

Nuclei of the Abducens, Facial and Vestibulocochlear Nerves

The abducens nerve (VI) supplies the lateral rectus muscle of the eye. The fibres of the facial nerve (VII) arch around the abducens nucleus forming a bulge, the facial colliculus, in the floor of the fourth ventricle.

The facial nerve arises from three nuclei; the motor nucleus controls the muscles of facial expression; the superior salivatory nucleus supplies parasympathetic innervation for salivatory and lacrimal glands, and the solitary nucleus is a sensory nucleus for the sense of taste. In addition, the spinal nucleus of the trigeminal nerve receives a few facial nerve sensory fibres from the ear.

Six nuclei receive incoming sensory fibres in the vestibulocochlear nerve. These are the dorsal and ventral cochlear nuclei, associated with the cochlear division of the nerve and the sense of hearing, and the superior, inferior, medial and lateral vestibular nuclei associated with the vestibular division of the nerve and with the sense of equilibrium.

● *The medial longitudinal fasciculus links the oculomotor, trochlear and abducens nuclei with the vestibular nuclei. It enables eye movements to be coordinated with head position and movements.*

● *Facial movements are important in emotional expression and the facial motor nucleus probably has connections with the limbic areas of the cerebral cortex.*

I-J Histological sections to demonstrate the nuclei of the abducens and facial nerves.

I A section through the tegmental portion of the pons to show the nuclei and fibres of the abducens and facial nerves. Weigert stain. x8.3

1 Abducens nucleus
2 Abducens nerve (VI) fibres
3 Basilar portion of pons
4 Corticospinal tract
5 Facial colliculus
6 Facial motor nucleus
7 Facial nerve (VII) fibres
8 Fourth ventricle
9 Medial lemniscus
10 Medial longitudinal fasciculus
11 Pontine genu of facial nerve
12 Spinal nucleus of trigeminal nerve (V)
13 Spinal tract of trigeminal nerve
14 Superior salivatory nucleus
15 Tectospinal tract
16 Tegmental portion of pons
17 Transverse pontine fibres

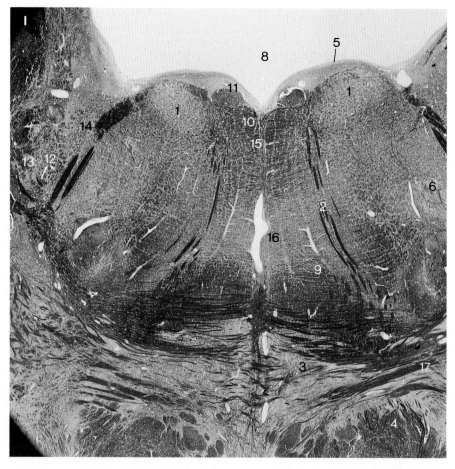

J A section of the floor of the fourth ventricle to demonstrate connections from the medial longitudinal fasciculus to the abducens nucleus. Luxol fast blue and acid fuchsin stain. x9

1 Abducens nucleus
2 Facial nerve (VII)
3 Fibres from medial longitudinal fasciculus to abducens nucleus (arrow)
4 Fourth ventricle
5 Medial longitudinal fasciculus
6 Median sulcus
7 Pontine genu of facial nerve
8 Sulcus limitans
9 Tectospinal tract

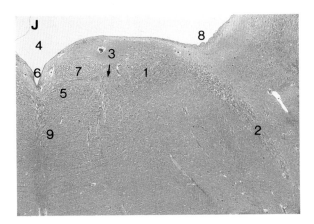

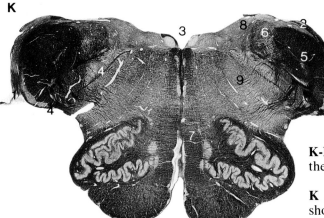

K-L Histological sections to illustrate the nuclei of the vestibulocochlear nerve.

K A transverse section of the medulla oblongata showing the dorsal and ventral cochlear nuclei and the medial and inferior vestibular nuclei. Weigert stain. x3.8

1 Cochlear nerve (VIII)
2 Dorsal cochlear nucleus
3 Fourth ventricle
4 Glossopharyngeal nerve (IX)
5 Inferior cerebellar peduncle
6 Inferior vestibular nucleus
7 Medial lemniscus
8 Medial vestibular nucleus
9 Reticular formation
10 Ventral cochlear nucleus

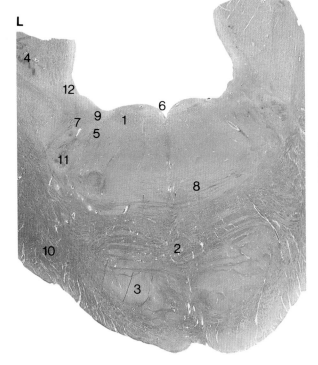

L A transverse section of the pons to demonstrate the superior, medial and lateral vestibular nuclei. Luxol fast blue and acid fuchsin stain. x3.4

1 Abducens nucleus
2 Basilar portion of pons
3 Corticospinal tract
4 Dentate nucleus
5 Facial nerve (VII)
6 Fourth ventricle
7 Lateral vestibular nucleus
8 Medial lemniscus
9 Medial vestibular nucleus
10 Middle cerebellar peduncle
11 Spinal nucleus of the trigeminal nerve
12 Superior vestibular nucleus

The Glossopharyngeal, Vagus, Accessory and Hypoglossal Nerves and their Nuclei

The glossopharyngeal (IX), vagus (X), and accessory (XI) nerves emerge in sequence from the medulla oblongata, in the longitudinal groove between the olive and the inferior cerebellar peduncle.

The glossopharyngeal is a mixed nerve. It contains motor fibres from the nucleus ambiguus to supply the stylopharyngeus muscle and parasympathetic fibres from the inferior salivatory nucleus for the parotid gland. Sensory fibres terminate in the solitary nucleus from taste buds on the posterior third of the tongue, from the oropharynx, from the carotid sinus (baroreceptor for the control of blood pressure), and the carotid body (chemoreceptor for the control of respiration). Sensory fibres from the middle ear terminate in the spinal trigeminal nucleus (see page **183-184**).

The vagus is also a mixed nerve. Sensory fibres from the aortic arch, aortic bodies, respiratory and gastrointestinal tract terminate in the solitary nucleus, forming part of the reflex mechanisms for cardiovascular function, respiration and gastrointestinal tract mobility. Taste fibres enter the solitary nucleus from taste buds on the epiglottis, and somatic sensory fibres from the external ear go to the spinal trigeminal nucleus.

Visceral efferent (parasympathetic) fibres in the vagus nerve from the nucleus ambiguus supply the heart. The dorsal motor nucleus supplies parasympathetic innervation to the respiratory and digestive tracts. The nucleus ambiguus supplies muscles of the larynx and pharynx.

The accessory nerve is a purely motor nerve. Its nucleus is an elongated column of cells extending in the anterior horn of the first five or six cervical segments of the spinal cord. These cells give rise to its spinal root. It also has a cranial root arising from the nucleus ambiguus (sometimes viewed as part of the vagus). The spinal root ascends through the foramen magnum to join the cranial root. The fibres in the accessory nerve arising from the accessory nucleus supply the trapezius and sternocleidomastoid muscles in the neck. Fibres from the nucleus ambiguus supply the muscles of the pharynx.

The hypoglossal nerve emerges from the medulla by multiple rootlets between the pyramid and the olive. It is a purely motor nerve that innervates the intrinsic and extrinsic muscles of the tongue.

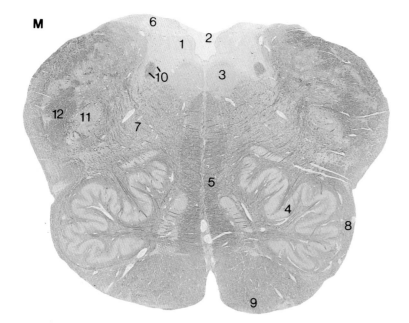

M A transverse section of the medulla oblongata to show the solitary nucleus, nucleus ambiguus, dorsal motor nucleus of the vagus and hypoglossal nucleus. Myelin stain. x6.7

  1 Dorsal motor nucleus of vagus nerve
  2 Fourth ventricle
  3 Hypoglossal nucleus
  4 Inferior olivary nucleus
  5 Medial lemniscus
  6 Medial vestibular nucleus
  7 Nucleus ambiguus
  8 Olive
  9 Pyramid
  10 Solitary nucleus and tract
  11 Spinal nucleus of trigeminal nerve
  12 Spinal tract of trigeminal nerve

CEREBELLUM

The cerebellum is the largest part of the hindbrain. It consists of two cerebellar hemispheres united by a central, median vermis. The surface of the cerebellum is deeply folded. Major folds, the fissures, subdivide the cerebellum into superior and inferior halves, and demarcate subdivisions, the anterior, posterior, and flocculonodular lobes within each hemisphere. The fissures and the lobes which they demarcate form early in the development of the cerebellum; they also have functional significance. The flocculonodular lobe forms first, is mainly concerned with equilibrium and is separated from the rest of the cerebellum by the posterior lateral fissure. The anterior lobe, lying rostral to the next fissure to form, the primary fissure, is mainly associated with proprioception (the sense of position) while the remainder of the cerebellum is concerned with complex processes of automatic motor control.

The cerebellum is similar in structure to the cerebral hemisphere: the cerebellar cortex (grey matter) forms folds (folia) on the surface and surrounds the white matter, within which are embedded the intracerebellar or deep nuclei i.e. the dentate, emboliform, globose and fastigial nuclei.

The cerebellar cortex has three cellular layers; the outermost molecular layer is mainly synaptic, containing sparse, small stellate and basket cells; the middle layer is composed of the giant Purkinje cells whose dendrites branch in the molecular layer and whose axons pass into the granular layer and enter the white matter; and the granular layer is innermost and is densely populated by small granule and larger but much sparser Golgi cells.

The white matter of the cerebellum resembles a tree with repeated branching. The trunk of the tree is the medullary centre while the branches are the arbor vitae. There are three types of fibres in the white matter; intrinsic, afferent and efferent. Intrinsic fibres connect different areas in the same hemisphere or the same area in both hemispheres.

The afferent and efferent fibres connect the cerebellum with other parts of the central nervous system. Their fibres are aggregated into three bundles in each hemisphere called the superior, middle and inferior peduncles. Afferent fibres make up the bulk of the white matter. They enter via the middle and inferior cerebellar peduncles and terminate in the cerebellar cortex, and many have collateral connections to the deep nuclei. A large proportion of the afferent fibres terminate as 'mossy fibres' in the granular layer. 'Climbing fibres' from the inferior olivary complex end on Purkinje cell dendrites. The Purkinje cells are the output cells of the cerebellar cortex. With the exception of a minority, located in the flocculonodular lobe, their axons do not leave the cerebellum but project to the deep cerebellar nuclei. It is from these deep nuclei that most cerebellar efferents arise. The axons of the minority group of Purkinje cells project directly to the brainstem.

The cerebellum coordinates muscular activity and controls the force, direction and extent of voluntary movements. It is also important as a centre for body equilibrium (flocculonodular lobe) and in the maintenance of posture. Its sensory input along its afferent pathways is from the eyes, ears, cutaneous sensory receptors and proprioceptors. In turn the efferent connections pass to motor control centres in the brainstem some of which in turn are linked to the cerebral cortex. There is no direct output to cerebral cortex.

Functionally the cerebellum can be considered as three parts; the archicerebellum, paleocerebellum and neocerebellum. The first consists of the flocculonodular lobe, the second includes the anterior lobe, pyramid and uvula, the third is the remainder of the hemisphere. The fastigial nucleus is the deep nucleus associated with the archicerebellum, the globose and emboliform nuclei are linked to the paleocerebellum and the dentate nucleus is the deep nucleus of the neocerebellum.

• *Each cerebellar hemisphere assists in the control of movement on its own side of the body.*

• *In spite of its large sensory input no conscious sensations are perceived in the cerebellum.*

• *The inhibitory neurotransmitter for basket, stellate, Purkinje and Golgi cells is gamma-aminobutyric acid (GABA). The excitatory transmitter of the granule cells is glutamate.*

For cerebellar connections see pages **245-252**.

A-C The cerebellum *in situ*.

A Midsagittal section of the brainstem and cerebellum. x.59
1 Choroid plexus of fourth ventricle
2 Fourth ventricle
3 Hemisphere of cerebellum
4 Medulla oblongata
5 Midbrain
6 Pons
7 Vermis of cerebellum

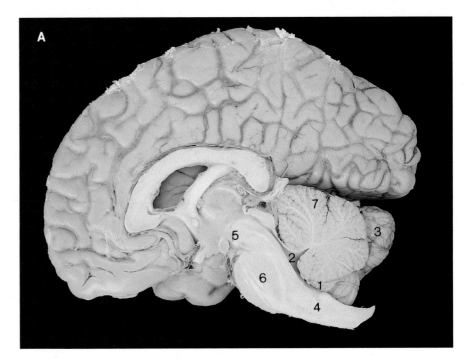

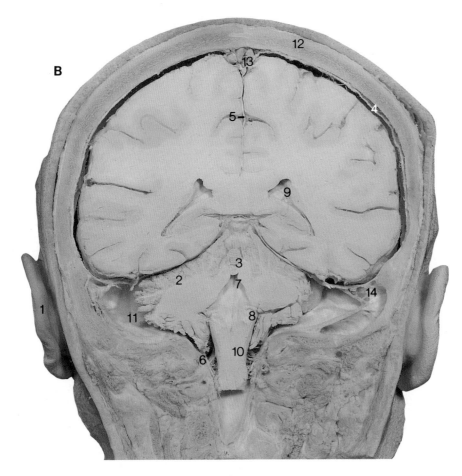

B Coronal section passing through the posterior cranial fossa. x.7
1 Auricle
2 Cerebellar hemisphere
3 Cerebellar vermis
4 Dura mater
5 Falx cerebri
6 Foramen magnum
7 Fourth ventricle
8 Inferior cerebellar peduncle (restiform body)
9 Lateral ventricle
10 Medulla oblongata
11 Posterior cranial fossa
12 Skull vault
13 Superior sagittal sinus
14 Transverse sinus

RCS

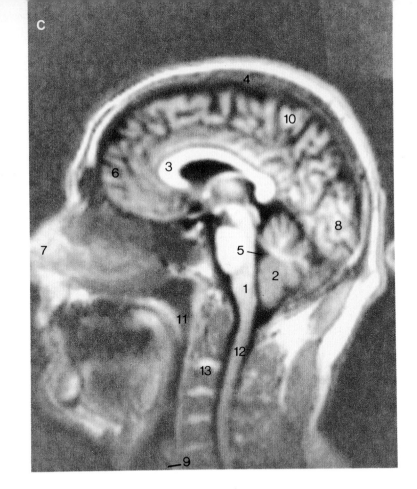

C Sagittal image of the normal adult brain as visualized by nuclear magnetic resonance technique (NMR).

1 Brainstem
2 Cerebellum
3 Corpus callosum
4 Cranial vault
5 Fourth ventricle
6 Frontal lobe
7 Nose
8 Occipital lobe
9 Oesophagus
10 Parietal lobe
11 Pharynx
12 Spinal cord
13 Vertebral column

Dr G. Bydder

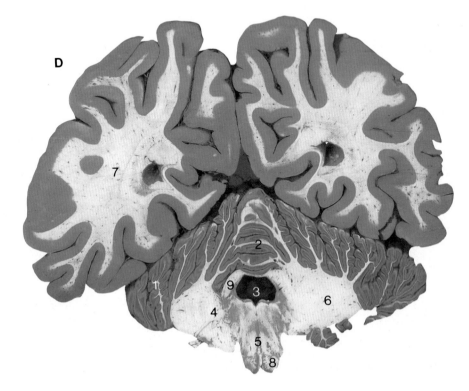

D Thick transverse slice through the brainstem, cerebellum and both cerebral hemispheres to show the relationship of the cerebellum to the fourth ventricle. Mulligan stain. x1.04

1 Cerebellar hemisphere
2 Cerebellar vermis
3 Fourth ventricle
4 Inferior cerebellar peduncle
5 Medulla oblongata
6 Middle cerebellar peduncle
7 Occipital lobe
8 Pyramid of medulla
9 Superior cerebellar peduncle

163

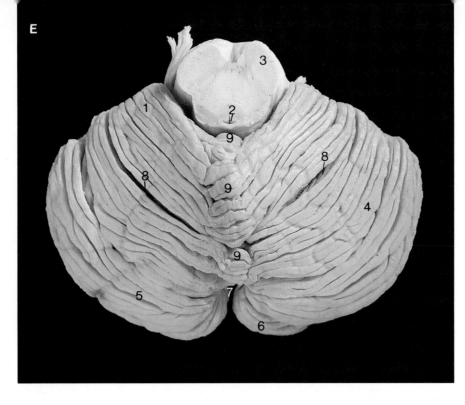

E-F The cerebellum and brainstem.

E Superior surface of cerebellum attached to the brainstem. The blood vessels have been removed. x1.05
1 Anterior lobe
2 Cerebral aqueduct
3 Crus cerebri
4 Hemisphere of cerebellum
5 Horizontal fissure
6 Posterior lobe
7 Posterior notch
8 Primary fissure
9 Superior vermis

F Cerebellum and brainstem from below. The blood vessels have been removed. x1.1
1 Flocculus
2 Hemisphere
3 Inferior cerebellar peduncle (restiform body)
4 Medulla oblongata
5 Middle cerebellar peduncle (brachium pontis)
6 Pons
7 Posterolateral fissure
8 Posterior notch
9 Pyramid of medulla
10 Tonsil
11 Transverse pontine fibres
12 Trigeminal nerve (V)
13 Vallecula
14 Vermis

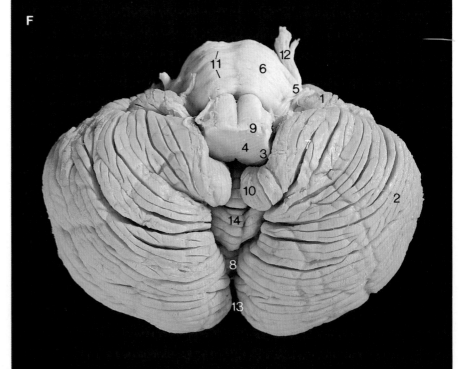

G-M The white matter of the cerebellum. Fibres form the medullary centre and the branching arbor vitae.

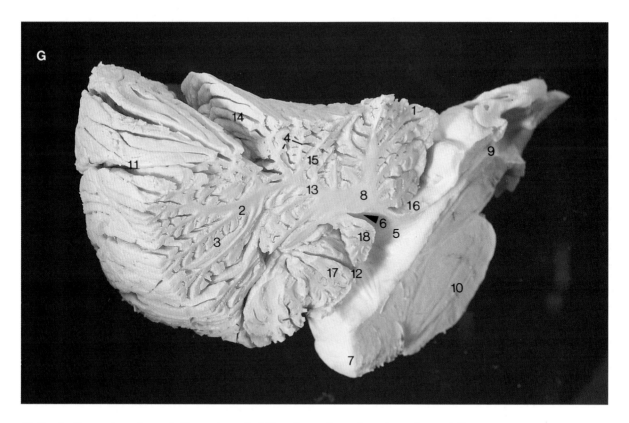

G Sagitally sectioned cerebellum viewed obliquely to show the arbor vitae. x1.7

1 Anterior lobe	**7** Medulla oblongata	**13** Primary lamina of arbor vitae
2 Arbor vitae	**8** Medullary centre	**14** Primary fissure
3 Cortex	of cerebellum	**15** Secondary lamina of arbor vitae
4 Folia	**9** Midbrain	**16** Lingula
5 Fourth ventricle	**10** Pons	**17** Uvula } of vermis
6 Lateral recess of fourth	**11** Posterior lobe	**18** Nodule
ventricle (arrow)	**12** Posterolateral fissure	

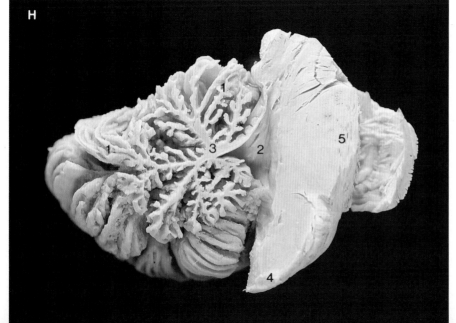

H The fibrous skeleton of the cerebellum. (The cellular structure has been removed on the sectioned face of the cerebellum.) x1.3

1 Arbor vitae
2 Fourth ventricle
3 Medullary centre
4 Medulla oblongata
5 Pons

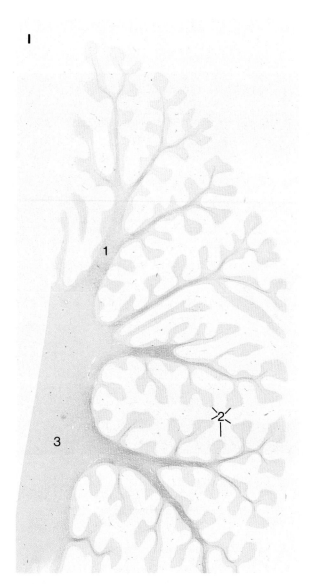

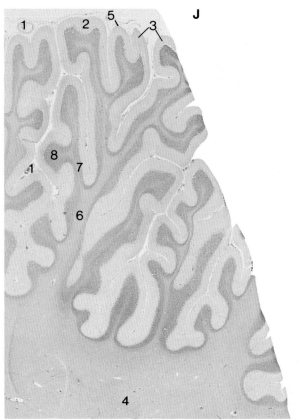

I Histological section of the arbor vitae. Luxol fast blue and cresyl violet stain. x3.7
1 Arbor vitae
2 Folia
3 Medullary centre

J An histological section to show the arbor vitae in relation to the cerebellar cortex. Bodian stain and neutral red stain. x6.6
1 Blood vessels
2 Cortex
3 Folia
4 Medullary centre
5 Pia mater
6 Primary lamina of arbor vitae
7 Secondary lamina of arbor vitae
8 Tertiary lamina of arbor vitae

K-M Afferent, efferent and intracortical fibres of arbor vitae and the cerebellar cortex.

1 Climbing fibres (afferent) around Purkinje cells
2 Basket cell processes
3 Fibres (intracortical) parallel to cortical surface
4 Granular layer
5 Molecular layer
6 Myelinated fibres of arbor vitae
7 Myelinated fibres in granular layer
8 Purkinje cell bodies
9 Purkinje cell layer

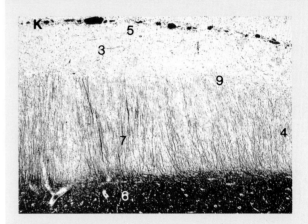

K Weigert-Pal stain. x55

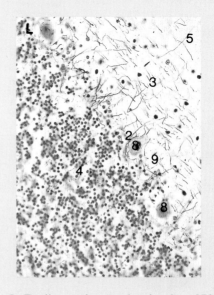

L Bodian and neutral red stain. x270

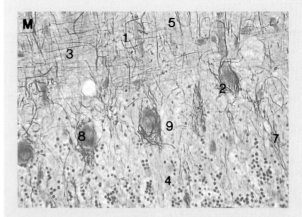

M Palmgren stain. x356

N-P The cellular structure of the cerebellar cortex. The cortex consists of three cellular layers; granular, Purkinje and molecular.

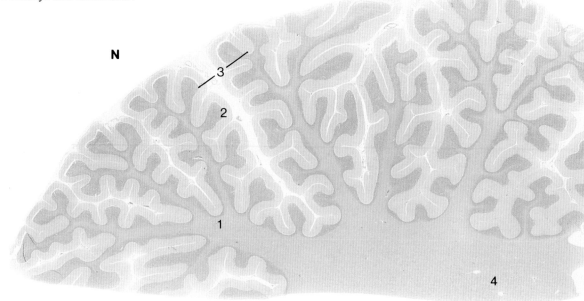

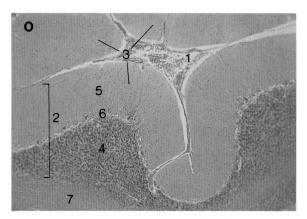

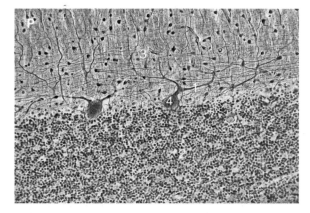

N Paraffin wax section to show the cerebellar cortex. Haematoxylin and eosin stain. x4.4
1 Arbor vitae
2 Cerebellar cortex
3 Folia
4 Medullary centre

O Higher magnification of folia showing full thickness of cortex. Haematoxylin and eosin stain. x71
1 Blood vessels in arachnoid mater
2 Cortex
3 Folia
4 Granular layer
5 Molecular layer
6 Purkinje layer
7 White matter of arbor vitae

P Purkinje cells and their processes between the granular and molecular layers of the cerebellar cortex. Silver stain. x223
1 Dendrites
2 Granular layer
3 Molecular layer
4 Purkinje cell body

Q-T The intracerebellar or deep nuclei. The major nuclei are the dentate, emboliform, globose and fastigial nuclei. Axons from the dentate, emboliform and globose nuclei leave the cerebellum via the superior cerebellar peduncle. Axons from the fastigial nucleus leave via the inferior cerebellar peduncle.

Fibres from the dentate nucleus run to the red nucleus and thalamus.

The emboliform and globose nuclei send fibres to the red nucleus.

The fastigial nucleus is connected to the lateral vestibular nucleus and reticular formation.

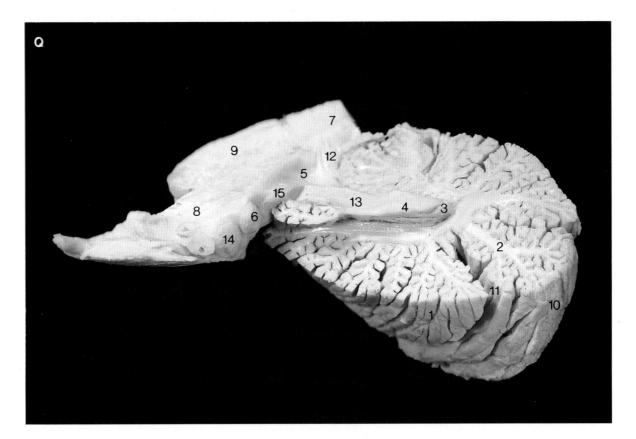

Q Sagittally sectioned cerebellum and brainstem to show the dentate nucleus and superior cerebellar peduncle. x1.4
   1 Anterior lobe
   2 Arbor vitae
   3 Dentate nucleus
   4 Fibres joining superior peduncle
   5 Fourth ventricle
   6 Inferior colliculus
   7 Medulla oblongata
   8 Midbrain
   9 Pons
   10 Posterior lobe
   11 Primary fissure
   12 Striae medullares
   13 Superior cerebellar peduncle
   14 Superior colliculus
   15 Superior medullary velum

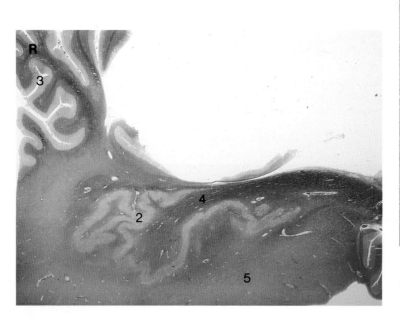

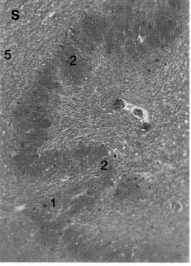

R Paraffin wax section of the dentate nucleus. Myelin stain and counterstain. x3.33

MHMS

S Higher magnification of part of the dentate nucleus. Luxol fast blue and cresyl violet stain. x55

1 Cell bodies
2 Dentate nucleus
3 Folia
4 Hilus of dentate nucleus
5 Medullary centre

CXWMS

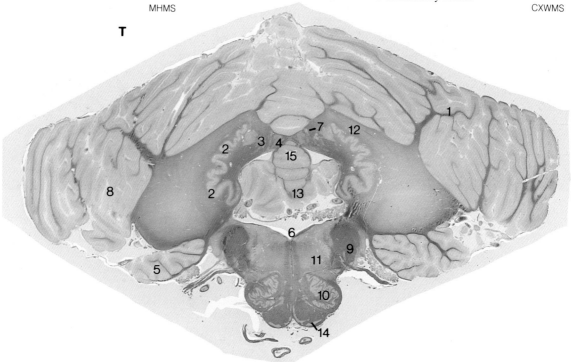

T Celloidin section through cerebellum and medulla oblongata to show the deep cerebellar nuclei. Weigert-Pal stain and celloidin embedded section cut by Mr P.A. Runnicles. x1.49

1 Arbor vitae	7 Globose nucleus	13 Nodule
2 Dentate nucleus	8 Hemisphere	14 Pyramid of medulla
3 Emboliform nucleus	9 Inferior cerebellar peduncle	15 Uvula of vermis
4 Fastigial nucleus	10 Inferior olivary nucleus	
5 Flocculus	11 Medulla oblongata	
6 Fourth ventricle	12 Medullary centre	

MHMS

SPINAL CORD

The spinal cord lies in the vertebral canal and is continuous with the medulla oblongata. Distally it tapers into the conus medullaris which ends at a variable level between the twelfth thoracic vertebra (T12) and the disc between the first and second lumbar vertebrae (L1-L2). Thirty-one pairs of spinal nerves arise from the cord and leave the vertebral column through the intervertebral foramina. Due to differential growth between the spinal cord and the vertebral column, the lower lumbar and sacral segments of the spinal cord lie opposite the lower thoracic and upper lumbar vertebrae in the adult. Their nerves run obliquely downwards to the foramina. Those lying beyond the conus medullaris form a leash of nerves called the cauda equina or 'horse's tail'. Every nerve has an anterior or ventral (motor) and a posterior or dorsal (sensory) root, except that some individuals lack the dorsal root of the first cervical nerve (C1). The cord is surrounded and protected by all three layers of the meninges and by the cerebrospinal fluid, all of which are continuous with those around the brain. A longitudinal groove, the anterior (or ventral) median fissure, runs the entire length of the cord. Although there is no fissure posteriorly, a posterior (dorsal) median septum is seen in cross-section.

The spinal cord can be divided into cervical, thoracic, sacral and coccygeal regions according to the parts of the body its nerves supply. Each of these can be further subdivided into segments, each giving rise to a pair of spinal nerves i.e. eight cervical (C1-C8), twelve thoracic (T1-T12), five lumbar (L1-L5), five sacral (S1-S5) and one coccygeal. The grey matter of the cord is enlarged where the nerves of the brachial and lumbosacral plexuses arise; these swellings are called the cervical (C5-T1) and lumbar (L2-S3) enlargements.

In cross-section the spinal cord consists of an external layer of white matter and an inner core of grey matter, within which there is a minute central canal continuous with the fourth ventricle of the brain. The grey matter is shaped like a butterfly with the wings on each side being the anterior (ventral) and posterior (dorsal) horns. From T1 or T2 to L2 a lateral horn is discernible. The anterior horn is motor in function, the posterior horn is sensory and the lateral horn is sympathetic. Different levels of the cord can easily be distinguished in transverse sections because there is a preponderance of grey matter at lower (lumbar and sacral) levels and of white matter at thoracic or cervical levels. Sections through the first cervical segment (C1) show a transitional arrangement between the spinal cord and the lower levels of the medulla oblongata.

The white matter is arranged around the grey matter into anterior, posterior and lateral white columns (or funiculi) and anterior and posterior white commissures. The columns contain nerve fibres grouped in tracts. Cell groupings within the grey matter may be described as nuclei or as layers, the laminae of Rexed. These have indistinct borders, and much intermingling, and are difficult to demarcate in human material. The long ascending and descending tracts link the spinal cord with the brain. The fasciculi proprii are short tracts for local connections within the cord. The white commissures contain some fibres which remain on their own side and others which cross (decussate) from one side of the cord to the other.

Very simple nervous activity, for example the reflex arc, is possible in the spinal cord without involving the brain. More complex activity, voluntary movement and conscious sensations, involve communication with the brain. Ascending tracts carry impulses up to the brain and are sensory in function. Descending tracts carry impulses down from the brain to the spinal cord and are motor.

Ascending tracts in the spinal cord are part of the ascending, sensory, nervous pathways which convey information about the general or somatic senses from the trunk and limbs to the brain. The somatic senses are touch, pain, temperature, pressure and vibration and proprioception, the sense of position. All are consciously perceived except for proprioception, which exists in two forms, unconscious from muscles, and conscious from joints and tendons. Pathways concerned with conscious sensations ultimately terminate in the primary sensory cortex, that is, the post-central gyrus, Brodmann's areas 1, 2 and 3. They do so on the opposite side to that on which the sensation is received by a peripheral sensory receptor, for example a nerve ending in the skin. This is because the ascending pathways concerned with these sensations decussate *en route* to the sensory cortex. They are also interrupted at one or more points along their course. A pathway consists of a chain of neurons and their processes linked together by synapses. The impulse passes from one neuron to the next along the course of the pathway; the successive neurons in the sequence being known as first, second and third order neurons. The tracts in the spinal cord concerned with conscious sensations are the anterior spinothalamic tract, for crude, non-discriminating touch, the lateral spinothalamic tract for pain and temperature, and the fasciculus gracilis and fasciculus cuneatus, jointly known as the posterior columns, for fine touch, pressure, vibration and conscious proprioception. Unconscious proprioception is exceptional in that the tracts conveying this sensory information, the spinocerebellar tracts, terminate in the cerebellum, and are predominantly uncrossed.

A number of structures in the brain are motor in function. These include the primary motor cortex (Brodmann's areas 4 and 6), the red nucleus, substantia nigra, corpus striatum, cerebellum, vestibular nuclei, inferior olivary nucleus, midbrain tectum and reticular formation. They give origin to descending tracts, which form motor pathways between some of the motor centres in the brain and the motor neurons in the anterior horn of the spinal cord. The former are known as upper motor neurons and the latter as lower motor neurons. Lower motor neuron stimulation alone will cause a muscle to contract, but purposeful voluntary movements and the co-ordination of the actions of different muscles requires the participation of upper motor neurons via the descending motor pathways. Like a sensory pathway, a motor pathway may decussate along its course and be interrupted by one or more synaptic relays. The major pathway for the control of voluntary movement of the trunk and limbs is the lateral corticospinal tract. It decussates in the brainstem, so bringing movements on each side of the body under the control of the opposite (contralateral) side of the brain. Along with its companion tract, the corticobulbar tract, which controls voluntary movement in the head through its connections with motor cranial nerve nuclei, it forms the pyramidal tract. The name refers to its passage through the pyramid of the medulla oblongata during its descent. The remaining pathways do not pass through the medullary pyramid and are referred to as 'extrapyramidal'. They control postural and automatic movements of the neck, trunk and limbs.

The main ascending and descending tracts are summarized in the table below; for details see the appropriate chapters in the second section of the book.

• *The names of tracts indicate the origin and termination of the tract and the direction in which impulses flow, for example:* **spinocerebellar**: *from* **spinal** *cord to* **cerebellum** *(ascending);* **corticospinal**: *from motor* **cortex** *to* **spinal** *cord (descending).*

ASCENDING AND DESCENDING TRACTS

	ASCENDING TRACTS	**DESCENDING TRACTS**
ANTERIOR COLUMN	Anterior (ventral) spinothalamic	Anterior (ventral) corticospinal (pyramidal)
		Vestibulospinal Tectospinal Reticulospinal
LATERAL COLUMN	Spinocerebellar Lateral spinothalamic	Lateral corticospinal Rubrospinal Olivospinal
	Spinotectal	
POSTERIOR COLUMN	Fasciculus gracilis Fasciculus cuneatus	Fasciculus interfascicularis Septomarginal fasciculus
DIFFUSE IN ANTERIOR AND LATERAL COLUMNS	Spinoreticular	

• *The most medially placed cells in the anterior horn supply axial muscles, more laterally placed cells supply the limbs.*

• *Due to intermingling of adjacent tracts disease processes rarely affect one tract exclusively.*

• *Vertebral column injuries between T12 and L1 damage segment S1 of the spinal cord and paralyse the bladder.*

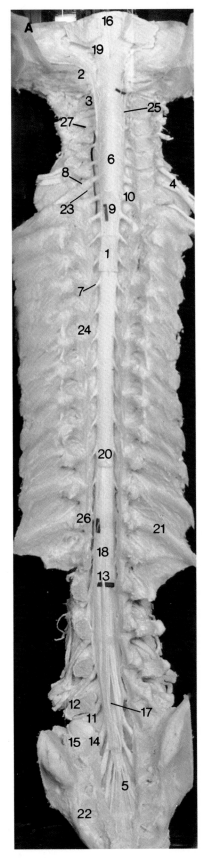

A A dissection of the adult spinal cord *in situ* to demonstrate its anatomy and relationships. x.28

1 Arachnoid mater
2 Atlas
3 Axis
4 Brachial plexus
5 Cauda equina
6 Cervical enlargement
7 Dorsal (posterior) root
8 Dorsal (posterior) root ganglion
9 Dura mater
10 Eighth cervical nerve root (C8)
11 Fifth lumbar nerve root (L5)
12 Fifth lumbar vertebra
13 Filum terminale
14 First sacral nerve root (S1)
15 First sacral vertebra (S1)
16 Fourth ventricle
17 Lumbar cistern
18 Lumbar enlargement
19 Medulla oblongata
20 Pia mater
21 Ribs
22 Sacrum
23 Seventh cervical vertebra (C7)
24 Sixth thoracic vertebra (T6)
25 Spinal root of accessory nerve
26 Twelfth thoracic vertebra (T12)
27 Ventral (anterior) root

OXF

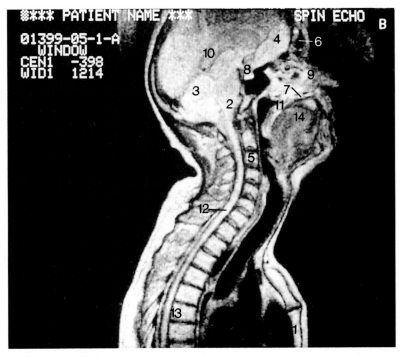

B An NMR image to illustrate the brain and spinal cord *in situ* and to demonstrate the pliability of the spinal cord.

1 Body of sternum
2 Brainstem
3 Cerebellum
4 Cerebral hemisphere
5 Cervical vertebrae
6 Frontal sinus
7 Hard palate
8 Hypophysis
9 Nose
10 Position of lateral ventricle
11 Soft palate
12 Spinal cord
13 Thoracic vertebrae
14 Tongue

Elscint Ltd

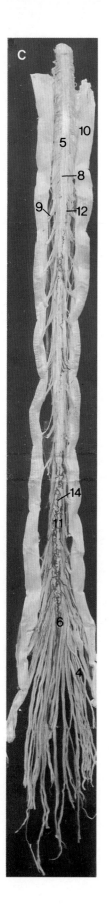

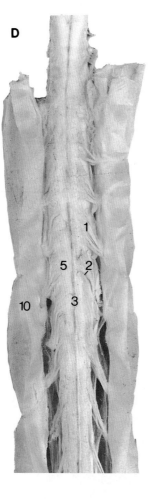

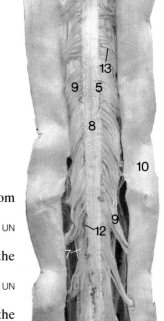

C-G Dissections and histological preparations to demonstrate the spinal cord in its meningeal coverings. Spinal meninges differ from those around the brain in two important respects: first, the pia mater is more robust and sometimes is described as having two layers. There is a thick outer layer, the epi-pia, and a thin inner layer, the pia intima. Second, an epidural space containing fatty areolar tissue and a venous plexus lies between the dura mater and the bone of the vertebral canal.

C Isolated spinal cord and meninges viewed from the dorsal (posterior) aspect. x.35

UN

D The cervical enlargement viewed from the ventral (anterior) aspect. x.89

UN

E The cervical enlargement viewed from the dorsal (posterior) aspect. x.85

1 Anterior (ventral) nerve roots
2 Anterior radicular artery
3 Anterior spinal artery
4 Cauda equina
5 Cervical enlargement
6 Conus medullaris
7 Denticulate ligament of the pia mater
8 Dorsal (posterior) columns
9 Dorsal (posterior) nerve roots
10 Dura and arachnoid mater, opened
11 Lumbar enlargement
12 Posterior spinal artery
13 Posterior radicular artery
14 Venous plexus

UN

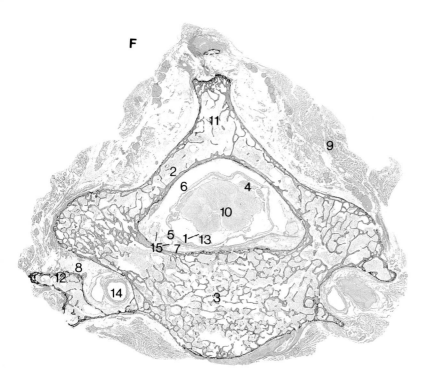

F Histological section through a cervical vertebra and the spinal cord *in situ*, to show the relationship between the spinal cord, bone and meninges. Block-stained with silver nitrate, section stained with light green and Orange G. x1.9

1 Arachnoid and pia mater
2 Arch or lamina of vertebra
3 Body of vertebra
4 Dorsal (posterior) nerve root
5 Dura mater
6 Epidural space
7 Fat within epidural space
8 Foramen transversarium
9 Neck muscles
10 Spinal cord
11 Spine of vertebra
12 Transverse process
13 Ventral (anterior) nerve roots
14 Vertebral artery
15 Vessels in epidural space

Mr D. Adams

G A section to show the structure of pia mater covering the spinal cord. Weigert-Pal stain. x31.4

1 Arachnoid mater
2 Blood vessels
3 Dorsal (posterior) horn
4 Dorsal (posterior) nerve root
5 Dorsal (posterior) white columns
6 Grey matter
7 Lateral white column
8 Pia mater

CAM

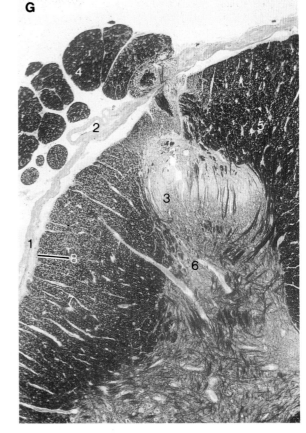

● *In spinal anaesthesia, anaesthetic solution may be introduced into either the epidural space or the sub-arachnoid space, where it mixes with the CSF.*

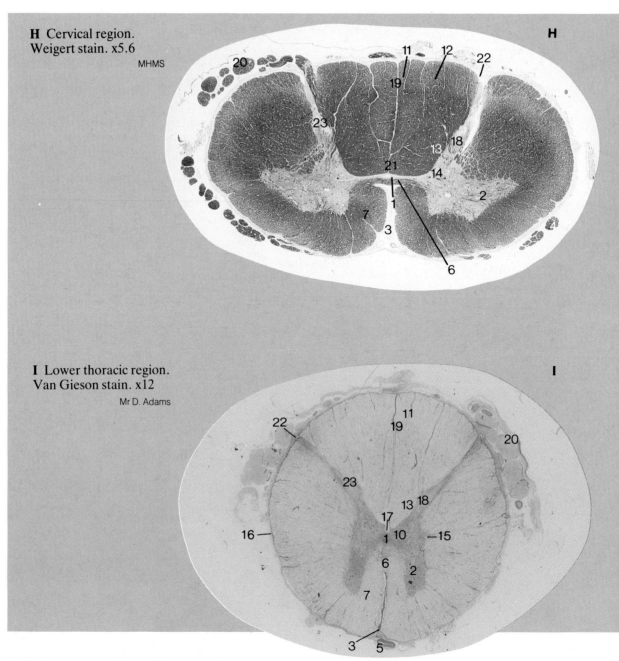

H Cervical region.
Weigert stain. x5.6

MHMS

I Lower thoracic region.
Van Gieson stain. x12

Mr D. Adams

H-K A sequence of paraffin wax sections to show regional variations in the arrangement of grey and white matter in the spinal cord.

1 Anterior (ventral) grey commissure (part of Rexed's lamina X)
2 Anterior (ventral) horn (Rexed's laminae VIII and IX)
3 Anterior (ventral) median sulcus
4 Anterior (ventral) nerve roots
5 Anterior (ventral) spinal vessels
6 Anterior (ventral) white commissure
7 Anterior (ventral) white funiculus (or column)
8 Cauda equina
9 Central canal
10 Nucleus dorsalis; Clarke's nucleus, (Rexed's lamina VI)
11 Fasciculus gracilis ⎱ Dorsal or posterior
12 Fasciculus cuneatus ⎰ white columns
13 Fasciculi proprii
14 Intermediate zone (Rexed's laminae VI and VII)
15 Lateral (intermediolateral) horn

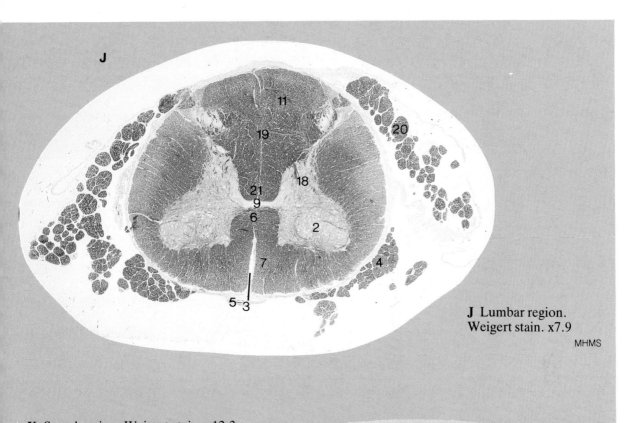

J Lumbar region.
Weigert stain. x7.9

K Sacral region. Weigert stain. x12.3

16 Pia mater
17 Posterior (dorsal) grey commissure
18 Posterior (dorsal) horn (Rexed's laminae I to V)
19 Posterior median septum
20 Posterior (dorsal) nerve roots
21 Posterior (dorsal) white commissure
22 Posterolateral (dorsolateral) sulcus
23 Substantia gelatinosa (Rolandi) (Rexed's laminae II and III)

● *Enkephalins and substance-P are found in the substantia gelatinosa. Pain fibres in dorsal roots terminate there and throughout laminae I to III.*

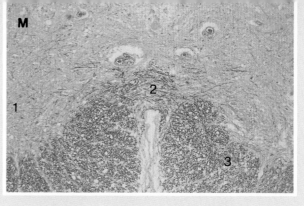

L-P Histological sections to show the cells and fibres of the spinal cord.

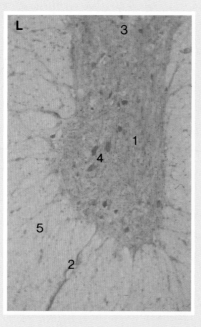

M A paraffin wax section of the anterior white commissure of the sacral spinal cord showing decussating fibres. Myelin stain. x55
1 Anterior (ventral) horn
2 Anterior (ventral) white commissures
3 Anterior (ventral) white funiculus

L The anterior (ventral) horn of the spinal cord at lower thoracic levels. Van Gieson stain. x22

1 Anterior (ventral) horn	3 Grey matter
2 Anterior (ventral) root fibres	4 Motor neurons
	5 White matter

Mr D. Adams

● *The large α motor neurons which supply skeletal muscle are cholinergic.*

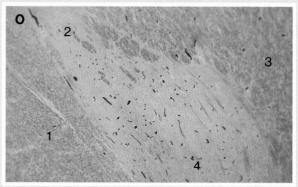

O A paraffin wax section of the substantia gelatinosa of the lumbar spinal cord. Weigert stain. x55
1 Lateral white funiculus
2 Posterolateral fasciculus (Lissauer's Tract)
3 Posterior (dorsal) columns
4 Substantia gelatinosa (Rolandi)

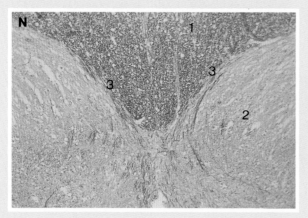

N An histological section showing fibres leaving the dorsal (posterior) horn to enter fasciculi proprii in the sacral spinal cord. Myelin stain. x55
1 Dorsal (posterior) column
2 Dorsal (posterior) horn
3 Fasciculi proprii

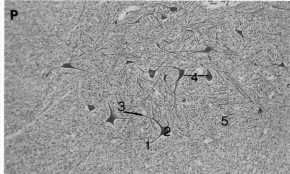
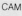

P Motor neurons in the anterior horn of the cervical spinal cord. Silver stain. x89

1 Axon	4 Motor neuron
2 Cell body	5 Neuropil
3 Dendrite	

Cauda Equina

The cauda equina (horse's tail) consists of the filum terminale, a pial and neuroglial strand, and the dorsal and ventral roots of the lumbar and sacral nerves. It lies in the lumbar cistern of the subarachnoid space.

● *Lumbar punctures below the level of L3-L4 will not encounter spinal cord. The needle passes between the spinal nerves which are displaced.*

A-B Dissections to show the structure of the cauda equina.

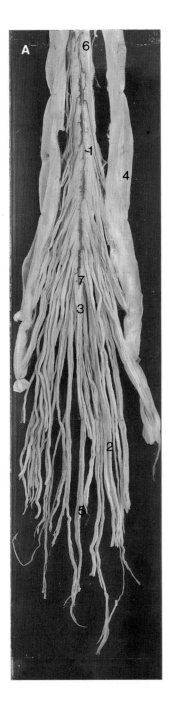

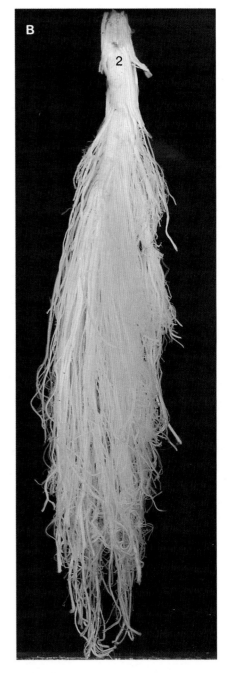

A The lumbar and sacral regions of the spinal cord and the cauda equina, in their meningeal coverings. The cauda equina has been spread to demonstrate individual nerve roots. The filum terminale has been severed in removing the spinal cord from the vertebral canal. x.68

1 Anterior spinal artery
2 Cauda equina
3 Conus medullaris
4 Dura and arachnoid mater
5 Filum terminale
6 Lumbar region of spinal cord
7 Sacral region of spinal cord

UN

B An 18th-century dissection of the cauda equina prepared by John Hunter, from the Hunterian Museum of the Royal College of Surgeons of England. x.75

1 Frayed nerves of cauda equina
2 Spinal cord

FUNCTIONAL SYSTEMS OF THE CENTRAL NERVOUS SYSTEM

REFLEX ARC

The nervous system is able to make involuntary motor responses to sensory stimuli which are either painful or potentially damaging. This type of response is termed a reflex and it is dependent upon the integrity of a nervous pathway known as a reflex arc. The simplest type of arc consists of a receptor organ, an afferent neuron, an efferent neuron and an effector organ.

The sensory receptor organs are located in skin, mucous membranes, connective tissue or muscles. They are innervated by primary sensory neurons whose cell bodies lie in the dorsal (posterior) root ganglia. These cells are unipolar, but their axons divide into two processes; a central process connecting the cell to the spinal cord and a peripheral one connecting it to the receptor. The peripheral processes of the axons form the sensory (afferent) fibres in peripheral nerves and the central processes form the nerve roots. When the receptor is stimulated an impulse travels along the two processes of the axon to the dorsal (posterior) horn of the spinal cord.

The afferent fibres entering the cord frequently synapse with one or more internuncial neurons which act as intermediate or messenger neurons. These in turn synapse with motor (efferent) neurons. The axons of the motor neurons pass out through the ventral root and to the effector organ (muscle or gland). Fibres from the internuncial neurons may ascend or descend in the cord to stimulate motor neurons at different segmental levels of the spinal cord. They may also cross to the opposite side of the cord and stimulate motor neurons.

Although such reflex arcs are at the spinal cord level they may be influenced by the brain via the olivospinal, rubrospinal, reticulospinal, corticospinal, tectospinal, and vestibulospinal tracts. These are all motor pathways or descending tracts. The effect of these motor connections is to suppress the activity of many reflex arcs in the spinal cord. These reflexes, many of which are primitive defence responses, are present in babies before the descending tracts are mature. They may reappear in adults if the descending pathways are interrupted by injury or disease. An example of this release from inhibition is Babinski's sign. In a normal adult the toes flex when the sole of the foot is stimulated. In babies or in adults with lesions of the corticospinal tract the toes extend.

● *Reflex arcs in the spinal cord play an important role in maintaining muscle tone and posture.*

● *Flexor and extensor muscles of the same limb do not simultaneously contract in a reflex. There are connections between the afferent flexor nerve fibres which synapse with extensor motor neurons of the same limb and inhibit them. This effect is called the law of reciprocal innervation.*

● *Stimulation of one lower limb may result in extension of the contralateral limb. This response is known as the crossed extensor reflex. Its anatomical basis is the connection of incoming sensory fibres to contralateral motor neurons in the spinal cord, via internuncial neurons whose axons cross the midline.*

A diagram of the reflex arc.

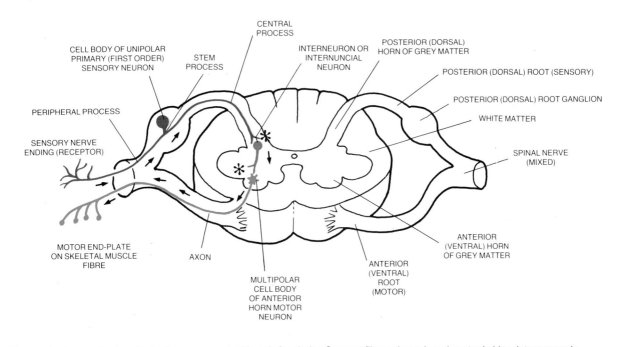

CELL BODY OF UNIPOLAR
PRIMARY (FIRST ORDER)
SENSORY NEURON

STEM
PROCESS

CENTRAL
PROCESS

INTERNEURON OR
INTERNUNCIAL
NEURON

POSTERIOR (DORSAL)
HORN OF GREY MATTER

POSTERIOR (DORSAL) ROOT (SENSORY)

POSTERIOR (DORSAL) ROOT GANGLION

WHITE MATTER

PERIPHERAL PROCESS

SENSORY NERVE
ENDING (RECEPTOR)

SPINAL NERVE
(MIXED)

MOTOR END-PLATE
ON SKELETAL MUSCLE
FIBRE

AXON

MULTIPOLAR
CELL BODY
OF ANTERIOR
HORN MOTOR
NEURON

ANTERIOR
(VENTRAL)
ROOT
(MOTOR)

ANTERIOR
(VENTRAL) HORN
OF GREY MATTER

Diagram to show a simple spinal reflex arc, on one side only for clarity. Sensory fibres shown in red, motor in blue, interneuron in green. Arrows show the direction of impulse flow.
* Indicates synapses.

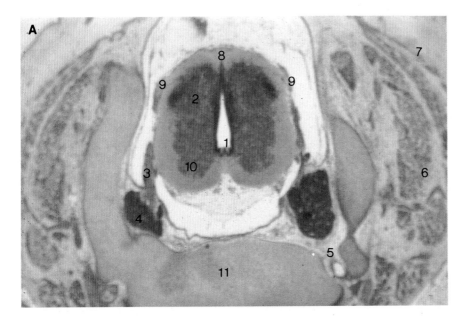

A A transverse paraffin wax section of the spinal cord and vertebral canal of a 27 mmCR embryo to show the components of a reflex arc. Haematoxylin and eosin stain. x61

1 Central canal
2 Dorsal horn (grey matter)
3 Dorsal root
4 Dorsal root ganglion
5 Intervertebral foramen
6 Muscle
7 Skin
8 Spinal cord
9 Spinal nerve (position of)
10 Ventral horn (grey matter)
11 Vertebral body

MHMS

SENSORY AND MOTOR PATHWAYS

Sensory pathways convey information from a peripheral sensory receptor via lower sensory centres to higher sensory centres in the brain. The pathways for the somatic senses (touch, pain, temperature and proprioception or position sense) are known as ascending tracts because information is transmitted in an ascending direction from the spinal cord or brainstem to the cerebral cortex.

Conversely a motor pathway conveys information from higher centres to muscles or glands. Because of the direction in which information passes, the motor pathways are also known as descending tracts. The descriptions of the ascending and descending tracts reflect the direction of these pathways.

Somatic Sensory Pathways

The somatic or general senses comprise the categories (modalities) of touch, pain, temperature, pressure, vibration and proprioception. All are consciously perceived. In addition, there is an unconscious form of proprioception.

Sensory receptors for touch, pressure, vibration and temperature are present in the skin. Receptors for proprioception, the sense of position, lie in muscles, tendons and joints. Pain receptors are widely distributed throughout the body.

The surface of the trunk and limbs can be imagined as being divided into a series of strips. Each strip or dermatome contains sensory receptors which transmit information predominantly to one segment of the spinal cord along the segmental spinal nerve. There is some overlap in the distribution of sensory nerves along the borders of adjacent dermatomes, so that interruption of a single spinal nerve root may cause relatively little sensory loss.

From the spinal cord the sensory information is conveyed to the brain by ascending sensory pathways, each specifically associated with one or more sensory modalities.

The sensory pathways each consist of a chain of neurons, connected by synapses. Impulses pass from neuron to neuron along the pathway. Neurons are designated first order, second order, etc., according to their position in the chain. First order neurons are also referred to as primary sensory neurons. The passage of the impulse across a synapse from one neuron to the next constitutes a synaptic relay.

Sensory receptors in the head are innervated by cranial nerves, primarily the trigeminal (V) nerve, but also the facial (VII), glossopharyngeal (IX) and vagus (X) nerves. Ascending tracts from the brainstem accompany those from the spinal cord.

Sensory pathways for conscious sensations are crossed so that sensory information reaches the cerebral hemisphere contralateral to the stimulus. The pathway for unconscious proprioception is uncrossed. Pathways for conscious sensations terminate in the primary sensory cortex, that is, the postcentral gyrus of the parietal lobe, Brodmann's areas 1, 2 and 3. Pathways for unconscious proprioception terminate in the cerebellum. The cortex of both the postcentral gyrus and the proprioceptive areas of the cerebellum is organized somatotopically, with particular areas of the cortex receiving sensory information from particular areas of the body.

Further processing and interpretation of conscious sensory information received in the primary sensory cortex is the function of adjacent somatic sensory association cortex, Brodmann's areas 5 and 7.

Pain and temperature

Receptors
Cutaneous pain and temperature receptors are free nerve endings in the dermis and epidermis. They also exist in mucous membranes, for example, in the oral mucosa and in the cornea and in the walls of hollow viscera, for example, the digestive tract, where they are stimulated by over-distension. The free nerve endings are the terminal branches of the axons of the first order neurons.

The pathway from the trunk and limbs: the lateral spinothalamic tract
The first order neurons lie in the dorsal root ganglia of the spinal nerves. When the receptor is stimulated sensory information passes along the axon of the first order neuron into the dorsal horn of the spinal cord. There the axon synapses with a second order neuron, whose axon crosses the midline and ascends in the lateral spinothalamic tract on the opposite side of the body. The axons of second order neurons synapse in the ventral posterolateral nucleus of the thalamus with the third order neurons. The axons of the third order neurons pass via the internal capsule to the postcentral gyrus.

The primary sensory neurons also have branches which ascend or descend one segment of the cord in the dorsolateral fasciculus (column or tract) of Lissauer before entering the dorsal horn and synapsing with the second order neurons. Consequently the tract carrying sensory information to the brain from a particular dermatome may arise one segment above or below the segment actually corresponding to that dermatome. Lesions of the spinal cord may therefore abolish sensations from dermatomes below those supplied by the injured segments.

Some axons from Lissauer's tract enter the substantia gelatinosa of the spinal cord and there may be additional synaptic relays in the substantia gelatinosa. This arrangement enables the substantia gelatinosa to act as a 'gate' or 'filter' regulating the entry of impulses into the spinothalamic tract.

● *One cause of pain from phantom limbs following amputation is that nerve axons in the stump are squeezed by scar tissue. The stimulus is perceived by the sensory cortex as not from the stump, but the missing area of limb.*

● *If pain becomes intractable it may, very rarely, be necessary to obtain relief by cordotomy, an operation in which the lateral spinothalamic tract is cut on the contralateral side to the source of the pain. Due to spinal overlap the surgeon will cut the cord at a segmental level one or two segments higher than the relevant sensory input.*

The pathway from the head
Sensory receptors for pain and temperature are free nerve endings of fibres in all three divisions of the trigeminal (V) nerve. The facial (VII) nerve carries some pain and temperature fibres from the external ear. The glossopharyngeal (IX) and vagus (X) nerves supply the mucosa of the back of the tongue, pharynx, larynx, auditory tube and middle ear. The scalp behind the vertex of the skull is supplied by cervical spinal nerves. The cranial dura mater has a plentiful supply of pain-sensitive nerve endings supplied by the trigeminal nerve, the vagus nerve and the upper cervical nerves.

The cell bodies of the first order trigeminal sensory neurons are located in the semilunar or Gasserian ganglion of the trigeminal nerve. The first order neurons for the facial, glossopharyngeal and vagus nerves lie in the sensory ganglia of those nerves. The ganglia are, therefore, homologous to the dorsal root ganglia of spinal nerves. The central processes of the axons of the first order neurons descend through the brainstem in the spinal trigeminal tract to the spinal trigeminal nucleus where they synapse with the second order neurons. The axons of the second order neurons decussate to the contralateral side and ascend in the ventral trigeminal tract to synapse in the ventral posteromedial nucleus of the thalamus with the third order neurons. The ventral trigeminal tract or ventral secondary ascending tract of V is analogous to the lateral spinothalamic tract. The axons of the third order neurons pass through the internal capsule to the postcentral gyrus (Brodmann's areas 1, 2, 3).

The entry of nerve fibres into the spinal tract and nucleus of the trigeminal nerve is highly organized. It can be described in terms of an imaginary picture of the head being projected onto the nucleus like a slide on a screen. This is called a somatotopic organization and is common in sensory systems. If the nucleus is envisaged as a fingerlike object lying parallel to the neuraxis then sensations from successive strips of tissue in the head are fed into successive slices of the nucleus. This is called the 'onion-skin' concept. In addition, in a transverse section of that part of the nucleus connected to the trigeminal nerve itself, three tiers of cells are associated with the ophthalmic, maxillary and mandibular divisions of the nerve respectively.

A diagram to demonstrate the sensory input into the spinal tract and nucleus of the trigeminal nerve. On the left is the onion-skin concept of the longitudinal organization of the nucleus. On the right is the relationship between a cross-section of the tract and nucleus and the peripheral distribution of the trigeminal nerve.

The colours indicate areas of the face linked to their area of sensory input in the spinal trigeminal nucleus and tract.

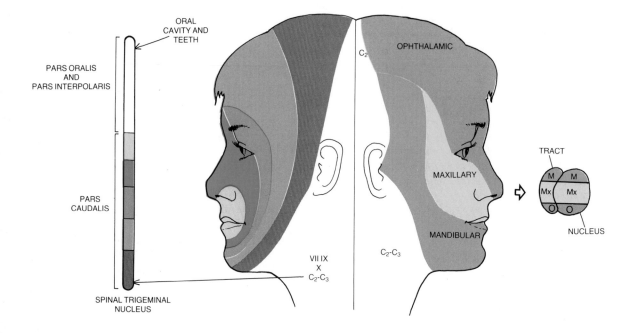

A diagram of the lateral spinothalamic (red) and ventral trigeminothalamic (green) pathways conveying pain and temperature information from the body and head respectively. Each is shown on one side only for clarity. Fibres from pain and temperature receptors in the head enter in all three divisions of the trigeminal nerve but for clarity only one is drawn.

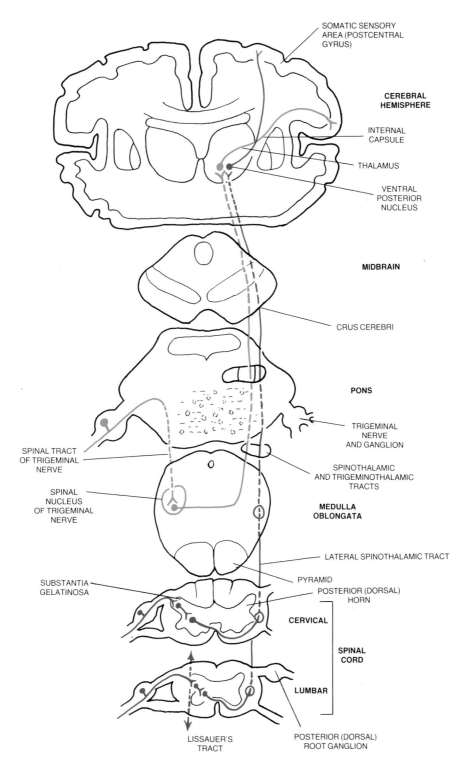

SOMATIC SENSORY AREA (POSTCENTRAL GYRUS)

CEREBRAL HEMISPHERE

INTERNAL CAPSULE

THALAMUS

VENTRAL POSTERIOR NUCLEUS

MIDBRAIN

CRUS CEREBRI

PONS

TRIGEMINAL NERVE AND GANGLION

SPINAL TRACT OF TRIGEMINAL NERVE

SPINOTHALAMIC AND TRIGEMINOTHALAMIC TRACTS

SPINAL NUCLEUS OF TRIGEMINAL NERVE

MEDULLA OBLONGATA

LATERAL SPINOTHALAMIC TRACT

PYRAMID

SUBSTANTIA GELATINOSA

POSTERIOR (DORSAL) HORN

CERVICAL

SPINAL CORD

LUMBAR

LISSAUER'S TRACT

POSTERIOR (DORSAL) ROOT GANGLION

Simple (light or crude) touch and pressure

Receptors

The cutaneous receptors for light touch are varied. They include free nerve endings, nerve endings associated with hair follicles, and nerve endings associated with specialised epidermal cells, the Merkel discs. The pressure receptors are complex structures, the Pacinian corpuscles, in which the nerve endings are enclosed in a multilayered capsule. They are deeply situated in the dermis, and are also found in periosteum, around joints and in mesenteries.

The pathway from the trunk and limbs: the anterior (ventral) spinothalamic tract

Cutaneous receptors for crude touch and pressure are located in the dermal layer of skin. They are innervated by the primary sensory neurons (first order neurons) which lie in the dorsal root ganglia. When the receptor is stimulated sensory information passes along the axon of the primary sensory neuron to the dorsal white column where the axons bifurcate. One branch enters the dorsal horn grey matter at the same level whilst the second branch ascends in the dorsal column ipsilaterally for as many as ten spinal segments. Both branches synapse with second order neurons in the dorsal horn grey matter. Axons from the second order neurons decussate and enter the ventral white column where they ascend as the ventral spinothalamic tract. Passing through the brainstem, these axons form part of the spinal lemniscus. This tract ascends to the ventral posterolateral nucleus of the thalamus. Here the neurons synapse with third order neurons whose axons pass via the internal capsule to the postcentral gyrus (Brodmann's areas 1, 2, 3).

The pathway from the head

The primary (first order) sensory neurons are situated in the semilunar ganglion of the trigeminal (V) nerve with a few in the geniculate ganglion of the facial nerve (VII) and the superior ganglion of the glossopharyngeal (IX) and vagus (X) nerves (see Pain and temperature above).

When a receptor supplied by the trigeminal (V) nerve is stimulated, impulses flow along the axon of the primary sensory neuron in the nerve. After the axon traverses the semilunar ganglion it enters the pons and may synapse with second order neurons in either the spinal or the principal (chief) sensory nucleus of the trigeminal nerve. The axons of second order neurons travel as either the crossed (ventral) trigeminothalamic tract or the uncrossed (dorsal) trigeminothalamic tract to synapse in the ventral posteromedial nucleus of the thalamus with the third order neurons. Axons of the third order neurons pass through the internal capsule to the primary sensory cortex of the postcentral gyrus.

Fibres in the facial, glossopharyngeal and vagus nerves synapse with second order neurons in the spinal trigeminal nucleus only, having no input into the principal nucleus. From the spinal nucleus onward the pathway continues alongside the second order neurons of the trigeminal pathways.

Fine touch, vibration and conscious proprioception

Receptors

Proprioception is the sense of position or movement. Conscious proprioception is associated with ligaments and joints. The sensory receptors are free nerve endings, Pacinian corpuscles, which respond to pressure, and Ruffini endings, which respond to stretch.

Fine or discriminating touch is a precise form of touch sensitivity mainly associated with the hands, especially the fingers. The sensory receptors are encapsulated nerve endings known as Meissner's corpuscles which lie in the dermis immediately deep to the epidermis.

The sensors for vibration are the Pacinian corpuscles. These are also numerous in the hand. Vibration is not a specific sensory modality but a tactile sense that is discontinuous and rapid.

All three sensations are carried by the same pathway from the trunk and limbs, but travel separately from the head.

The pathway from the trunk and limbs: the dorsal (posterior) columns and medial lemniscus

The receptors are innervated by the primary sensory neurons (first order neurons) which lie in the dorsal root ganglion. When the receptor is stimulated, sensory information passes along the axon of the primary sensory neuron into the ipsilateral dorsal white column where it ascends to the medulla oblongata. Axons from the cervical and upper thoracic levels enter the lateral part of the dorsal column and ascend there as the fasciculus cuneatus whilst axons from the lower thoracic, lumbar and sacral levels enter the medial part of the dorsal column and ascend there as the fasciculus gracilis.

Each fasciculus ascends to its own nucleus in the medulla. Here the first order neuron synapses with a second order neuron whose axon crosses the midline in the sensory decussation and ascends in the contralateral medial lemniscus to the ventral posterolateral nucleus of the thalamus. At this site

A diagram of the pathways for simple touch and pressure.

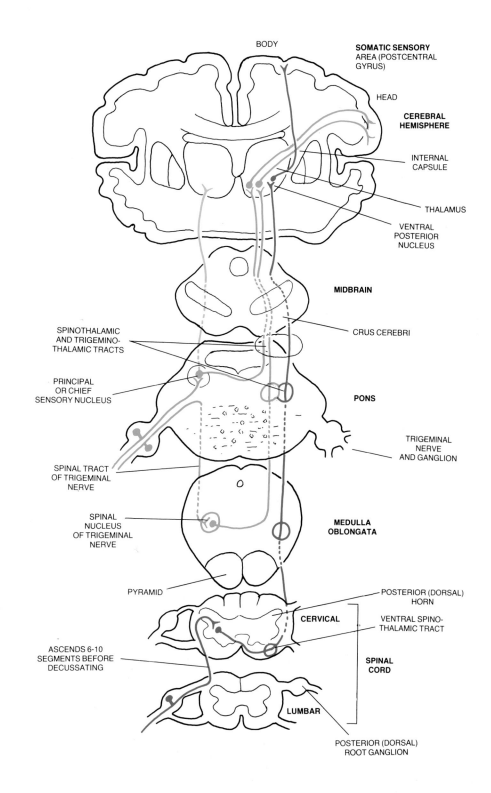

Pathways conveying simple, light or crude touch and pressure sensations from the body (red) and head (green). The pathways are shown on one side only for clarity. Fibres from touch receptors in the head travel in all three divisions of the trigeminal nerve, but for clarity only one is shown. Uncrossed fibres from the head are shown in light green.

the second order neuron synapses with third order neurons whose axon passes through the internal capsule to the primary sensory cortex i.e. the postcentral gyrus of the parietal lobe, Brodmann's areas 1, 2, 3.

● *Two point discrimination is the ability to distinguish between two sharp points placed on the skin close together. It is a measure of the level of discriminating touch perception in an area of skin. It is best developed where Meissner's corpuscles are most numerous.*

The pathways from the head

As already explained the pathways from the head differ for the sensory modalities.
i) **Fine Touch and Vibration:** the face is well-supplied with fine touch receptors especially around the lips. When they are stimulated impulses flow in the trigeminal nerve. The first order neurons lie in the semilunar ganglion. These cells synapse with second order neurons in the principal or chief sensory nucleus in the pons. The axons of the second order neurons run in either the ventral (crossed) or dorsal (uncrossed) trigeminothalamic tract to the ventral posteromedial nucleus of the thalamus where they synapse with the third order neurons. Third order neuron axons pass via the internal capsule to the postcentral gyrus.

The existence of both crossed and uncrossed pathways for crude and fine touch provides for awareness of touch from each side of the head in both cerebral hemispheres.

ii) **Conscious proprioception:** proprioceptive axons in the mandibular division of the trigeminal (V) nerve supply the capsule of the temporomandibular joint (TMJ), as well as facial and extra-ocular muscles and the muscles of mastication. The first order neurons have their cell bodies located in the mesencephalic nucleus of the midbrain. This is an exception to the pattern of first order sensory neurons being in a ganglion outside the central nervous system. The fibres of the first order neurons enter the pons in the sensory and motor roots of the trigeminal nerve. In the brainstem they form the mesencephalic tract of the trigeminal (V) nerve. The destination of the central processes is poorly understood, but they are believed to have connections to the contralateral thalamus and to the cerebellum (see below, Unconscious proprioception).

● *If the semilunar ganglion is damaged all facial sensations on the same side will be lost.*

● *If one side of the sensory cortex is damaged, pressure and touch on the same side of the face will be unaffected. However, pain and temperature sensations will be lost on the contralateral side.*

Unconscious Proprioception

Receptors

The sensory receptors for unconscious proprioception are the muscle spindles of skeletal muscles and Golgi tendon organs in tendons.

The pathway from the trunk and limbs: the anterior and posterior spinocerebellar tracts and the cuneocerebellar tracts

The muscle spindles and Golgi tendon organs are innervated by the terminal branches of axons from the first order neurons in the dorsal root ganglia. Sensory information reaches the cerebellum through three pathways.

i) The Anterior (Ventral) Spinocerebellar Tract

This tract transmits unconscious proprioceptive information from the lower limbs and the lower part of the trunk. Axons of the first order neurons synapse with the second order neurons in the intermediate zone of the spinal grey matter. These cells also receive afferent fibres from the internuncial neurons of spinal reflexes. Second order neurons' processes ascend in the lateral funiculus of the spinal cord to the brainstem, where they enter the cerebellum via its superior peduncle and terminate in the vermis. Some fibres in this tract decussate in the spinal cord before ascending.

ii) The Posterior (Dorsal) Spinocerebellar Tract

Unconscious proprioception from the lower limb, trunk and upper limb is carried to the ipsilateral side of the cerebellar vermis. First order neurons enter the spinal cord and synapse with the second order neurons in Clarke's nucleus, which extends from segments C8 to L3 of the spinal grey matter. Second order neurons' axons from Clarke's nucleus ascend in the lateral funiculus of the spinal cord to the brainstem, then enter the cerebellum through the inferior peduncle. Some of these axons are the largest in the body.

iii) The Cuneocerebellar Tract

Axons of first order neurons innervating proprioceptors in the neck and upper limb ascend from segments above C8 in the spinal cord with the fasciculus cuneatus. The second order neurons lie in the nucleus cuneatus. Their axons enter the cerebellum via the inferior cerebellar peduncle, ipsilaterally.

A diagram of the pathways for fine touch and conscious proprioception. Fine touch from the lumbar and lower thoracic regions (red), the upper thoracic and cervical regions (orange) and the head (green). With the exception of the head, conscious proprioception is carried by the same pathways. Proprioception from the head (grey) both conscious and unconscious is also shown. Proprioceptive information from the head is carried only in the mandibular division of the trigeminal (V) nerve while touch receptors in the head contribute to all three divisions. For clarity, only one is drawn.

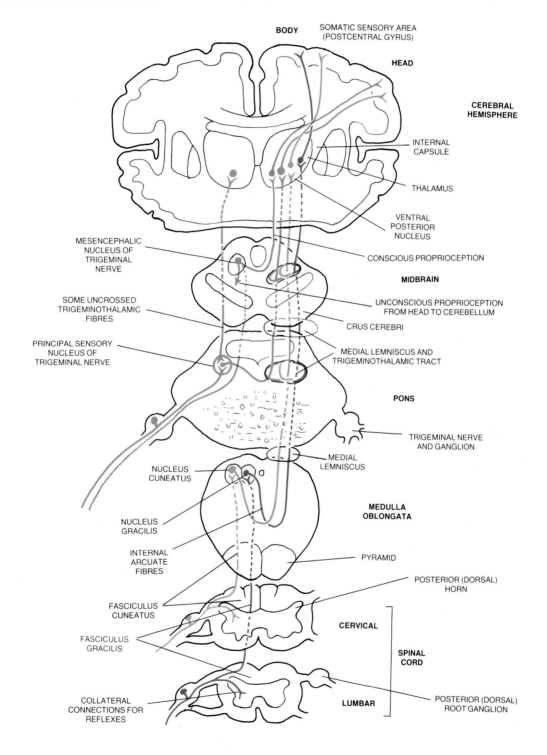

The pathway from the head

The pathway for unconscious proprioception from the head follows that for conscious proprioception (see above) to the mesencephalic tract of the trigeminal (V) nerve. Fibres then pass to the cerebellum.

A diagram to illustrate the pathways for unconscious proprioception. The anterior (ventral) in red, and posterior (dorsal) in green, spinocerebellar tracts for unconscious proprioception from the body. Each is shown on one side only for clarity. Note that because the anterior spinocerebellar tract decussates twice both tracts project to the ipsilateral side of the cerebellum.

Other sensory tracts

Several other ascending spinal pathways are recognized. These include the spinoreticular, spinocortical, spinopontine, spinovestibular and spino-olivary tracts.

● *The reader is referred to page **241** for further detail on the cerebellum and its connections and to pages **154-155** for detail of the sensory nuclei of the trigeminal nerve.*

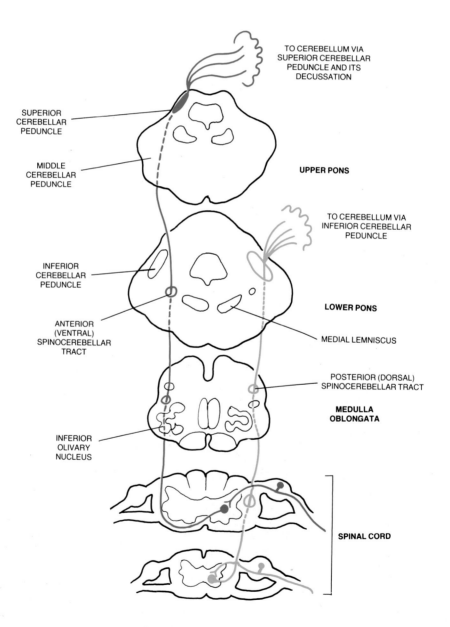

TO CEREBELLUM VIA SUPERIOR CEREBELLAR PEDUNCLE AND ITS DECUSSATION

SUPERIOR CEREBELLAR PEDUNCLE

MIDDLE CEREBELLAR PEDUNCLE

UPPER PONS

TO CEREBELLUM VIA INFERIOR CEREBELLAR PEDUNCLE

INFERIOR CEREBELLAR PEDUNCLE

LOWER PONS

ANTERIOR (VENTRAL) SPINOCEREBELLAR TRACT

MEDIAL LEMNISCUS

POSTERIOR (DORSAL) SPINOCEREBELLAR TRACT

MEDULLA OBLONGATA

INFERIOR OLIVARY NUCLEUS

SPINAL CORD

A-L A series of specimens to show the course of the ascending tracts from the spinal cord to the primary sensory cortex.

A A transverse section through the upper thoracic levels of the spinal cord to show the position of the ascending tracts. Myelin stain. x8.9

1 Central canal
2 Dorsal (posterior) horn of grey matter
3 Dorsal (posterior) spinocerebellar tract
4 Dorsolateral fasciculus (Lissauer's tract)
5 Dorsolateral sulcus
6 Fasciculus cuneatus
7 Fasciculus gracilis
8 Fasciculi proprii
9 Lateral horn of grey matter
10 Lateral spinothalamic tract
11 Ventral (anterior) horn of grey matter
12 Ventral (anterior) spinocerebellar tract
13 Ventral (anterior) spinothalamic tract

OXF

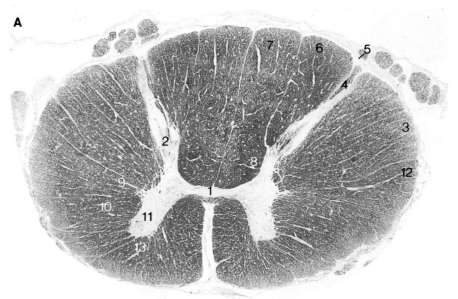

B A transverse section through the first cervical segment (C1) of the spinal cord to show the position of the ascending tracts. Weigert stain. x7.4

1 Arachnoid mater
2 Anterolateral system (spinothalamic and spinotectal tracts)
3 Dorsal (posterior) horn
4 Dorsal (posterior) spinocerebellar tract
5 Fasciculus cuneatus
6 Fasciculus gracilis
7 Spinal nucleus of trigeminal nerve
8 Spinal tract of trigeminal nerve
9 Ventral (anterior) horn
10 Ventral (anterior) spinocerebellar tract
11 Vertebral artery

191

C Transverse section through the caudal end of the medulla oblongata to show the internal arcuate fibres passing from the nucleus gracilis and nucleus cuneatus into the medial lemniscus. Weigert stain. x7.4

1 Anterolateral system (spinothalamic and spinotectal tract)
2 Dorsal (posterior) spinocerebellar tract
3 Fasciculus cuneatus
4 Fasciculus gracilis
5 Internal arcuate fibres
6 Medial lemniscus and its decussation
7 Nucleus cuneatus
8 Nucleus gracilis
9 Pyramid of medulla oblongata
10 Spinal nucleus of trigeminal nerve
11 Spinal tract of trigeminal nerve
12 Ventral (anterior) spinocerebellar tract

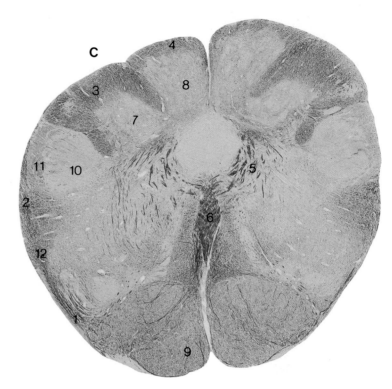

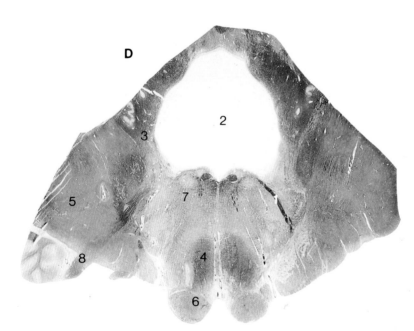

D Transverse section through the junction between the medulla oblongata and the pons to show the midline position and vertical orientation of the medial lemniscus. Weigert stain. x3

1 Facial nerve (VII)
2 Fourth ventricle
3 Inferior cerebellar peduncle
4 Medial lemniscus
5 Middle cerebellar peduncle
6 Pyramid of medulla oblongata
7 Reticular formation
8 Vestibulocochlear nerve (VIII)

MHMS

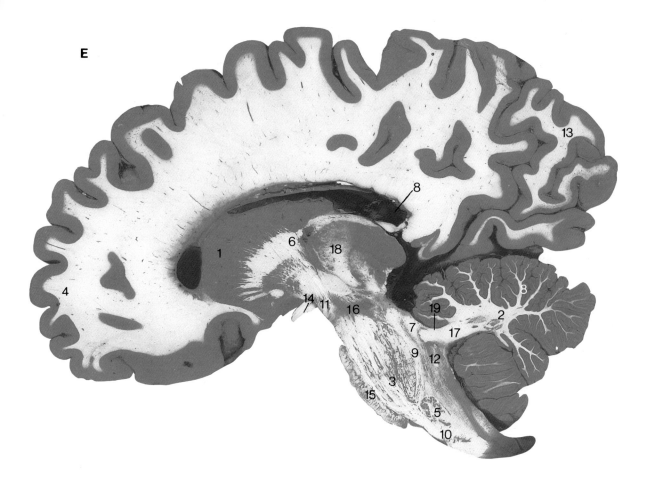

E A longitudinal thick slice through the brain to show the medial lemniscus ascending through the brainstem. Mulligan stain. x.96

1 Caudate nucleus
2 Cerebellum
3 Corticospinal tract
4 Frontal lobe
5 Inferior olivary nucleus
6 Internal capsule
7 Lateral lemniscus
8 Lateral ventricle
9 Medial lemniscus
10 Medulla oblongata
11 Midbrain
12 Motor, principal sensory and mesencephalic nuclei of trigeminal nerve
13 Occipital lobe
14 Optic chiasma
15 Pons
16 Substantia nigra
17 Superior cerebellar peduncle
18 Thalamus
19 Ventral (anterior) spinocerebellar tract

F A transverse section of pons at the level of the facial and abducens nerves to show the ascending tracts. Weigert stain. x2.81

1 Abducens nerve (VI)
2 Abducens nucleus
3 Anterolateral system (spinothalamic and spinotectal tracts)
4 Corticospinal tract
5 Facial nerve (VII)
6 Fourth ventricle
7 Medial lemniscus
8 Middle cerebellar peduncle
9 Reticular formation
10 Spinal tract and nucleus of trigeminal nerve
11 Transverse pontine fibres
12 Trigeminal nerve (V)
13 Ventral (anterior) spinocerebellar tract
14 Vestibular nuclei

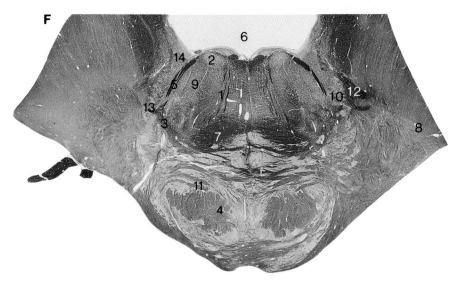

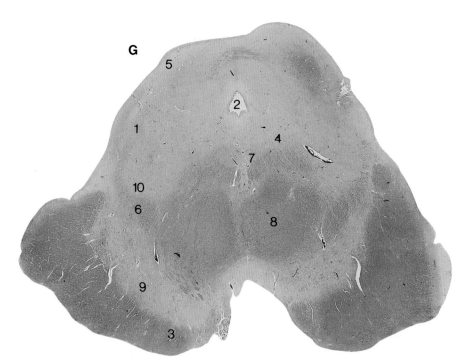

G A transverse section through the midbrain showing the medial lemniscus, anterolateral system and trigeminothalamic tracts. Myelin stain. x3.9

1 Anterolateral system (spinothalamic and spinotectal tracts)
2 Cerebral aqueduct
3 Crus cerebri
4 Dorsal trigeminothalamic tract
5 Inferior colliculus
6 Medial lemniscus
7 Oculomotor nucleus
8 Red nucleus
9 Substantia nigra
10 Ventral trigeminothalamic tract

H-J Sections to show the ventral posterior nuclei of the thalamus.

H A coronal section through one cerebral hemisphere, and half the diencephalon and brainstem to show the thalamus in relation to the internal capsule. Higher magnification at asterisk in L. Solochrome cyanin and nuclear fast red stain. x1

1	Caudate nucleus	**9**	Midbrain
2	Corpus callosum	**10**	Parietal lobe
3	Crus cerebri	**11**	Pons
4	Hippocampus	**12**	Primary sensory cortex
5	Insula	**13**	Red nucleus
6	Internal capsule	**14**	Substantia nigra
7	Lateral ventricle	**15**	Temporal lobe
8	Lentiform nucleus	**16**	Thalamus

I An enlargement of the thalamus from **H** to show the ventral posterolateral and ventral posteromedial nuclei. Solochrome cyanin and nuclear fast red stain. x1.6

1	Caudate nucleus	**10**	Red nucleus
2	Cerebral peduncle	**11**	Reticular nucleus of thalamus
3	Corpus callosum	**12**	Third ventricle
4	Dorsomedial nucleus of thalamus	**13**	Ventral posterolateral nucleus of thalamus
5	Fornix	**14**	Ventral posteromedial nucleus of thalamus
6	Hippocampus		
7	Insula		
8	Internal capsule		
9	Medial lemniscus, spinothalamic and trigeminothalamic tracts		

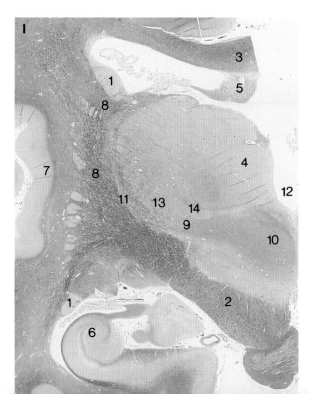

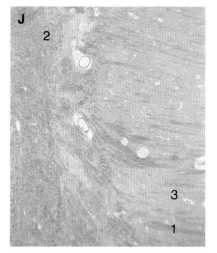

J An high magnification view of ascending tract fibres entering the ventral posterolateral nucleus. Solochrome cyanin and nuclear fast red stain. x14

1 Ascending tract fibres
2 Internal capsule
3 Ventral posterolateral nucleus

K-L The primary sensory cortex.

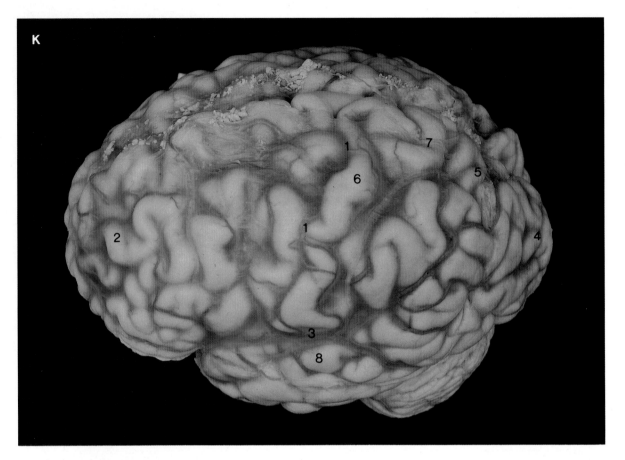

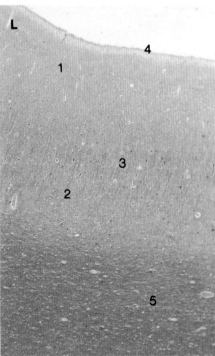

K A lateral view of the cerebral hemisphere to show the postcentral gyrus. x.85
1 Central sulcus
2 Frontal lobe
3 Lateral sulcus
4 Occipital lobe
5 Parietal lobe
6 Postcentral gyrus
7 Sensory association cortex
8 Temporal lobe

L An histological section of part of the postcentral gyrus from **H** (asterisk) showing the bands of Baillarger, caused by incoming afferent fibres from the thalamus. Solochrome cyanin and nuclear fast red stain. x27
1 Cortex
2 Inner band of Baillarger
3 Outer band of Baillarger
4 Pia mater
5 White matter

Special Senses

Vision

The visual pathways

Vision is a complex phenomenon involving not only the eye itself, but also the visual pathway connecting the eye to the cerebral cortex and associated pathways for visual reflexes. The retina develops as an outgrowth of the embryonic forebrain (diencephalon), and interacts with surrounding tissues, inducing them to form the other parts of the eye.

The cornea, lens and vitreous body are transparent and focus light onto the retina. The iris and ciliary body are muscular and pigmented. The choroid is a vascular nutritive layer and the sclera is a firm protective coat.

The retina contains the photoreceptive rods and cones and is the only component of the eye actually sensitive to light. Rods are more numerous than cones, peripherally situated, function best in dim light, and cannot resolve detail or perceive colour. Cones are more centrally situated, especially concentrated in the macula lutea. They function in bright light and give high acuity and colour vision.

Rods and cones contain visual pigments, which undergo chemical change when exposed to light. They are unique among sensory receptors in that their activity is inhibited, rather than increased, when they are stimulated. The response of rods and cones to light initiates the transmission of information through the visual pathway. Photoreceptors synapse with the retinal bipolar cells and these in turn synapse with the retinal ganglion cells. Horizontal and amacrine cells are retinal interneurons, found in the same layer as bipolar cells in the inner nuclear layer. They enable neighbouring bipolar or ganglion cells to interact.

Unmyelinated ganglion cell axons converge across the retinal surface to the optic disc. They then become myelinated as they leave the eye to form the optic nerve. Each optic nerve contains about one million fibres. It is not a true nerve but a drawn-out brain tract, hence its supporting cells are neuroglia (including oligodendrocytes) and not Schwann cells.

Left and right optic nerves meet at the optic chiasma. Fibres from the nasal side of each retina decussate into the contralateral optic tract, while fibres from the temporal side continue in the ipsilateral optic tract. About 90 per cent of optic tract fibres end by synapsing with neurons in the lateral geniculate body. The remaining 10 per cent enter the midbrain and pass both to the superior colliculus and pretectal area (see page **204**).

Cells in the lateral geniculate body are arranged in six layers. Each layer receives contralateral or ipsilateral optic tract fibres but not both. From the lateral geniculate body the visual pathway continues as the visual radiation or the geniculocalcarine tract. Visual pathway fibres entering the cortex form a band, the stria of Gennari. The fibres end in the striate cortex (Brodmann's area 17) which is the primary visual cortex located along the lips of the calcarine fissure in the occipital lobe.

Impulses from the macula lutea are received in the most posterior part of the depths and borders of the calcarine fissure. Neurons in the primary visual cortex are aligned in columns with alternate columns receiving pathways from left and right retinae. Visual information received in the primary visual cortex is further processed and interpreted in visual association cortex, also known as secondary and tertiary visual cortex. This surrounds the primary visual cortex. It forms Brodmann's areas 18 and 19 in the occipital lobe and cuneus.

At rest the two eyes face forwards so that their visual fields overlap giving binocular vision. They are moved in the orbits by six extraocular muscles, supplied by the oculomotor (III), trochlear (IV), and abducens (VI) nerves. In the frontal lobe there is a cortical centre for the control of eye movements.

- *The anterior part of the optic chiasma may be compressed by hypophyseal tumours, causing a visual field defect in the nasal side of each eye (bitemporal hemianopia).*

- *The central artery of the retina is an end artery. It supplies superficial layers of the retina, deeper layers being nourished by the choroidal vessels.*

- *Association tracts connect the visual association cortex to the angular gyrus of its own side; other fibres connect one angular gyrus to the one on the opposite side by passing through the corpus callosum. These connections are essential for reading.*

- *If a person views a visual stimulus, for example a pattern on a screen, electrical activity called the 'visual evoked potential' can be recorded by electrodes stuck to the scalp.*

- *Damage to the nuclei of the oculomotor (III), trochlear (IV) or abducens (VI) nerves, or to the nerves themselves, will paralyse the extraocular muscles and may cause double vision (diplopia) by disturbing the normal overlap of the visual fields.*

- *Retinohypothalamic fibres project via the optic nerves and chiasma to the suprachiasmatic nucleus of the hypothalamus. They are responsible for the effects of light in hypothalamic function, important in many mammals in regulating reproductive activity.*

A diagram to show the course of decussating and non-decussating fibres in the visual pathway, and collateral pathways to the superior colliculus.

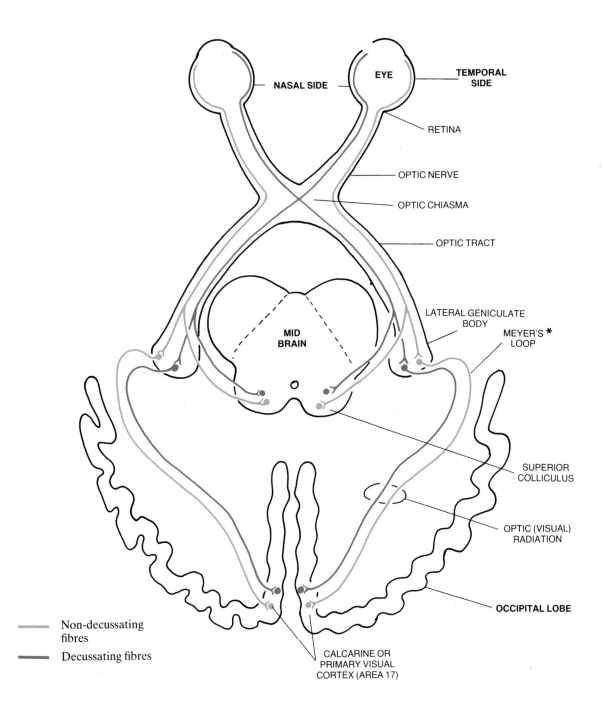

NASAL SIDE

EYE

TEMPORAL SIDE

RETINA

OPTIC NERVE

OPTIC CHIASMA

OPTIC TRACT

MID BRAIN

LATERAL GENICULATE BODY

MEYER'S * LOOP

SUPERIOR COLLICULUS

OPTIC (VISUAL) RADIATION

OCCIPITAL LOBE

CALCARINE OR PRIMARY VISUAL CORTEX (AREA 17)

——— Non-decussating fibres

——— Decussating fibres

Only fibres destined for the lower half of area 17 form Meyer's loop

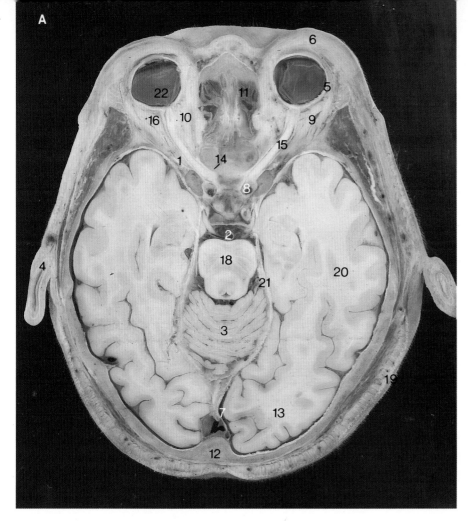

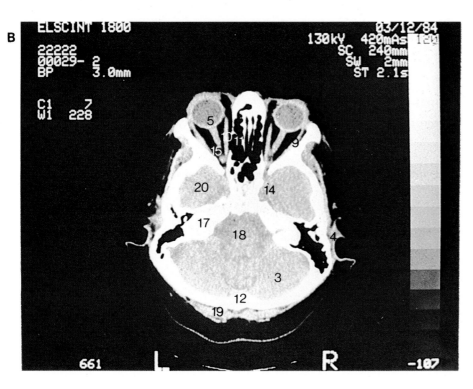

A-B Horizontal section through the head and CT scan image to show the eye *in situ*.

A UN x.75

1 Apex of orbit
2 Basilar artery
3 Cerebellum
4 Ear
5 Eye
6 Eyelid
7 Falx cerebri
8 Internal carotid artery
9 Lateral rectus muscle
10 Medial rectus muscle
11 Nasal cavity
12 Occipital bone
13 Occipital lobe
14 Optic canal
15 Optic nerve (II)
16 Orbital fat
17 Petrous temporal bone
18 Pons
19 Scalp
20 Temporal lobe
21 Tentorium cerebelli
22 Vitreous body

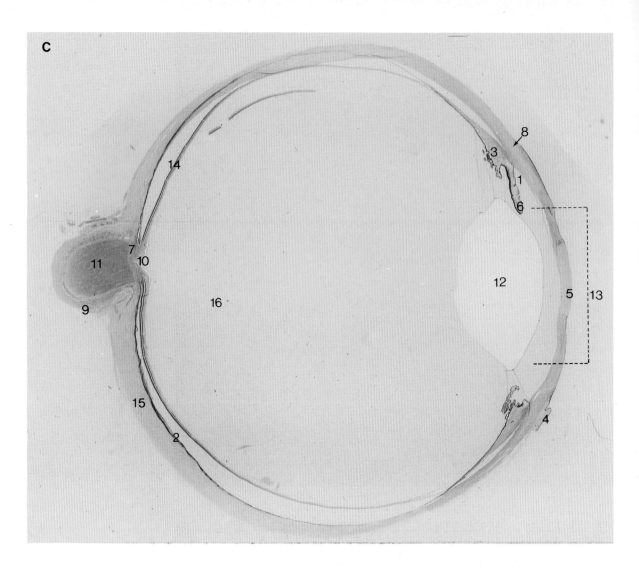

C A low power photomicrograph of an histological section through the whole eye to show its component parts. Celloidin section, haematoxylin and eosin stain. x5.8

1 Angle	**7** Lamina cribrosa	**13** Pupil
2 Choroid and pigment epithelium	**8** Limbus or corneoscleral junction	**14** Retina
3 Ciliary body	**9** Meningeal coverings of optic nerve	**15** Sclera
4 Conjunctiva	**10** Optic disc	**16** Vitreous body
5 Cornea	**11** Optic nerve (II)	
6 Iris	**12** Position of lens (lost in sectioning)	

Dr J. Southgate

● *This section is from the eye of a patient who had received a corneal graft.*

D-F Histological sections to show the structure of the retina.

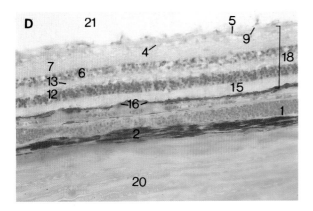

D Low power photomicrograph of a paraffin wax section through the choroid, sclera and retina, to show the retinal layers. Masson's trichrome stain. x111

OXF

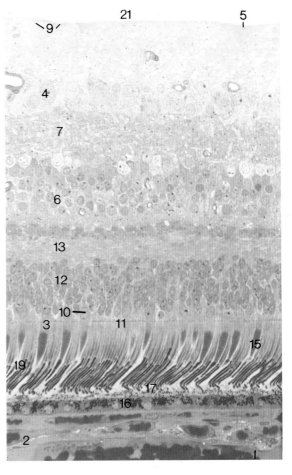

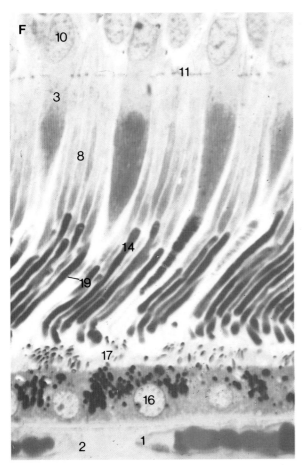

E Medium power photomicrograph of a plastic section through the retina of a 19-year-old. Toluidine blue stain. x478

Prof. J. Marshall

F High power photomicrograph of a plastic section through the retina to show details of the pigment epithelium and photoreceptors. Toluidine blue stain. x1915

1 Blood vessel	**12** Outer nuclear layer
2 Choroid	**13** Outer plexiform layer
3 Cone	**14** Outer segment
4 Ganglion cell layer	**15** Photoreceptor layer
5 Inner limiting membrane	**16** Pigment epithelium
6 Inner nuclear layer	**17** Processes of pigment
7 Inner plexiform layer	epithelial cells
8 Inner segment	**18** Retina
9 Nerve fibre layer	**19** Rod
10 Nucleus of	**20** Sclera
photoreceptor cell	**21** Vitreous body
11 Outer limiting	
'membrane'	

Prof. J. Marshall

- *The outer limiting 'membrane' is a line of deeply staining cell-to-cell adhesions. The inner limiting membrane is similar to a basement membrane.*

G-J Sections to demonstrate the structure of the optic nerve.

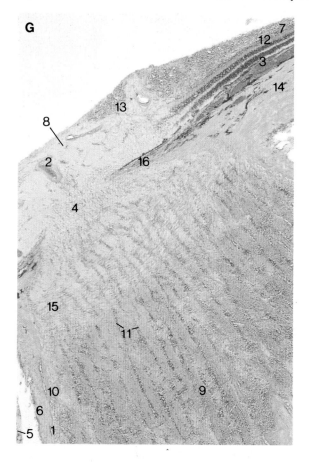

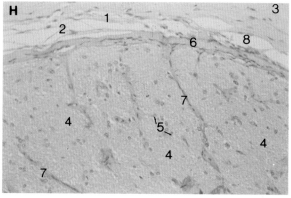

H A transverse section showing the meningeal coverings of the optic nerve. Haematoxylin and eosin stain. x56

1 Arachnoid mater
2 Arachnoid trabeculae
3 Dura mater
4 Nerve fibre bundles
5 Neuroglial nuclei
6 Pia mater
7 Pial septa
8 Subarachnoid space

OXF

G A low power photomicrograph showing the exit of the optic nerve from the eye. Masson's trichrome stain. x56

1 Arachnoid mater and subarachnoid space
2 Central retinal vessels
3 Choroid
4 Choroidal part of lamina cribrosa
5 Dura mater
6 Dural sheath of optic nerve
7 Nerve fibre layer of retina
8 Optic disc
9 Optic nerve (II)
10 Pia mater
11 Pial septa in optic nerve
12 Retina
13 Retinal part of optic nerve head
14 Sclera
15 Scleral part of lamina cribrosa
16 Spur of collagenous tissue between choroid and lamina cribrosa

OXF

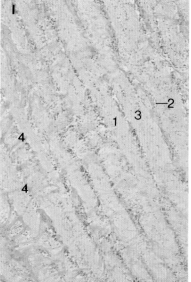

I A longitudinal section of optic nerve showing the distribution of neuroglial cells. Masson's trichrome stain. x81

1 Nerve fibre bundle
2 Neuroglial nuclei around fibre bundle
3 Neuroglial nuclei within fibre bundle
4 Pial septa

OXF

Individual nerve fibre bundles within the optic nerve are separated by pial septa and ensheathed by layers of glial cells. Glial cells also lie within the bundles, between the nerve fibres.

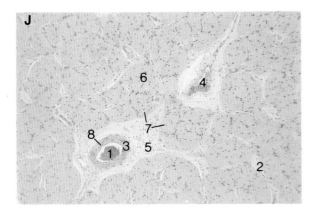

J Section showing the central retinal artery and vein inside the optic nerve. Haematoxylin and eosin stain. x175

1 Blood cells in vessel lumen
2 Capillary
3 Central retinal artery
4 Central retinal vein
5 Fibroblast nuclei
6 Neuroglial cell nuclei
7 Optic nerve fibre bundles
8 Smooth muscle of arterial wall

Dr J. Southgate

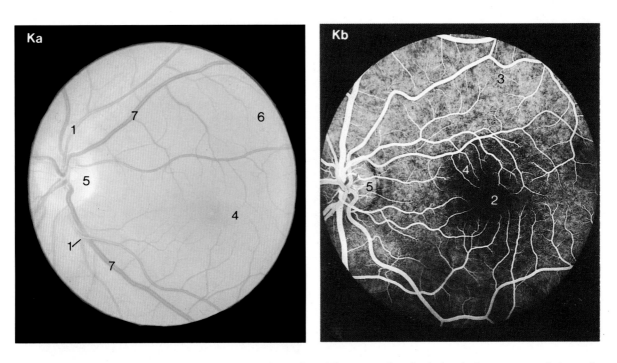

K Preparations to show the blood supply to the retina. The normal retinal circulation compared through an ophthalmoscope and in a fluorescein angiogram.

a Ophthalmoscope

b Fluorescein angiogram

1 Branches of central retinal artery
2 Capillary free zone
3 Choroidal fluorescence
4 Macular area

5 Optic disc
6 Retina
7 Tributaries of central retinal vein

Prof. A. Fielder and Mr H. Harris

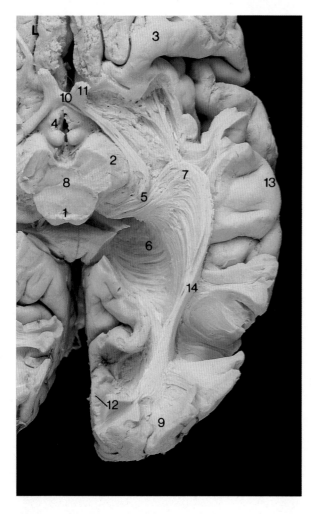

L-S Dissections and histological preparations to show the visual pathway.

L The brain dissected from below to show the pathway from the optic nerve to the occipital lobe. x1.08
1 Cerebral aqueduct (of Sylvius)
2 Cerebral peduncle
3 Frontal lobe
4 Hypothalamus
5 Lateral geniculate body
6 Lateral ventricle wall
7 Meyer's loop
8 Midbrain
9 Occipital lobe
10 Optic chiasma
11 Optic nerve
12 Primary visual or calcarine cortex
13 Temporal lobe
14 Visual radiation

● *Meyer's loop consists of visual radiation fibres looping anteriorly around the lateral ventricle in the temporal lobe.*

M A paraffin wax section of diencephalon and midbrain showing the optic chiasma. Weigert stain. x1.9
1 Cerebral aqueduct becoming third ventricle
2 Cerebral peduncle
3 Fornix
4 Hypothalamus
5 Lateral geniculate body
6 Medial geniculate body
7 Optic chiasma
8 Optic nerve
9 Optic tract
10 Pulvinar of thalamus
11 Red nucleus
12 Superior colliculus

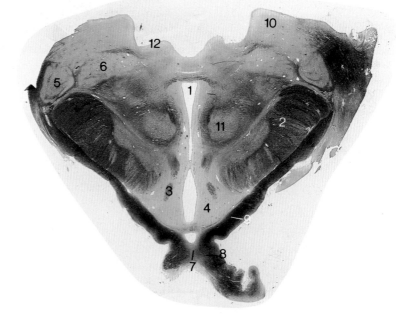

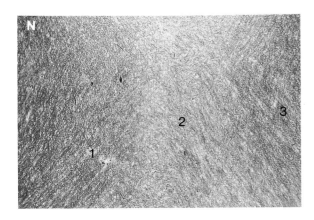

N An histological section to show decussating fibres in the optic chiasma. Weigert stain. x56
1 Blood vessel
2 Decussating fibres
3 Non-decussating fibres

O An histological section to show the structure of the lateral geniculate body. Weigert stain. x11
1 Cerebral peduncle
2 Hilum of lateral geniculate body
3 Lateral geniculate body
4 Medial geniculate body
5 Optic tract
6 Pulvinar
7 Retrolentiform part of internal capsule
8 Visual radiation
9 I-VI cellular layers of lateral geniculate body

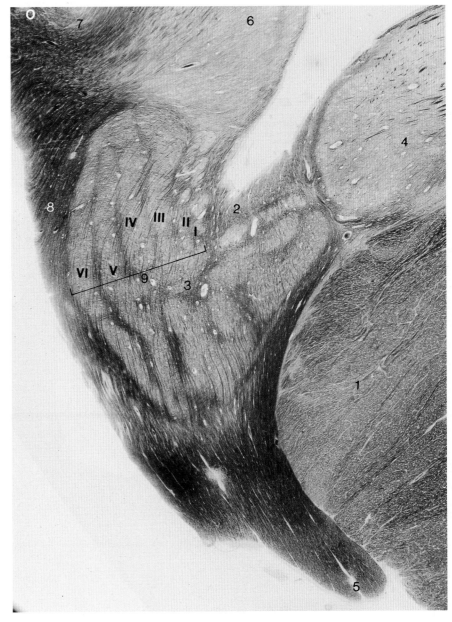

P-S Dissections and histological preparations to show the visual pathway between the lateral geniculate body and the primary visual cortex in the occipital lobe.

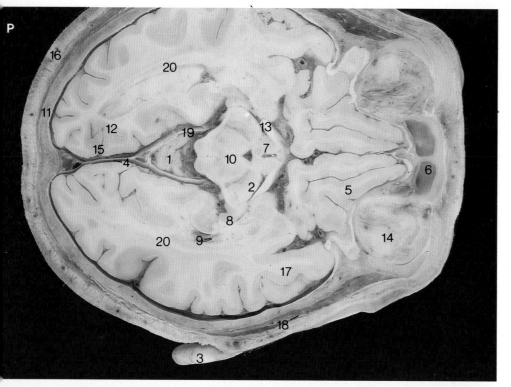

P An horizontal section through the head showing the visual radiation (optic radiation, geniculo-calcarine tract). x.75

1 Cerebellum
2 Cerebral peduncle
3 Ear
4 Falx cerebri
5 Frontal lobe
6 Frontal sinus
7 Hypothalamus
8 Lateral geniculate body
9 Lateral ventricle
10 Midbrain
11 Occipital bone
12 Occipital lobe
13 Optic tract
14 Orbit
15 Primary visual (calcarine) cortex
16 Scalp
17 Temporal lobe
18 Temporalis muscle
19 Tentorium cerebelli
20 Visual radiation

UN

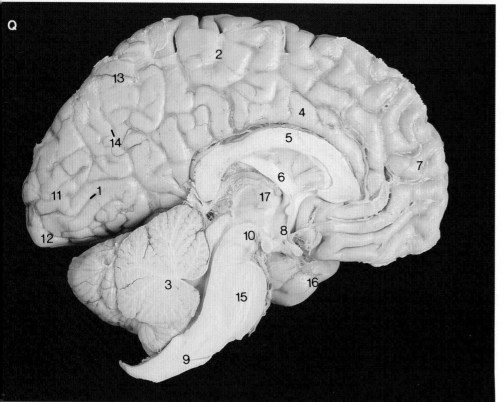

Q A sagittal section of the brain showing the calcarine sulcus and the primary visual cortex on the medial aspect of the occipital lobe. x.79

1 Calcarine sulcus
2 Central sulcus
3 Cerebellum
4 Cingulate gyrus
5 Corpus callosum
6 Fornix
7 Frontal lobe
8 Hypothalamus
9 Medulla oblongata
10 Midbrain
11 Occipital lobe
12 Occipital pole
13 Parietal lobe
14 Parieto-occipital sulcus
15 Pons
16 Temporal lobe
17 Thalamus

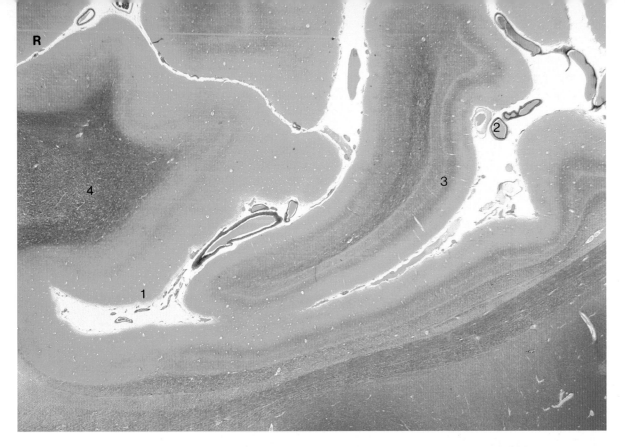

R Low power photomicrograph of part of an horizontal section through the primary visual cortex to show cortex, white matter and posterior cerebral vessels. Solochrome cyanin and light green stain. x5.6

1 Cortex
2 Posterior cerebral vessels
3 Stria of Gennari
4 White matter

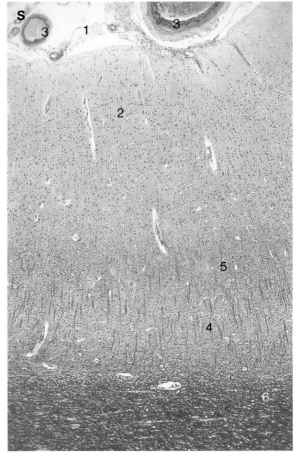

S An histological section through the full thickness of the primary visual cortex to show the stria of Gennari. Myelin stain. x34

1 Arachnoid mater
2 Cortex
3 Posterior cerebral vessels
4 Projection fibres from visual radiation
5 Stria of Gennari
6 White matter

CAM

● *Franceso Gennari (1750-1796?) discovered and described the stria named after him while still a medical student in Italy.*

Structures Associated with the Visual Pathway

At the rostral end of the midbrain lie two important visual structures, the superior colliculus and the pretectal area. Both receive fibres from the optic tract which do not pass to the lateral geniculate body i.e. about 10 per cent of the fibres of the optic tract.

The superior colliculus has evolved from the optic lobe, which is a part of the midbrain, and in lower vertebrates is the highest visual centre. This is reflected in its varied connections to other parts of the brain including the cerebral cortex and other sensory systems. It has a cortex composed of several layers of cells. It controls visual reflexes, such as the coordinated movements of the eyes in tracking moving objects or in scanning a static scene.

The pretectal area, including the pretectal nucleus, is an extensive, complex region with many nuclei in front of the superior colliculus. One of these, the olivary pretectal nucleus, controls the light reflex, adjusting pupil size to environmental light levels. At least three pretectal nuclei receive some input from the eyes.

A-E Dissections and histological preparations to show the superior colliculus and pretectal area.

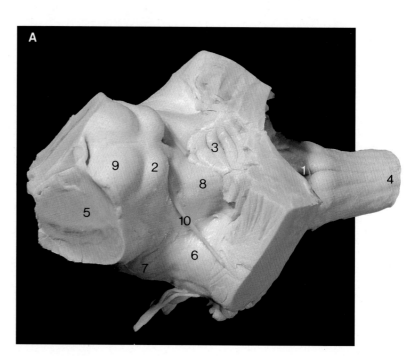

A The brainstem viewed from the dorsal surface to show the superior and inferior colliculi. x1.5
1 Fourth ventricle
2 Inferior colliculus
3 Lingula of cerebellum
4 Medulla oblongata
5 Midbrain
6 Middle cerebellar peduncle
7 Pons
8 Superior cerebellar peduncle
9 Superior colliculus
10 Trochlear nerve (IV)

B Sagittal histological section of brainstem showing the superior and inferior colliculi and the pretectal area. Solochrome cyanin and nuclear fast red stain. x2.1
1 Brachium of superior colliculus
2 Cerebral aqueduct
3 Corticospinal fibres
4 Crus cerebri
5 Fourth ventricle
6 Inferior colliculus
7 Inferior olivary nucleus
8 Medulla oblongata
9 Midbrain
10 Pons
11 Posterior column nuclei
12 Pretectal area
13 Superior cerebellar peduncle
14 Superior colliculus
15 Superior medullary velum
16 Tegmentum
17 Trigeminal nerve fibres (V)

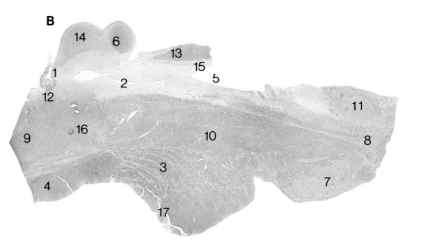

C A coronal section through the tectum of the midbrain showing the superior colliculus. Weigert stain. x5.8

1 Brachium of inferior colliculus
2 Central grey matter
3 Cerebral aqueduct
4 Commissure of superior colliculus
5 Medial lemniscus
6 Oculomotor nerve fibres
7 Oculomotor nucleus
8 Reticular formation
9 Spinothalamic tract
10 Superior colliculus
11 Strata of superior colliculus

● *As well as visual input into its superficial layer, the superior colliculus receives auditory and somatosensory connections into its deep strata. It gives rise to the tectospinal tract, an extrapyramidal motor pathway (see page 234). It is a sensory/motor integrating centre, particularly in relation to orientating stimuli.*

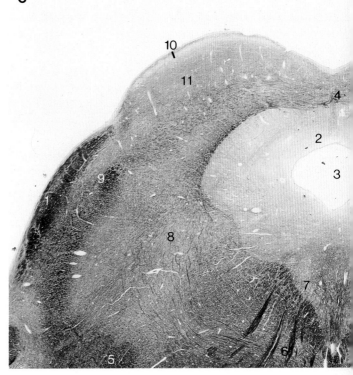

D A coronal section through part of the transition between midbrain and diencephalon showing the position and relationships of the pretectal area. Myelin stain and counterstain. x2.8

1 Central grey matter
2 Cerebral aqueduct/third ventricle transition
3 Crus cerebri
4 Fornix
5 Habenular commissure
6 Habenulopeduncular tract
7 Hypothalamus
8 Lateral geniculate body
9 Mamillothalamic tract
10 Medial geniculate body
11 Optic radiation
12 Optic tract
13 Pineal organ
14 Posterior commissure
15 Pretectal area including pretectal nucleus
16 Pulvinar of thalamus

MHMS

● *Efferent fibres from the olivary pretectal nucleus pass to the parasympathetic (Edinger-Westphal) part of the oculomotor nucleus which supplies the pupillary sphincter muscles.*

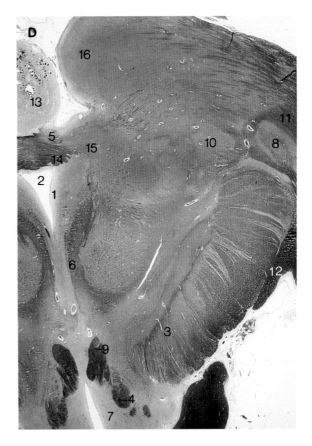

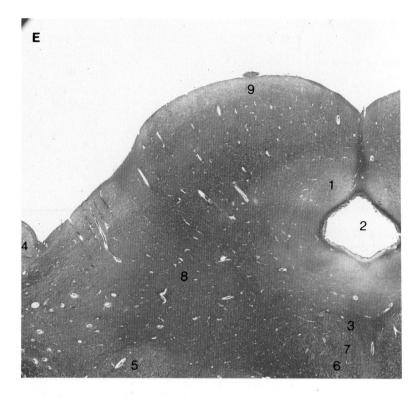

E Low power photomicrograph of part of an histological section of midbrain at the level of the superior colliculus, to show the Edinger-Westphal nucleus. Luxol fast blue and fuchsin stain. x7.6

1 Central grey matter
2 Cerebral aqueduct
3 Edinger-Westphal nucleus
4 Medial geniculate body
5 Medial lemniscus
6 Medial longitudinal fasciculus
7 Oculomotor nucleus
8 Reticular formation
9 Superior colliculus

A diagram to show the nervous connections of the pupillary light reflex.

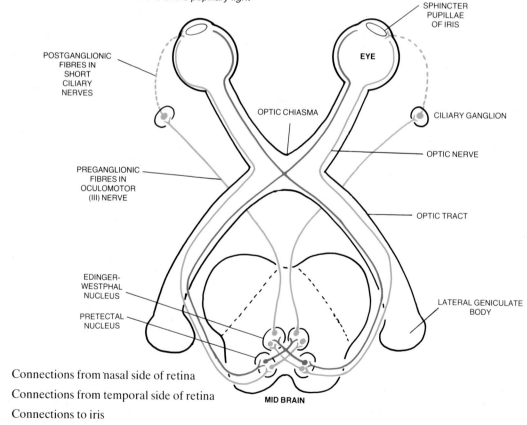

POSTGANGLIONIC FIBRES IN SHORT CILIARY NERVES

SPHINCTER PUPILLAE OF IRIS

EYE

OPTIC CHIASMA

CILIARY GANGLION

OPTIC NERVE

PREGANGLIONIC FIBRES IN OCULOMOTOR (III) NERVE

OPTIC TRACT

EDINGER-WESTPHAL NUCLEUS

PRETECTAL NUCLEUS

LATERAL GENICULATE BODY

MID BRAIN

—— Connections from nasal side of retina
—— Connections from temporal side of retina
—— Connections to iris

Hearing

The auditory (VIII) nerve transmits information to the brain from the auditory and vestibular apparatus of the inner ear; each apparatus is supplied with its own division of the nerve. The auditory pathway will be dealt with in this section and the vestibular in the next.

The auditory pathway is initiated when hair cells in the cochlea (inner ear) are stimulated by sound transmitted as vibrations by the external and middle ear.

The hair cells are innervated by bipolar primary sensory neurons whose cell bodies are located in the spiral ganglion in the cochlea. The central processes of these cells run in the cochlear division of the vestibulocochlear (VIII) nerve to the pontomedullary junction. On entering the brainstem they separate into two divisions, some passing to the dorsal cochlear nucleus and some to the ventral cochlear nucleus. From the cochlear nuclei the auditory pathway becomes diverse and sensory information is carried by a variety of routes to the primary auditory cortex in the temporal lobe (Brodmann's areas 41 and 42). It is important to note that each auditory cortex will receive fibres from the left and right cochlear nuclei. This means that if one auditory cortex is damaged, hearing will still occur from both ears.

The dorsal and ventral cochlear nuclei are connected to the inferior colliculus by the lateral lemniscus. Some axons from the cochlear nuclei ascend in the lateral lemniscus on their own side whilst others decussate in the trapezoid body and ascend in the contralateral lateral lemniscus. Other axons have an additional synapse in the superior olivary nucleus before entering the lateral lemniscus either with or without decussating. To mediate auditory reflexes internuncial (messenger) neurons connect the nucleus of the inferior colliculus to various motor centres. For example, when startled by a loud noise, the eyes close and the body jumps in response.

The nuclei of the inferior colliculi are also connected to one another by commissural fibres.

From the nucleus of the inferior colliculus, fibres pass via the brachium of the inferior colliculus to the medial geniculate body where they synapse with neurons. The axons of these neurons form the auditory radiations which end in the cortex of the superior temporal gyrus. This is known as the primary auditory cortex (Brodmann's areas 41 and 42).

The olivocochlear bundle is an efferent component of the auditory pathway. It runs from the superior olivary nucleus to the cochlea. It improves the perception of low intensity sounds by influencing hair cell sensitivity.

• *In conduction (middle ear) deafness a vibrating tuning fork can only be partly heard (or not at all) unless placed on the patient's skull, bypassing the middle ear.*

• *In sensorineural deafness a vibrating tuning fork can only be partly heard (or not at all) when placed on the skull.*

• *Cochlear atrophy is one of the most common causes of deafness in the elderly.*

• *One cause of congenital deafness is maternal infection with rubella.*

• *Large doses of antibiotics (neomycin and streptomycin) may cause deafness and vestibular disturbances.*

• *The posterior part of the insula is connected to the primary auditory cortex.*

A diagram to show how the auditory cortex on each side receives ipsilateral and contralateral auditory pathways, so receiving information from both ears. (For clarity additional synapses that may occur in the trapezoid body and lateral lemniscus have not been drawn, nor have the efferent pathways.)

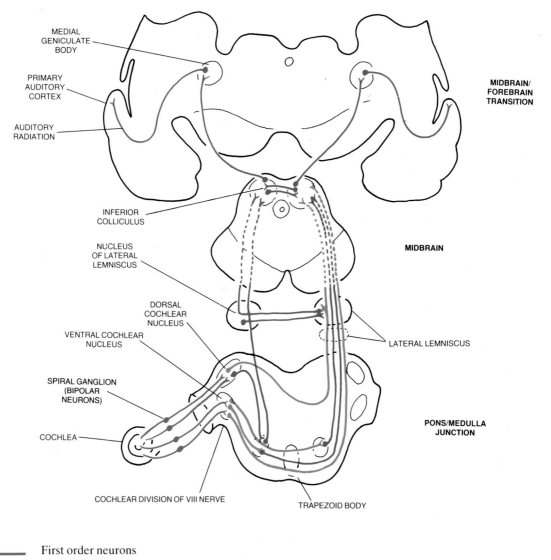

MEDIAL
GENICULATE
BODY

PRIMARY
AUDITORY
CORTEX

AUDITORY
RADIATION

MIDBRAIN/
FOREBRAIN
TRANSITION

INFERIOR
COLLICULUS

MIDBRAIN

NUCLEUS
OF LATERAL
LEMNISCUS

DORSAL
COCHLEAR
NUCLEUS

VENTRAL COCHLEAR
NUCLEUS

LATERAL LEMNISCUS

SPIRAL GANGLION
(BIPOLAR
NEURONS)

COCHLEA

PONS/MEDULLA
JUNCTION

COCHLEAR DIVISION OF VIII NERVE

TRAPEZOID BODY

⎯⎯ First order neurons

⎯⎯ Second order neurons

⎯⎯ Fibres arising after synaptic relay

A A CAT scan image to show the position of the petrous temporal bone.

1 Brainstem
2 Cerebellum
3 Fourth ventricle
4 Hypophyseal fossa
5 Nose
6 Occipital bone
7 Orbit
8 Petrous temporal bone
9 Posterior clinoid process
10 Sphenoidal sinus
11 Temporal lobe

Dr N. Messios

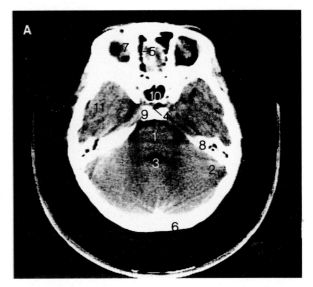

B A model of the ear viewed from above.
x.28

1 Auditory (Eustachian) tube
2 Auricle (pinna) ⎫
3 External auditory meatus ⎬ External ear
4 Cochlea
5 Incus
6 Inner ear
7 Internal carotid artery
8 Malleus
9 Middle ear
10 Semicircular canals
11 Skin
12 Statoacoustic (vestibulocochlear, VIII) nerve
13 Temporal bone (petrous part)
14 Temporal bone (squamous part)
15 Tympanic membrane

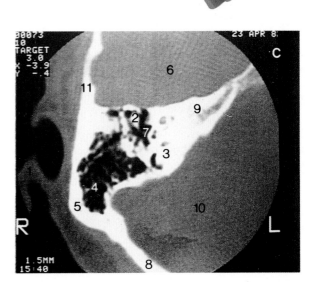

C An high bone definition CAT scan image of the temporal bone to demonstrate the middle ear cavity.

1 External ear
2 Head of malleus
3 Inner ear
4 Mastoid air cells
5 Mastoid process
6 Middle cranial fossa
7 Middle ear cavity
8 Occipital bone
9 Petrous temporal bone
10 Posterior cranial fossa
11 Squamous part of temporal bone

Dr N. Messios

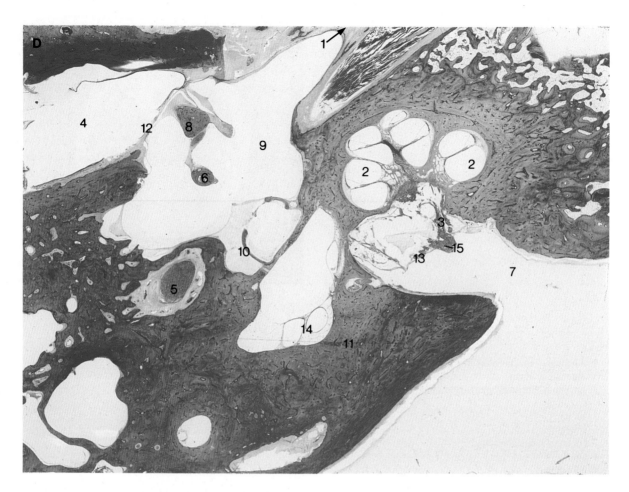

D An horizontal section through the temporal
bone to show the external, middle and inner ear.
Haematoxylin and eosin stain. x5.9

 1 Auditory (Eustachian) tube (direction, arrow)
 2 Cochlea
 3 Cochlear nerve
 4 External auditory meatus
 5 Facial nerve
 6 Incus
 7 Internal auditory meatus
 8 Malleus
 9 Middle ear
10 Stapes
11 Temporal bone
12 Tympanic membrane
13 Vestibular nerve
14 Vestibule
15 Vestibulocochlear nerve (VIII)

Mr N. Badham

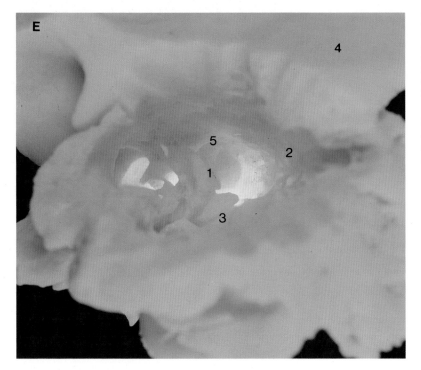

E The temporal bone dissected open to illustrate the orientation of the semicircular canals. The lateral wall of the temporal bone has been removed as well as the middle ear. x2.3

1 Lateral semicircular canal
2 Petrous temporal bone
3 Posterior semicircular canal
4 Squamous temporal bone
5 Superior semicircular canal

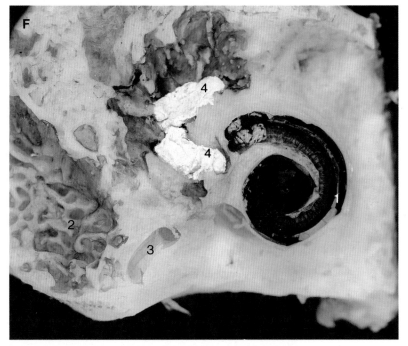

F The petrous temporal bone dissected to demonstrate the spiral form of the cochlea in the inner ear. The bony cochlea has been opened and the membranous cochlear duct stained with osmium tetroxide. x4.3

1 Cochlear duct
2 Cancellous bone
3 Semicircular canal
4 Supporting material

Dr M. Ingle Wright

G-K Histological preparations of the inner ear.

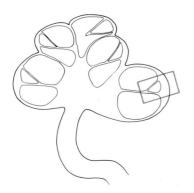

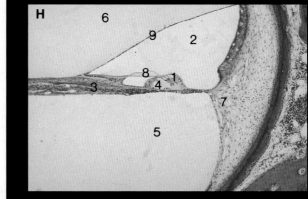

G A section and accompanying diagram through the cochlea and cochlear nerve. Haematoxylin and eosin stain. x7.1
1 Basilar membrane
2 Cochlea
3 Cochlear nerve (VIII)
4 Temporal bone
5 Vestibule

Dr M. Ingle Wright

H A radial section through one turn of the fetal cochlea showing the cochlear duct, organ of Corti, and tectorial membrane. An higher magnification as outlined in the diagram of **G**. Haematoxylin and eosin stain. x69
1 Cells of Hensen
2 Cochlear duct
3 Cochlear nerve (VIII)
4 Organ of Corti
5 Scala tympani
6 Scala vestibuli
7 Spiral ligament
8 Tectorial membrane
9 Vestibular membrane

Mr N. Badham

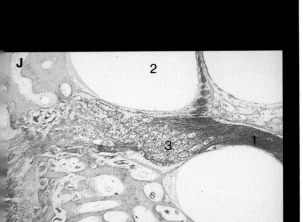

I An higher magnification of the Organ of Corti. x278

1 Basilar membrane	**7** Internal spiral sulcus
2 Border cells	**8** Outer hair cells
3 Cells of Hensen	**9** Pillar cells
4 Cochlear duct	**10** Scala tympani
5 Cochlear nerve	**11** Tectorial membrane
6 Inner hair cell	**12** Tunnel

Mr N. Badham

J The adult spiral ganglion and auditory (VIII) nerve. Haematoxylin and eosin stain. x69

1 Auditory nerve (VIII)
2 Cochlea
3 Spiral ganglion

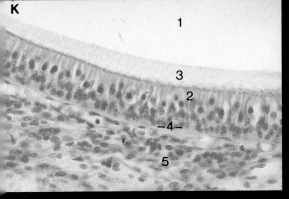

K An histological section through the macula of the fetal vestibule. Haematoxylin and eosin stain. x223

1 Endolymph in lumen
2 Hair cells
3 Otolithic membrane
4 Supporting cells
5 Wall of the vestibule

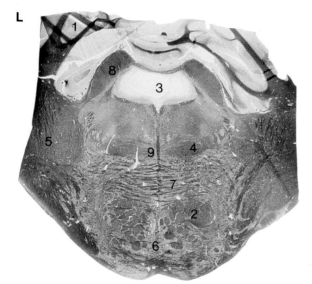

L The trapezoid body in the pons. Weigert stain. x2.3
1 Cerebellum
2 Corticospinal tract
3 Fourth ventricle
4 Medial lemniscus
5 Middle cerebellar peduncle
6 Pons
7 Pontine nuclei
8 Superior cerebellar peduncle
9 Trapezoid body

M A transverse section of the mid-medulla oblongata to demonstrate the cochlear nuclei and the medial and inferior vestibular nuclei. Weigert stain. x3.3
1 Dorsal cochlear nucleus
2 Fourth ventricle
3 Inferior cerebellar peduncle
4 Inferior olivary nucleus
5 Inferior vestibular nucleus and vestibulospinal tract
6 Medial lemniscus
7 Medial longitudinal fasciculus
8 Medial vestibular nucleus
9 Pyramid
10 Ventral cochlear nucleus

N A transverse section of the pons to show the position of the superior olivary nucleus and superior and lateral vestibular nuclei and their relations. Weigert stain. x3.4
1 Abducens nerve (VI)
2 Abducens nucleus
3 Central tegmental tract
4 Cerebellum
5 Corticospinal tract
6 Facial nerve (VII)
7 Facial nucleus
8 Fourth ventricle
9 Medial lemniscus
10 Middle cerebellar peduncle
11 Pons
12 Spinal tract and nucleus of V
13 Superior olivary nucleus
14 Superior and lateral vestibular nuclei

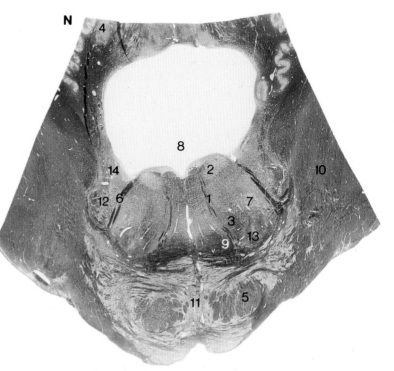

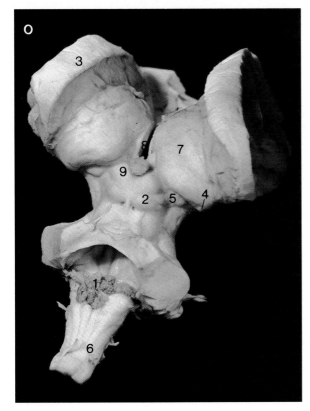

O A dissection of the brainstem and diencephalon to show inferior colliculus and medial geniculate body. Dorsal surface view. x.98
1 Choroid plexus of fourth ventricle
2 Inferior colliculus
3 Internal capsule
4 Lateral geniculate body
5 Medial geniculate body
6 Medulla oblongata
7 Thalamus
8 Third ventricle
9 Superior colliculus

P A transverse thick slice through the upper third of the pons to show the lateral lemniscus and inferior colliculus. Mulligan stain. x1.1
 1 Cerebellum
 2 Corticospinal tract
 3 Fourth ventricle
 4 Inferior colliculus
 5 Lateral lemniscus
 6 Lateral ventricle
 7 Medial lemniscus
 8 Medial longitudinal fasciculus
 9 Middle cerebellar peduncle
10 Parietal lobe
11 Reticular formation
12 Superior cerebellar peduncle
13 Transverse pontine fibres

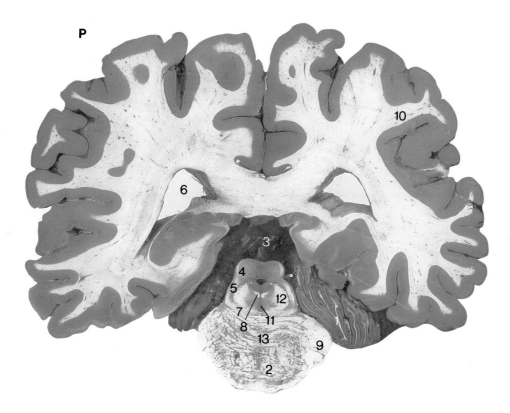

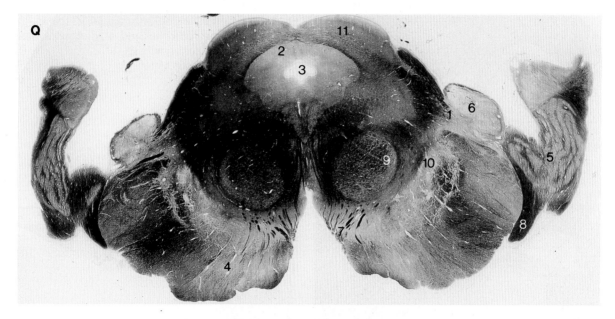

Q A transverse section through the rostral end of the midbrain to show the medial geniculate body and the brachium of the inferior colliculus. Weigert stain. x3

 1 Brachium of inferior colliculus
 2 Central grey matter
 3 Cerebral aqueduct
 4 Crus cerebri
 5 Lateral geniculate body
 6 Medial geniculate body
 7 Oculomotor nerve (III)
 8 Optic tract
 9 Red nucleus
 10 Substantia nigra
 11 Superior colliculus

R An higher magnification view of a portion of an adjacent section to **Q** showing the medial geniculate body. Weigert stain. x12.6

 1 Cerebral peduncle
 2 Lateral geniculate body
 3 Medial geniculate body
 4 Midbrain
 5 Substantia nigra
 6 Thalamus

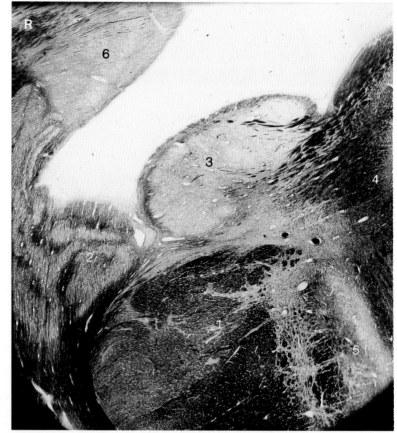

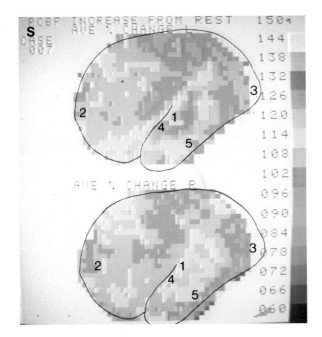

S The regional cerebral bloodflow of the auditory
cortex during listening as shown by the Xenon-133
intracarotid technique. Highly active areas with an
increased blood flow are shown in red.
1 Brodmann's areas 41 and 42
2 Frontal lobe
3 Occipital lobe
4 Superior gyrus of the temporal lobe
5 Temporal lobe

Dr N. Lassen

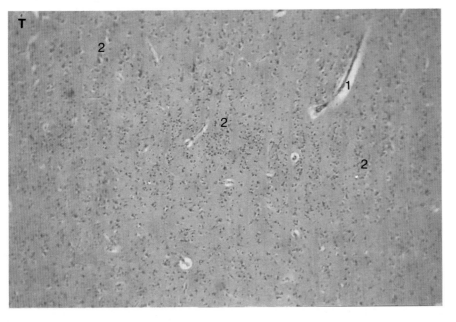

T The auditory cortex
of the temporal lobe to
illustrate the parallel
columns of cells. Haem-
atoxylin and eosin stain.
x108
1 Blood vessel
2 Columns of neurons

Equilibrium

The three receptor organs for equilibrium are found in the inner ear. These fluid-filled organs are located in all three spatial planes and are called the utricle, saccule, and the semicircular canals. Projecting into the fluid (endolymph) are hair cells which are sensitive to the movements of the endolymph.

From the inner ear the stimulus is transmitted to the vestibular bipolar ganglion situated in the internal acoustic meatus where the primary neuron cell bodies are aggregated. Their axons enter the brainstem at the pontomedullary junction and terminate in four vestibular nuclei in the area acoustica of the floor of the fourth ventricle. These nuclei have five major connections: vestibulocerebellar, vestibulospinal, vestibulo-ocular, vestibulocortical, and accessory.

Vestibulocerebellar connections

This is a cerebellar-vestibular feedback mechanism. The axons from the vestibular ganglion terminate in the superior and lateral vestibular nuclei. Second order neurons pass via the inferior peduncle to the flocculonodular lobe of the archi-cerebellum. Some first order neurons pass directly to this area.

The feedback stimulus travels to the fastigial nucleus and inferior peduncle, and hence to the vestibular nuclei of both sides.

Vestibulospinal tracts

Secondary neurons from the lateral vestibular nucleus descend ipsilaterally as the lateral vestibulospinal tract and synapse on lower motor neurons. These discharge reflexively to maintain equilibrium.

Secondary neurons from the superior, medial and inferior vestibular nuclei, both crossed and uncrossed descend as the medial vestibulospinal tracts to synapse on lower motor neurons. These neurons discharge reflexively to maintain equilibrium.

Vestibulo-ocular tracts

Besides maintaining the body equilibrium the vestibular system also plays a role in regulating eyeball movements. This tract functions when one's eyes are 'fixed' on an object and the head turns. Just before the medial vestibulospinal tract descends it branches and some axons ascend as the medial longitudinal fasciculus in the pons and midbrain where they synapse in the nuclei associated with eyeball movements (oculomotor III, trochlear IV, and abducens VI). The vestibular system is also connected to motor neuron pools responsible for head and neck movements.

Vestibulocortical connections

It is presumed that there are vestibular connections to the thalamus and cerebral cortex for consciousness. However, no morphological connections have yet been demonstrated.

Accessory pathway

In addition to the feedback mechanism of the vestibulocerebellar connections, there is another pathway. The fastigial nucleus is connected to the descending reticular areas and nuclei of the brainstem. These discharge via the multisynaptic reticulospinal tract to the lower motor neurons.

● *Nystagmus (the abnormal and constant movement of the eyes) and dizziness are common symptoms of vestibular injury.*

● *Lesions of the vestibular system often result in disturbances in walking and equilibrium.*

Diagram to show the vestibulocerebellar connections of the vestibular pathway. They are shown on one side only for clarity.

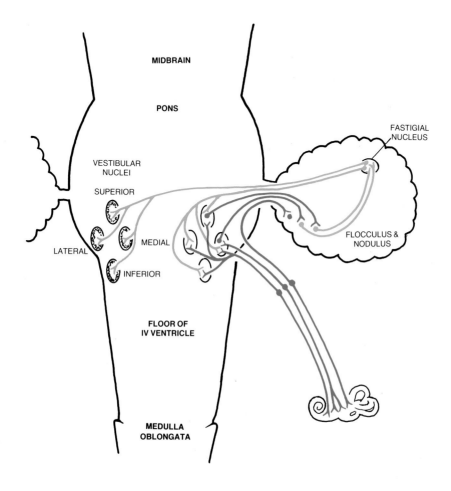

MIDBRAIN

PONS

FASTIGIAL
NUCLEUS

VESTIBULAR
NUCLEI

SUPERIOR

LATERAL

MEDIAL

INFERIOR

FLOCCULUS &
NODULUS

FLOOR OF
IV VENTRICLE

MEDULLA
OBLONGATA

— Primary stimulus
— Feedback

Smell

Smell can trigger various responses, both emotional and reflex (for example, the smell of bread baking evokes pleasure and induces salivation). Smell as well as taste plays a major role in our perception of substances in the mouth.

The yellowish-brown olfactory epithelium is located in the upper nasal cavity. Within the epithelium are bipolar olfactory receptor neurons which have apical microvilli. Receptor molecules on the microvilli bind specific odoriferent ('smell bearing') molecules. In the process, the cells are stimulated. The axons of these first-order unmyelinated bipolar neurons collect together into approximately 20 nerve bundles and pass up through the cribriform plate of the ethmoid bone into the olfactory bulb where they synapse with second-order neurons. The second-order axons form the olfactory tract. The tract passes posteriorly and upon reaching the anterior perforated substance of the frontal lobe bifurcates to form the medial and lateral olfactory tracts or striae.

The axons of the medial olfactory stria terminate in two ways: in the anterior perforated substance and paraolfactory (septal) area; or some enter the anterior commissure and cross to the contralateral septal area.

The axons of the lateral olfactory stria terminate in the uncus (prepiriform area) of temporal lobe cortex. This is not numbered as one of Brodmann's areas because it comprises the three-layered allocortex, not six-layered neocortex, with which Brodmann's study was concerned. Olfactory tract fibres also end in the amygdaloid nucleus (periamygdaloid area). Neuronal connections from the primary olfactory cortex pass to the secondary olfactory cortex (entorhinal area of the parahippocampal gyrus: Brodmann's area 28), lateral preoptic area, amygdaloid nucleus, and medial forebrain bundle. These cortical areas are responsible for the interpretation of smell.

Olfactory areas of the cerebral cortex have extensive connections with the hypothalamus. These, and also a pathway involving the habenular nuclei, form the basis for reflex visceral responses to olfactory stimuli controlled by the autonomic nervous system, for example salivating at the smell of food, vomiting in response to unpleasant odours.

Between the stimulus (the odour) and the response (increased visceral activity) the pathways are anatomically complex, often involving many synaptic relays, and are not always well understood. The major and best described ones are listed below and illustrated in the diagrams (see pages **225** and **228**).

1 From the amygdaloid nucleus to the hippocampus, then via the fornix to the hypothalamus.

2 From the amygdaloid nucleus to the hypothalamus by a connecting tract, the stria terminalis.

3 From the septal area to the hypothalamus. The hypothalamus itself is not directly linked to viscera. It is connected by reflex-discharge pathways to the reticular formation and visceral motor cranial nerve nuclei in the brainstem through which viscera are innervated. The most important of these tracts are the mamillotegmental tract and the dorsal longitudinal fasciculus.

The emotional reaction to many olfactory stimuli is evidence of links between the olfactory pathways and the limbic system (see page **258**).

The septal area is connected to the cingulate gyrus through the cingulum, and to the hippocampus and the entorhinal area (Brodmann's area 28) is also linked to the hippocampus. Indirectly the olfactory system is also connected to the cingulate gyrus by a complex pathway from the hypothalamus, mamillothalamic tract, and anterior thalamic nuclei.

- *There are seven primary odours (musky, floral, peppermint, pungent, putrid, camphor, ether-like) which combine to produce all other known odours.*

- *Anosmia is the loss of smell due to damage to the receptor cells, olfactory bulb or tract.*

- *Temporal lobe lesions in the area of the amygdala and uncus often produce olfactory hallucinations.*

- *The insula is believed to be connected to the lateral olfactory gyrus.*

- *For illustrations of the hypothalmus, autonomic nuclei in the brainstem and the limbic system, see pages **126-128, 160** and **258**.*

Diagram of the olfactory projection to the cerebral cortex.

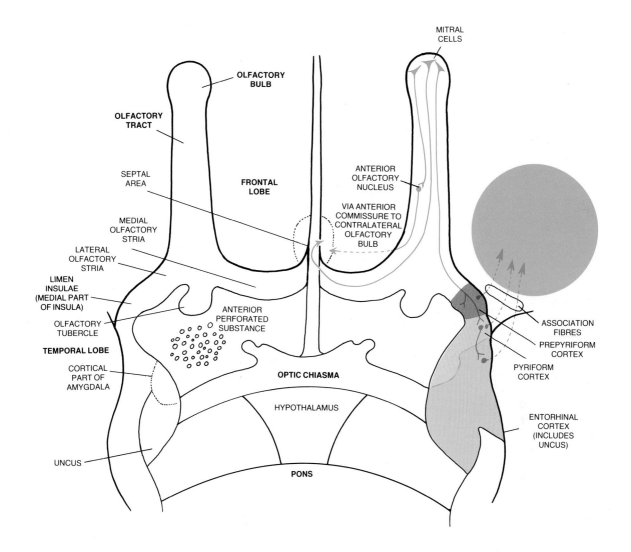

MITRAL CELLS

OLFACTORY BULB

OLFACTORY TRACT

SEPTAL AREA

FRONTAL LOBE

ANTERIOR OLFACTORY NUCLEUS

VIA ANTERIOR COMMISSURE TO CONTRALATERAL OLFACTORY BULB

MEDIAL OLFACTORY STRIA

LATERAL OLFACTORY STRIA

LIMEN INSULAE (MEDIAL PART OF INSULA)

OLFACTORY TUBERCLE

TEMPORAL LOBE

ANTERIOR PERFORATED SUBSTANCE

CORTICAL PART OF AMYGDALA

OPTIC CHIASMA

HYPOTHALAMUS

ASSOCIATION FIBRES

PREPYRIFORM CORTEX

PYRIFORM CORTEX

ENTORHINAL CORTEX (INCLUDES UNCUS)

UNCUS

PONS

All pathways

Primary olfactory cortex

Secondary olfactory cortex

Tertiary olfactory cortex

Pathways shown on one side only for clarity

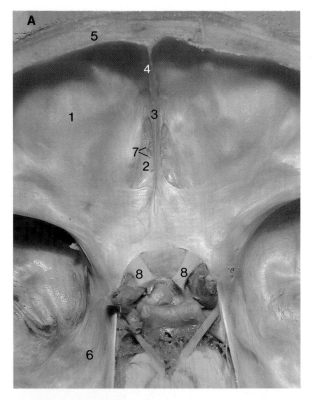

A The floor of the anterior cranial fossa showing the cribriform plate and the olfactory nerves passing through. x.98
1 Anterior cranial fossa
2 Cribriform plate
3 Crista galli
4 Falx cerebri
5 Frontal bone
6 Middle cranial fossa
7 Olfactory nerves
8 Optic nerves

B The frontal lobe on one half of the brain as seen from below with part of the temporal lobe removed. Note the olfactory tract and its bifurcation into the medial and lateral olfactory striae. x2.2
1 Anterior perforated substance
2 Frontal lobe
3 Gyrus rectus
4 Lateral olfactory stria
5 Medial olfactory stria
6 Middle cerebral artery
7 Olfactory bulb
8 Olfactory tract
9 Striate arteries and their openings
10 Temporal lobe (partly removed)

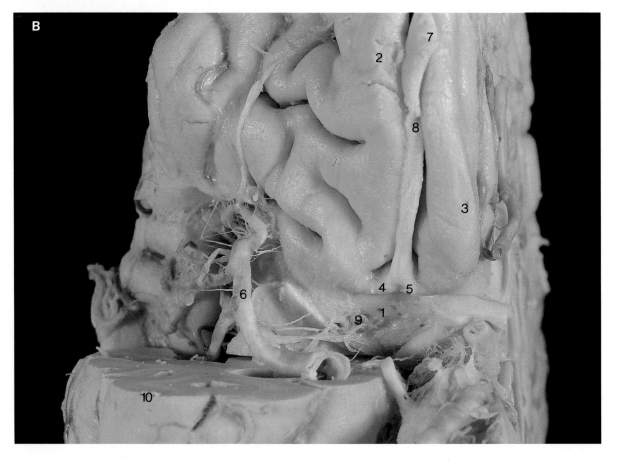

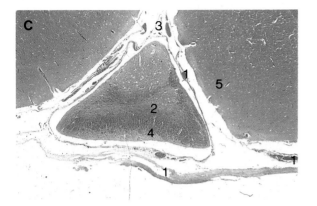

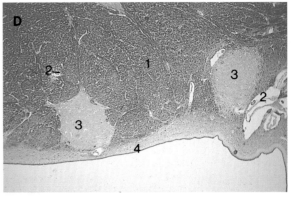

C A transverse section of the olfactory tract. Solochrome cyanin and nuclear fast red stain. x22
1 Blood vessels
2 Nucleus olfactorius anterior (grey matter)
3 Olfactory sulcus
4 Olfactory tract
5 Orbital surface of frontal lobe

Miss L. Ward

D Transverse section of the anterior perforated substance. Luxol fast blue and cresyl violet stain. x22
1 Anterior perforated substance
2 Blood vessels
3 Island of Calleja
4 Olfactory tract

● *Cell bodies in the anterior perforated substance form groups called Islands of Calleja.*

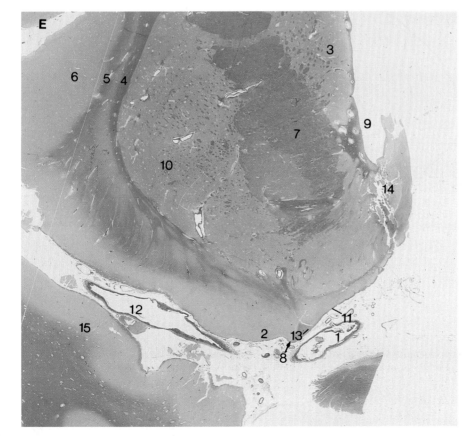

E A coronal section of the olfactory tract lying on the anterior perforated substance and dividing into the medial and lateral olfactory striae. Solochrome cyanin and nuclear fast red stain. x3.5
1 Anterior cerebral artery
2 Anterior perforated substance
3 Caudate nucleus
4 External capsule
5 Extreme capsule
6 Insula
7 Internal capsule
8 Lateral olfactory stria (origin of) (arrow)
9 Lateral ventricle
10 Lentiform nucleus
11 Medial olfactory stria
12 Middle cerebral artery
13 Olfactory tract
14 Septal area
15 Temporal lobe

F

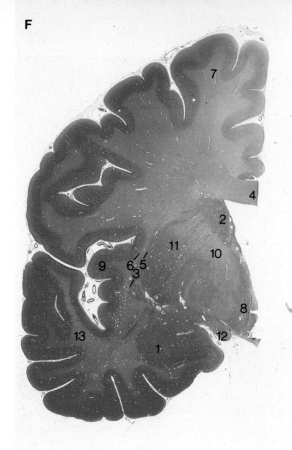

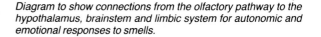

F Coronal section through one cerebral hemisphere to show the amygdaloid nucleus. Carmine stain. x.84

1 Amygdaloid nucleus	**8** Hypothalamus
2 Caudate nucleus	**9** Insula
3 Claustrum	**10** Internal capsule
4 Corpus callosum	**11** Lentiform nucleus
5 External capsule	**12** Optic tract
6 Extreme capsule	**13** Temporal lobe
7 Frontal lobe	

Diagram to show connections from the olfactory pathway to the hypothalamus, brainstem and limbic system for autonomic and emotional responses to smells.

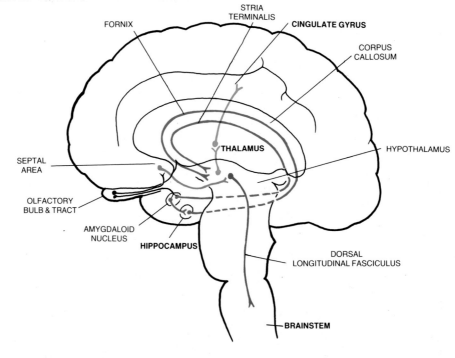

Connections to the hypothalamus via the stria terminalis and fornix, for autonomic and emotional responses.

Direct connections from the septal area to the hypothalamus.

From the hypothalamus to the brainstem via the dorsal longitudinal fasciculus, for reflexes e.g. salivation.

Via mamillothalamic tract to the thalamus, thence to the cingulate gyrus.

Taste

The overall sensation of taste is a complex of true taste, smell, texture and temperature. The true taste sensations include sourness, saltiness, sweetness, bitterness, and other tastes (for example metallic).

Taste buds are located on the tongue, palate, pharynx and epiglottis. The receptors for taste are specialised cells surrounded by nerve endings. The impulses from them are transmitted via three nerves: nervus intermedius, part of the facial nerve (VII) (chorda tympani) for the anterior two-thirds of the tongue; the glossopharyngeal (IX) for the posterior one-third and part of the pharynx; the vagus nerve (X) for the remaining taste buds in the pharynx and larynx.

When the impulses reach the ganglion associated with their nerve, they then pass to the rostral third of the nucleus solitarius. The pathway continues through the brainstem in the secondary ascending gustatory tract in the medial lemniscus to the contralateral ventral posteromedial nucleus in the thalamus. Some impulses may also travel to the hypothalamus. From the thalamus the pathway runs to the lowermost part of the postcentral gyrus and limen insulae of the insula (Brodmann's area 43).

- *The number of taste buds varies from one individual to another. It has been estimated that each of the 10-12 circumvallate papillae bears about 250 taste buds.*

- *Taste buds are more numerous in infants than adults, and decrease with age, at a rate of about 1 per cent per year.*

- *The caudal two-thirds of the nucleus solitarius (solitary nucleus) is a general visceral afferent nucleus receiving sensory information mainly from viscera supplied by the vagus (X) but also from the glossopharyngeal (IX) and facial (VII) nerves, in the digestive and respiratory tracts.*

A diagram of the taste or gustatory pathway.

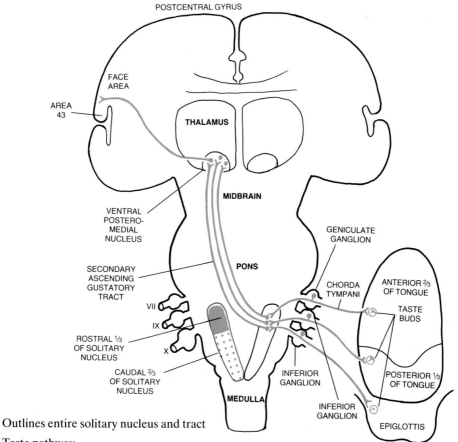

_____ Outlines entire solitary nucleus and tract

_____ Taste pathway

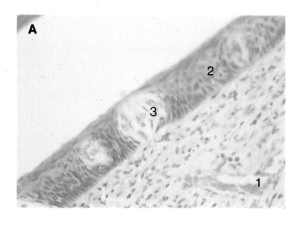

A Taste bud from the posterior part of the tongue. Haematoxylin and eosin stain. x73
1 Blood vessel
2 Epithelium of tongue
3 Taste bud

B Transverse section of the medulla oblongata to illustrate the solitary tract (tractus solitarius). Myelin stain. x5.1
  1 Anterior spinocerebellar tract
  2 Dorsal longitudinal fasciculus
  3 Fourth ventricle
  4 Hypoglossal nucleus
  5 Inferior olivary nucleus
  6 Medial lemniscus
  7 Medial longitudinal fasciculus
  8 Posterior spinocerebellar tract
  9 Pyramidal tract
10 Reticular formation
11 Solitary tract
12 Solitary nucleus (grey matter surrounding the tract)

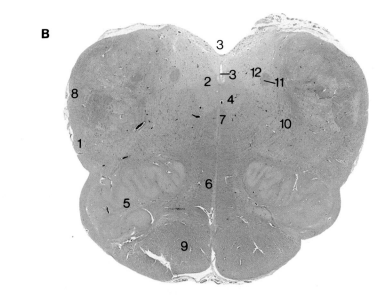

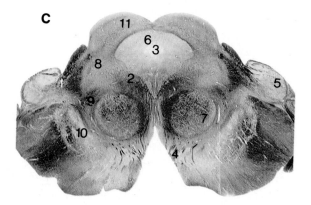

C Transverse section of the midbrain passing through the superior colliculi to demonstrate the secondary ascending gustatory tract. Weigert stain. x2
  1 Brachium of the inferior colliculus
  2 Central tegmental tract
  3 Cerebral aqueduct
  4 Fibres of oculomotor nerve (III)
  5 Medial geniculate body of the thalamus
  6 Periaqueductal grey substance
  7 Red nucleus
  8 Reticular formation
  9 Secondary ascending gustatory tract
10 Substantia nigra
11 Superior colliculus

Motor Pathways (Descending Tracts)

In its widest sense the term 'motor' embraces all forms of active response by the body, whether actual movement as a result of muscle contraction or secretomotor activity of a gland. Movements generated by skeletal muscle are termed somatic motor activity. Visceral motor activity involves smooth or cardiac muscle, and glandular secretion. This section is concerned with the neural pathways controlling somatic motor activity, both voluntary movement itself and the systems in the brain which ensure that it is smoothly co-ordinated.

Cells in a variety of structures in the brain are motor in function. They are connected by motor pathways or descending tracts to the cells that directly innervate muscles and cause them to contract. Cells in the first category are called upper motor neurons and those in the second are lower motor neurons.

Upper motor neurons which directly give rise to descending (motor) tracts are those in the precentral gyrus of the frontal lobe (Brodmann's area 4, the primary motor cortex), and those of the red nucleus, colliculi, vestibular nuclei, reticular formation and inferior olivary nucleus. Those which are indirectly connected to descending tracts are the cerebellum, the basal ganglia and the ventral nuclei of the thalamus.

Lower motor neurons comprise the anterior (ventral) horn cells of the spinal cord and the cells of motor cranial nerve nuclei supplying striated muscles. These are the oculomotor (III), trochlear (IV), trigeminal (V) (motor nucleus), abducens (VI), facial (VII) (motor nucleus), hypoglossal (XII) and the nucleus ambiguus, supplying glossopharyngeal (IX), vagus (X), and accessory (XI).

The corticospinal (pyramidal) and corticobulbar tracts

These tracts are the principal tracts responsible for voluntary movement. About one-third of their fibres arise from the motor cortex of the precentral gyrus (Brodmann's area 4), the remainder from premotor and precentral areas. There the cells are arranged in a very specific pattern. If you imagine a very small person (homunculus) hanging upside down with the feet positioned in the longitudinal fissure and their head at the edge of the lateral fissure, you have a general description of the pattern of distribution of the cell bodies for each part of the body (see page 233). The area supplying the hand is disproportionately large because of the fine movements required of the hand. Similarly the area supplying the face is increased and axons from this area descend in the internal capsule to the motor cranial nerve nuclei listed above. This tract is the corticobulbar pathway. The corticospinal tract, which supplies the trunk and limbs, descends via the internal capsule and the basis pedunculi of the midbrain. It then continues into the brainstem. In the medulla oblongata 80-90 per cent of the axons decussate to the contralateral side to form the lateral corticospinal tract. The remaining 10-20 per cent of the axons descend on their own side as the anterior (ventral) corticospinal tract.

On entering the spinal cord the lateral corticospinal tract lies in the lateral white column and the anterior corticospinal tract lies in the anterior (ventral) white column. The fibres of the anterior corticospinal tract decussate in the spinal cord at or close to the segmental level at which they terminate.

At each level of the spinal cord axons from the lateral and anterior corticospinal tracts enter the grey matter. Those from cells controlling the fine movements of the digits synapse directly on the lower motor neurons but the majority of corticospinal tract axons interact indirectly with the cells of the anterior horn via one or more internuncial neurons. Some axons in the corticospinal tract synapse on cells in the posterior (dorsal) horn of the spinal cord and the dorsal column nuclei that give rise to ascending sensory tracts. These may modulate transmission of sensory information.

Suppression of corticospinal activity

Though the majority of the axons in the tract arise from neurons in the precentral gyrus, there are some which originate from neurons anterior to the precentral gyrus (areas 4s and 6). These neurons inhibit the activity of the lower motor neurons, especially when responding reflexly to sensory stimuli.

- *A cerebrovascular accident (CVA) above the decussation will result in paralysis associated with an upper motor neuron lesion; the muscles on the opposite side of the body being affected. This is because both lateral and anterior corticospinal tracts decussate before reaching the lower motor neurons.*

- *If the axon of the upper motor neuron is damaged below the decussation, the muscles on the same side of the body will be affected causing paralysis. In addition, the suppressor neurons are no longer effective so that the lower motor neurons fire spontaneously or overdischarge to stimuli resulting in spasticity.*

● *A positive Babinski sign can be elicited with upper motor neuron lesions. If the outside of the sole of the foot is stroked from heel to toe, the toes will fan out and the big toe extends. A normal adult would respond by curling the toes in plantar flexion.*

● *Lower motor neuron paralysis is flaccid. This can occur, for example, in poliomyelitis when the ventral horn cells are selectively attacked.*

A diagram of the corticospinal and corticobulbar tracts.

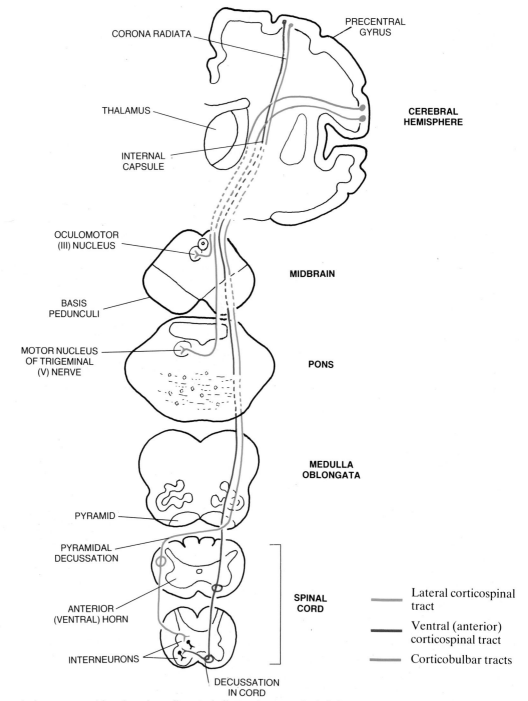

CORONA RADIATA

PRECENTRAL GYRUS

THALAMUS

INTERNAL CAPSULE

CEREBRAL HEMISPHERE

OCULOMOTOR (III) NUCLEUS

MIDBRAIN

BASIS PEDUNCULI

MOTOR NUCLEUS OF TRIGEMINAL (V) NERVE

PONS

MEDULLA OBLONGATA

PYRAMID

PYRAMIDAL DECUSSATION

ANTERIOR (VENTRAL) HORN

SPINAL CORD

INTERNEURONS

DECUSSATION IN CORD

——— Lateral corticospinal tract

——— Ventral (anterior) corticospinal tract

——— Corticobulbar tracts

For clarity each tract is drawn on one side only and not all corticobulbar pathways are included.

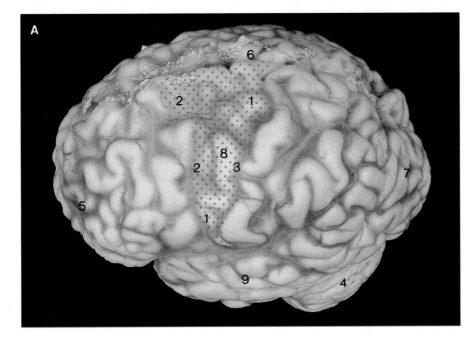

A A lateral view of the brain with a coloured overlay illustrating the corticospinal (pyramidal tract) region. x.63
1 Area 4
2 Area 6 and 4s
3 Central sulcus
4 Cerebellum
5 Frontal lobe
6 Longitudinal fissure
7 Occipital lobe
8 Precentral gyrus
9 Temporal lobe

B A coronal section of area 4 with a superimposed homunculus. x.87
1 Area 4
2 Corpus callosum
3 Homunculus
4 Lateral sulcus

• *A 'sensory homunculus' similar to the motor homunculus, relates the sensory innervation of the body to appropriate areas of the primary sensory cortex.*

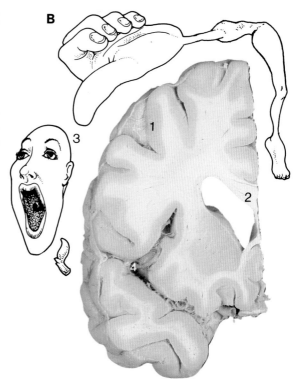

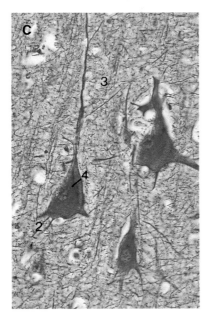

C An histological section to illustrate the pyramidal shape of the Betz cell bodies of the upper motor neurons. Silver stain. x334
1 Apical dendrite
2 Basal cell processes
3 Grey matter of the motor cortex
4 Upper motor neuron cell body

CAM

233

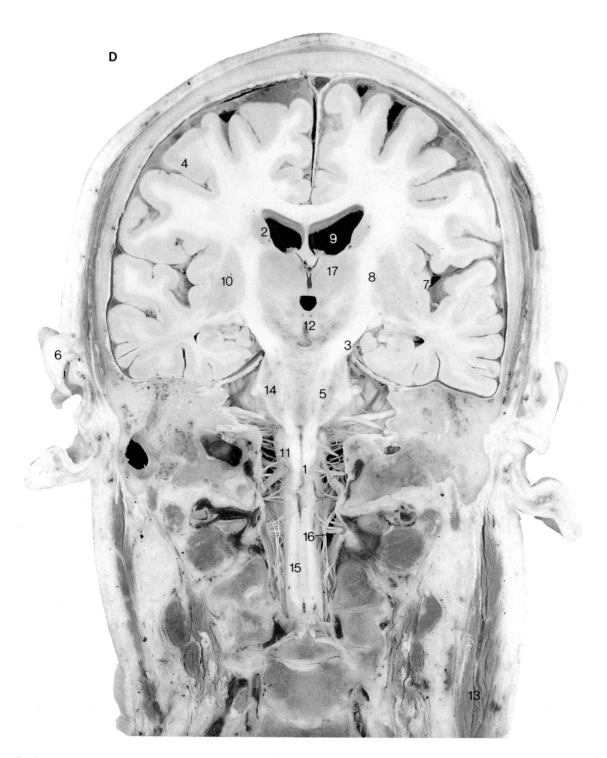

D A coronal section through the cerebral cortex, internal capsule and brainstem to illustrate the continuity of the corticospinal tract. x.89

1 Brainstem	**7** Insula	**13** Neck muscles
2 Caudate nucleus	**8** Internal capsule	**14** Pons
3 Cerebral peduncle	**9** Lateral ventricle	**15** Spinal cord
4 Cerebral cortex	**10** Lentiform nucleus	**16** Spinal nerves
5 Corticospinal tract	**11** Medulla oblongata	**17** Thalamus
6 Ear	**12** Midbrain	

UN

E A coronal section of the mid-brain to show the positions of the corticospinal tract. Van Gieson stain. x4.1

1 Blood vessel
2 Cerebral aqueduct
3 Corticospinal tract
4 Corticospinal tract fibres
5 Crus cerebri
6 Frontopontine tract
7 Medial longitudinal fasciculus
8 Periaqueductal grey substance
9 Reticular formation
10 Substantia nigra
11 Temporo-parieto-occipito-pontine tract

Mr D. Adams

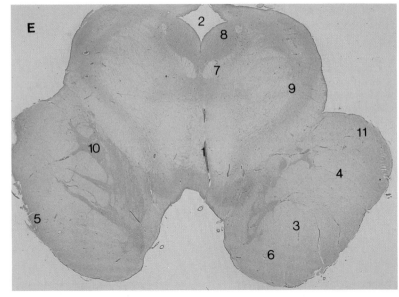

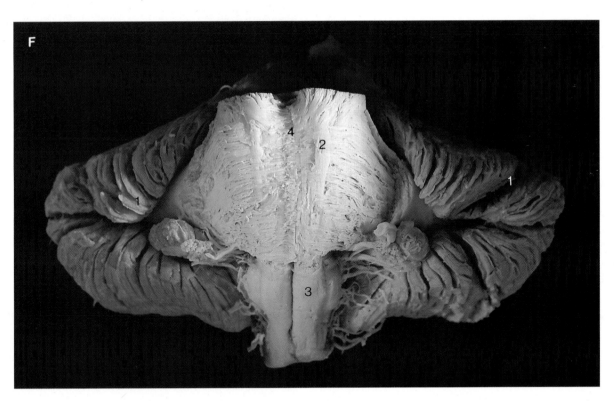

F The pons and cerebellum viewed from the anterior aspect to illustrate the corticospinal tract coursing through the pons. The anterior surface has been dissected to demonstrate the tracts. x1.5

1 Cerebellar hemispheres
2 Corticospinal tract
3 Medulla oblongata
4 Pons

G A coronal section of pons to show the position of the corticospinal tract fibre bundles. Weigert stain. x2.5

1 Basilar portion of pons
2 Corticospinal tract fibres
3 Fourth ventricle
4 Medial longitudinal fasciculus
5 Superior cerebellar peduncle
6 Superior medullary velum
7 Transverse pontine fibres

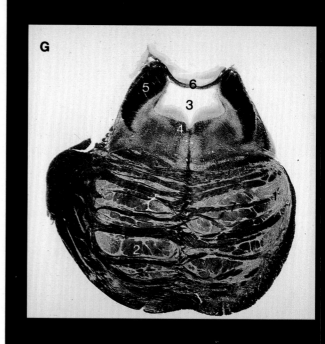

H A coronal section of medulla oblongata showing the pyramids. Myelin stain. x3.9

1 Fasciculus and nucleus cuneatus
2 Fourth ventricle
3 Inferior olivary nucleus
4 Medial lemniscus
5 Pyramid of medulla oblongata
6 Reticular formation

MHMS

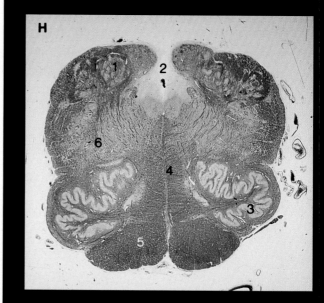

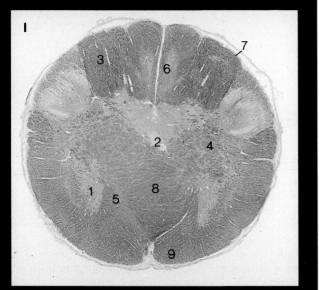

I A coronal section of medulla oblongata showing the motor decussation and the lateral and ventral corticospinal tracts. Weigert-Pal stain. x5.7
1 Anterior horn of the spinal cord
2 Central canal
3 Fasciculus cuneatus
4 Lateral corticospinal tract
5 Medial longitudinal fasciculus
6 Nucleus gracilis
7 Pia mater
8 Pyramidal (motor) decussation
9 Ventral corticospinal tract

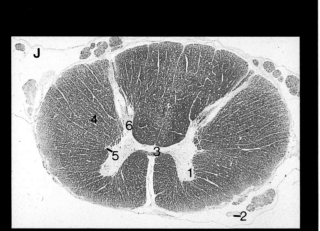

J A thoracic spinal cord cut transversely to illustrate the position of the corticospinal tract above thoracic spinal level T6. Weigert stain. x5.8
1 Anterior horn
2 Blood vessels
3 Central canal
4 Lateral corticospinal tract
5 Lateral horn
6 Posterior horn

OXF

Extrapyramidal Motor Pathways

A number of subcortical structures in the brain give rise to descending tracts that connect to lower motor neurons and are mainly concerned with automatic movements, such as walking, with posture, and with movements of muscle groups. These tracts do not pass through the pyramid of the medulla oblongata as they descend through the brainstem into the spinal cord, hence they are termed extrapyramidal pathways. They are the rubrospinal, tectospinal, vestibulospinal, reticulospinal and olivospinal tracts.

The rubrospinal and tectospinal tracts arise in the midbrain. The rubrospinal tract is a small tract which originates from the red nucleus, decussates almost immediately and terminates above the midthoracic level of the spinal cord. It predominantly controls the tone of the flexor muscles. The medial and lateral tectospinal tracts arise in the colliculi, decussate almost immediately and terminate in the cervical and upper thoracic regions of the spinal cord. The tectospinal tracts control reflex turning of the head and neck to auditory or visual stimuli. The vestibulospinal tract arises from the lateral vestibular nucleus (Dieter's nucleus) in the rostral part of the medulla oblongata and descends without decussating. It controls the muscles which maintain normal posture and balance. The reticulospinal tracts arise from the pontine and medullary reticular formation. They are partly crossed and concerned with regulating automatic movements in locomotion. The small olivospinal tract, originating in the inferior olivary nucleus, descends after decussating to cervical levels of the spinal cord and coordinates movements of the head and neck and upper limbs, contralateral to its origin.

The thalamus, red nucleus, vestibular nuclei, inferior olivary nucleus and reticular formation all receive substantial connections from the cerebellum. It is by means of these connections that the cerebellum influences lower motor neurons; the cerebellum has no descending tracts connecting to the spinal cord.

A diagram of the extrapyramidal motor pathways.

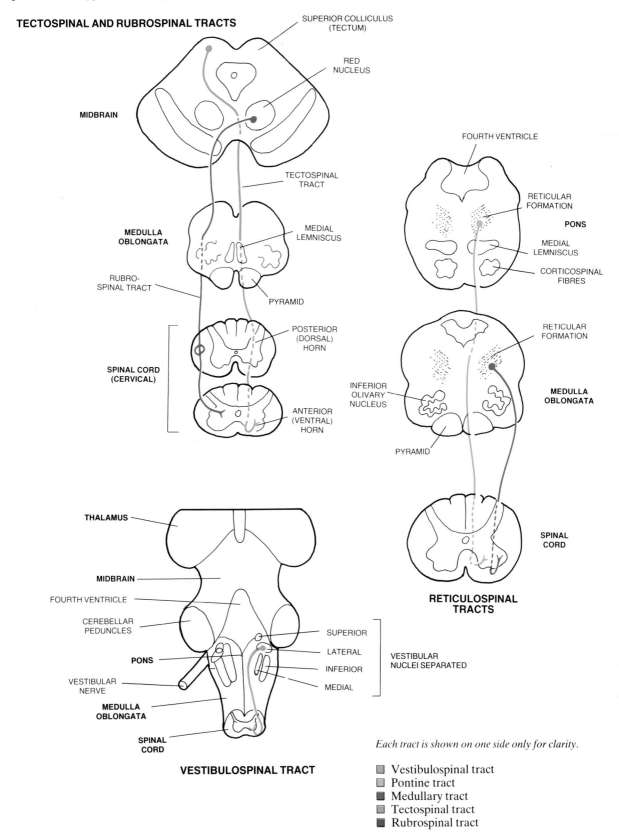

TECTOSPINAL AND RUBROSPINAL TRACTS

SUPERIOR COLLICULUS
(TECTUM)

RED
NUCLEUS

MIDBRAIN

TECTOSPINAL
TRACT

MEDULLA
OBLONGATA

MEDIAL
LEMNISCUS

RUBRO-
SPINAL TRACT

PYRAMID

POSTERIOR
(DORSAL)
HORN

SPINAL CORD
(CERVICAL)

ANTERIOR
(VENTRAL)
HORN

FOURTH VENTRICLE

RETICULAR
FORMATION

PONS

MEDIAL
LEMNISCUS

CORTICOSPINAL
FIBRES

RETICULAR
FORMATION

INFERIOR
OLIVARY
NUCLEUS

MEDULLA
OBLONGATA

PYRAMID

SPINAL
CORD

**RETICULOSPINAL
TRACTS**

THALAMUS

MIDBRAIN

FOURTH VENTRICLE

CEREBELLAR
PEDUNCLES

SUPERIOR

LATERAL

VESTIBULAR
NUCLEI SEPARATED

PONS

INFERIOR

VESTIBULAR
NERVE

MEDIAL

MEDULLA
OBLONGATA

SPINAL
CORD

VESTIBULOSPINAL TRACT

Each tract is shown on one side only for clarity.

☐ Vestibulospinal tract
☐ Pontine tract
☐ Medullary tract
☐ Tectospinal tract
☐ Rubrospinal tract

A-H Sections to illustrate the origin and course of all the extrapyramidal motor pathways in the brainstem and spinal cord.

A A section of midbrain showing the red nucleus and the rubrospinal tract. Myelin stain. x2.4

1 Cerebellorubrothalamic fibres
2 Cerebral aqueduct
3 Interpeduncular fossa
4 Medial lemniscus
5 Oculomotor nerve fibres
6 Periaqueductal grey matter
7 Red nucleus
8 Rubrospinal tract
9 Substantia nigra
10 Superior colliculus

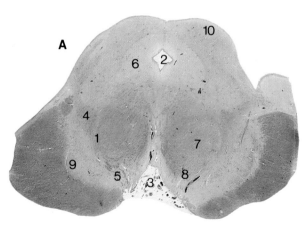

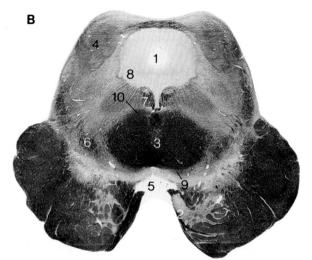

B A section of midbrain showing the tectospinal and rubrospinal tracts, at the level of the inferior colliculus. Weigert stain. x2.7

1 Cerebral aqueduct
2 Cerebral peduncle
3 Decussation of superior cerebellar peduncle
4 Inferior colliculus
5 Interpeduncular fossa
6 Medial lemniscus
7 Medial longitudinal fasciculus
8 Periaqueductal grey matter
9 Rubrospinal tract
10 Tectospinal tract

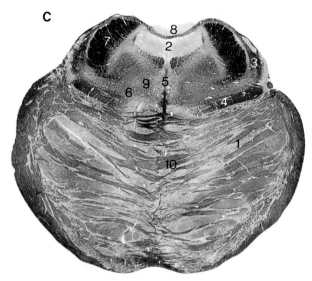

C A transverse section through the rostral part of the pons to demonstrate the position of the rubrospinal and tectospinal tracts as they descend through the brainstem. Weigert stain. x3

1 Basilar portion of pons
2 Fourth ventricle
3 Lateral lemniscus
4 Medial lemniscus
5 Reticular formation
6 Rubrospinal tract
7 Superior cerebellar peduncle
8 Superior medullary velum
9 Tectospinal tract
10 Transverse pontine fibres

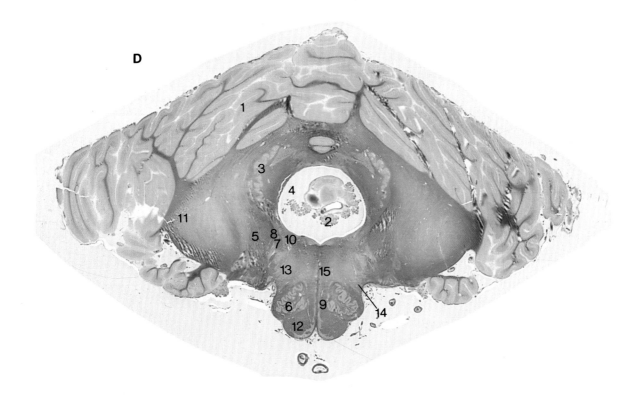

D

D A coronal section through the medulla oblongata and cerebellum to show the vestibular nuclei, inferior olivary nucleus and reticular formation: the origins of the vestibulospinal, olivospinal and reticulospinal tracts. Weigert-Pal stain. x1.6

  1 Cerebellum
  2 Choroid plexus
  3 Dentate nucleus
  4 Fourth ventricle
  5 Inferior cerebellar peduncle
  6 Inferior olivary nucleus
  7 Inferior vestibular nucleus
  8 Lateral vestibular nucleus
  9 Medial lemniscus
10 Medial vestibular nucleus
11 Middle cerebellar peduncle
12 Pyramid
13 Reticular formation
14 Rubrospinal tract
15 Tectospinal tract

MHMS

● *The rubrospinal tract, spinocerebellar tracts and spinothalamic tracts are crowded together in the area shown and cannot be demarcated clearly.*

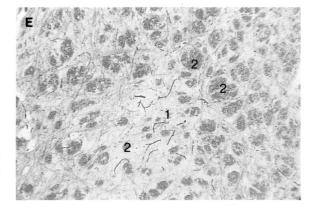

E Detail of the medial vestibular nucleus showing vestibulospinal tract fibres passing through the substance of the nucleus. Palmgren stain. x55

1 Medial vestibular nucleus
2 Vestibulospinal tract, fibre bundles

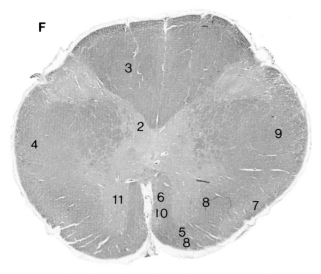

F

F-H Transverse sections of the spinal cord to demonstrate the position of extrapyramidal motor pathways and the different levels to which they descend in the cord.

F An histological section through the first cervical (C1) segment of the spinal cord. Weigert stain. x8.8

G An hemi-section through an upper thoracic segment. Van Gieson stain. x10

Mr D. Adams

H An histological section through a lower lumbar segment. Weigert stain. x9.4

1 Cauda equina
2 Dorsal (posterior) horn
3 Dorsal (posterior) white column
4 Lateral white column
5 Lateral vestibulospinal tract
6 Medial longitudinal fasciculus and medial
   vestibulospinal tract
7 Olivospinal tract
8 Reticulospinal tract
9 Rubrospinal tract
10 Tectospinal tract
11 Ventral (anterior) horn

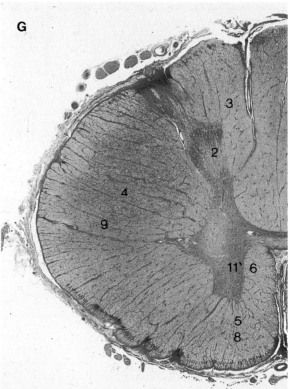

G

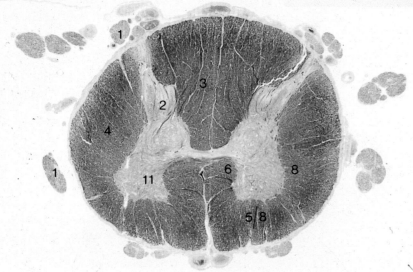

H

A Horizontal section of the brain to illustrate the level of the plane of section in **B** and **C**. x.6

1 Cerebellum
2 Frontal lobe
3 Insula
4 Lateral ventricle
5 Longitudinal fissure
6 Occipital lobe
7 Parietal lobe
8 Temporal lobe

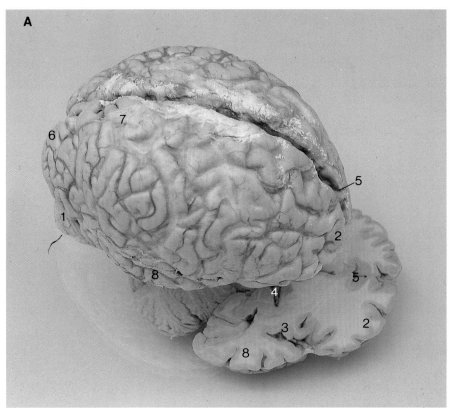

B A nuclear magnetic resonance (NMR) image of an horizontal section through the head to show the thalamus and basal ganglia.

1 Caudate nucleus
2 Corpus callosum
3 Frontal bone
4 Frontal lobe
5 Globus pallidus ⎫
6 Putamen   ⎬ Lentiform nucleus
7 Insula
8 Internal capsule
9 Lateral ventricle
10 Lentiform nucleus
11 Meninges
12 Occipital bone
13 Occipital lobe
14 Temporal lobe
15 Thalamus
16 Third ventricle

Dr G. Bydder

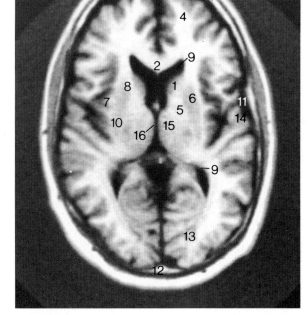

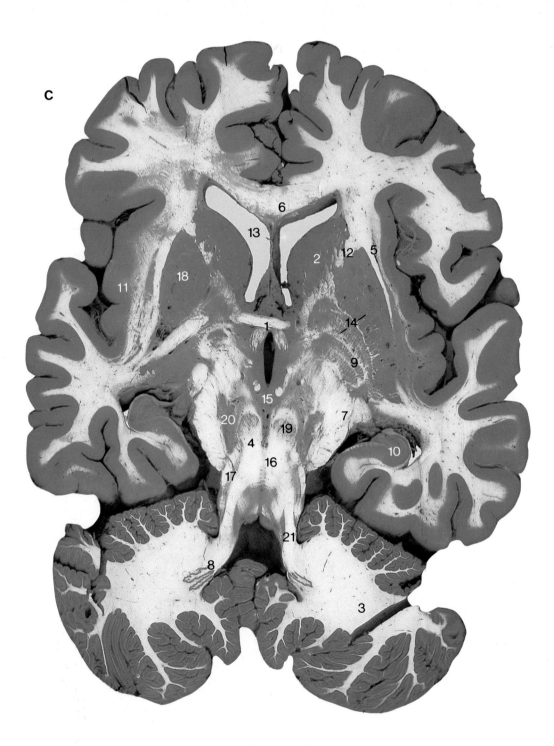

C Horizontal thick section of brain to show some structures important to the control of movement. Mulligan stain. x1.1

1 Anterior commissure	**8** Dentate nucleus	**15** Mamillary body
2 Caudate nucleus	**9** Globus pallidus	**16** Midbrain
3 Cerebellum	**10** Hippocampus	**17** Pons
4 Cerebellorubrothalamic fibres	**11** Insula	**18** Putamen
5 Claustrum	**12** Internal capsule	**19** Red nucleus
6 Corpus callosum	**13** Lateral ventricle	**20** Substantia nigra
7 Crus cerebri	**14** Lentiform nucleus	**21** Superior cerebellar peduncle

The Cerebellum in Movement Control

The cerebellum is one region where sensory and motor integration can take place. It may be likened to a reference library to which the motor cortex can 'refer'. As already explained, it has no direct link to lower motor neurons. There are two ways in which it influences movement indirectly. Firstly, it has connections to motor areas of the cerebral cortex via relay in the thalamus. Secondly, it also connects to the red nucleus, olivary complex, reticular formation and vestibular nuclei then through these to extrapyramidal motor pathways.

The cerebellum may be divided into three functional units—the archicerebellum, palaeocerebellum and neocerebellum. The archicerebellum is composed of the flocculonodular lobe and fastigial nucleus which are linked to the vestibular nuclei. The palaeocerebellum receives general sensory information, especially proprioception. Its extent is a little uncertain but it includes the anterior lobe, pyramid, uvula and the globose and emboliform nuclei. The neocerebellum is the largest part and comprises the remaining cortex which receives olivary afferents and a large input from the cerebral cortex via the pontine nuclei. Its deep nucleus is the dentate nucleus.

This functional subdivision parallels the order in which parts of the cerebellum have appeared in the course of evolution as movement control became more complex.

The inferior cerebellar peduncle connects cerebellum and medulla oblongata. It conveys the dorsal (posterior) spinocerebellar tract, olivocerebellar fibres from the contralateral inferior olivary complex, vestibulocerebellar fibres, trigeminocerebellar fibres, cuneocerebellar fibres from the accessory cuneate nucleus, and afferents from the reticular formation and arcuate nuclei (anterior external arcuate fibres and the striae medullares). Efferent fibres in the inferior peduncle pass to the vestibular nuclei and possibly to the reticular formation and olivary nuclei.

The middle peduncle is exclusively afferent. Its fibres originate from pontine nuclei. These receive afferents from wide areas of the contralateral cerebral cortex, thus connecting it to the cerebellum. This is the main route for sensory information to reach the cerebellum from cortical sensory areas, and also connects the motor cortex to the cerebellum. The pontine nuclei relay information to the cerebellar cortex.

The superior cerebellar peduncle contains only two afferent tracts, the anterior (ventral) spinocerebellar tract and tectocerebellar fibres from the midbrain colliculi. Efferent fibres run from the dentate nucleus to the contralateral red nucleus and ventrolateral nucleus of the thalamus, thence to the motor cortex of the cerebrum. Efferent fibres also link the fastigial nuclei to the lateral vestibular nucleus, and the globose and emboliform nuclei to the red nucleus and thalamus. The superior peduncle decussates in the midbrain.

The inferior olivary complex also receives afferent fibres from cerebral motor cortex, and the central tegmental tract from the corpus striatum and red nucleus.

The red nucleus projects to lower motor neurons via the rubrospinal tract. In addition to its connections from the cerebellum it receives afferent fibres from motor cortex and corpus striatum, sends efferents to the thalamus and is reciprocally linked to the substantia nigra.

No cells are lost from the inferior olivary nucleus in old age. Its cells accumulate lipofuscin (age pigment) in greater amounts and earlier in life than those in any other brain nucleus.

● *There may also be afferent adrenergic connections to the cerebellum from the locus coeruleus, of unknown functions.*

● *Animal studies suggest cerebellar connections with the autonomic system, possibly via the reticular formation.*

● *The flocculonodular lobe is the phylogenetically oldest part of the cerebellum, the archicerebellum which is present in all vertebrates.*

● *For further consideration of vestibular nuclei see pages 158-159.*

● *For further consideration of ventral lateral thalamic nuclei see pages 253-254.*

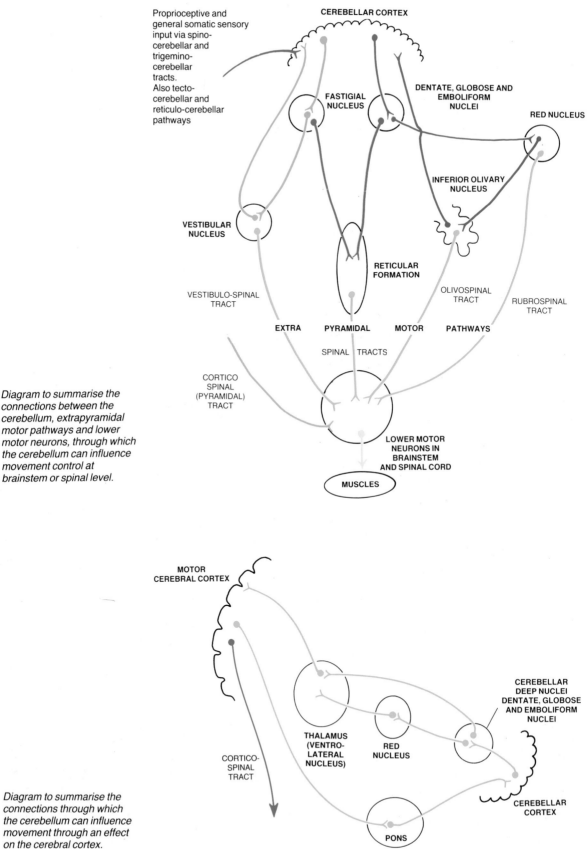

Proprioceptive and general somatic sensory input via spino-cerebellar and trigemino-cerebellar tracts.
Also tecto-cerebellar and reticulo-cerebellar pathways

CEREBELLAR CORTEX

FASTIGIAL NUCLEUS

DENTATE, GLOBOSE AND EMBOLIFORM NUCLEI

RED NUCLEUS

INFERIOR OLIVARY NUCLEUS

VESTIBULAR NUCLEUS

RETICULAR FORMATION

VESTIBULO-SPINAL TRACT

OLIVOSPINAL TRACT

RUBROSPINAL TRACT

EXTRA   PYRAMIDAL   MOTOR   PATHWAYS

SPINAL   TRACTS

CORTICO SPINAL (PYRAMIDAL) TRACT

LOWER MOTOR NEURONS IN BRAINSTEM AND SPINAL CORD

MUSCLES

Diagram to summarise the connections between the cerebellum, extrapyramidal motor pathways and lower motor neurons, through which the cerebellum can influence movement control at brainstem or spinal level.

MOTOR CEREBRAL CORTEX

CEREBELLAR DEEP NUCLEI DENTATE, GLOBOSE AND EMBOLIFORM NUCLEI

THALAMUS (VENTRO-LATERAL NUCLEUS)

RED NUCLEUS

CEREBELLAR CORTEX

CORTICO-SPINAL TRACT

PONS

Diagram to summarise the connections through which the cerebellum can influence movement through an effect on the cerebral cortex.

A-B Relationship between brainstem and cerebellum.

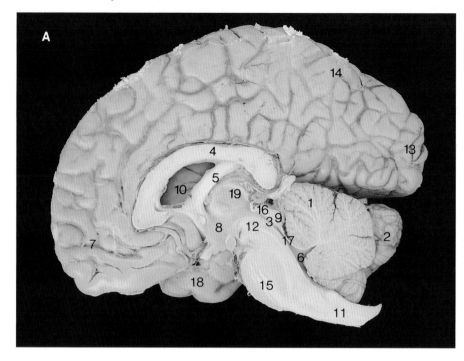

A A sagittal section of the brain to show the position and relationships of the cerebellum. x.7

 1 Arbor vitae
 2 Cerebellum
 3 Cerebral aqueduct
 4 Corpus callosum
 5 Fornix
 6 Fourth ventricle
 7 Frontal lobe
 8 Hypothalamus
 9 Inferior colliculus
10 Lateral ventricle
11 Medulla oblongata
12 Midbrain
13 Occipital lobe
14 Parietal lobe
15 Pons
16 Superior colliculus
17 Superior medullary velum
18 Temporal lobe
19 Thalamus

B Sagittal section of brainstem showing some structures with cerebellar connections. Myelin stain. x2.5

 1 Cerebellum
 2 Choroid plexus
 3 Corticospinal tract
 4 Fourth ventricle
 5 Inferior colliculus
 6 Inferior olivary nucleus
 7 Medulla oblongata
 8 Midbrain
 9 Pons
10 Superior cerebellar peduncle
11 Superior colliculus
12 Thalamus

CAM

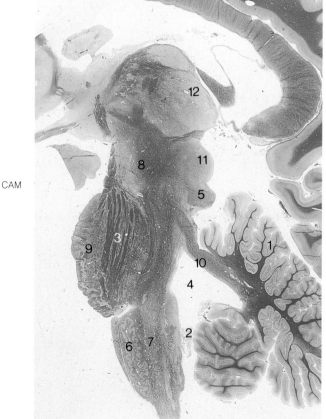

C-F Inferior and middle cerebellar peduncles and their connections.

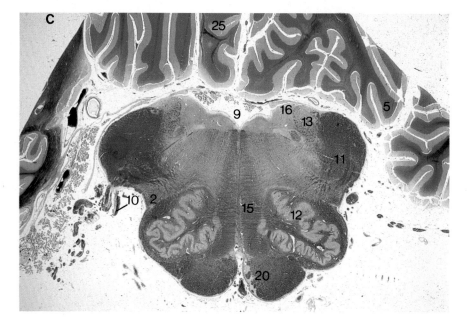

C Transverse section of medulla and cerebellum, showing vestibular nuclei and inferior cerebellar peduncle. Myelin stain and counterstain. x3

MHMS

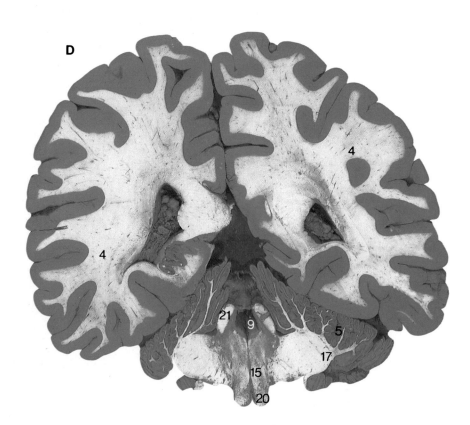

D A coronal thick slice of the cerebral hemispheres and brainstem to show the three cerebellar peduncles. Mulligan stain. x.84

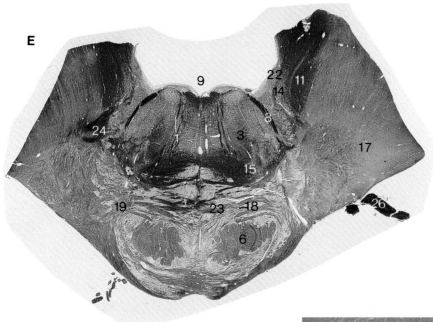

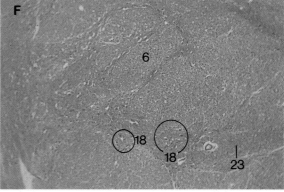

F Histology of the pontine nuclei and transverse pontine (pontocerebellar) fibres. Luxol fast blue and cresyl violet stain. x55

CXWMS

1 Abducens nerve (VI)
2 Anterior (ventral) spinocerebellar tract
3 Central tegmental tract
4 Cerebral hemispheres
5 Cerebellar hemisphere
6 Corticospinal tract
7 Dentate nucleus
8 Facial nerve (VII)
9 Fourth ventricle
10 Glossopharyngeal nerve (IX)
11 Inferior cerebellar peduncle
12 Inferior olivary nucleus
13 Inferior vestibular nucleus
14 Lateral vestibular nucleus
15 Medial lemniscus
16 Medial vestibular nucleus
17 Middle cerebellar peduncle
18 Pontine nuclei
19 Pontocerebellar fibres
20 Pyramid (of medulla oblongata)
21 Superior cerebellar peduncle
22 Superior vestibular nucleus
23 Transverse pontine fibres
24 Trigeminal nerve (V)
25 Vermis
26 Vestibulocochlear nerve (VIII)

G-K Sections to show the inferior olivary nucleus and some connecting structures.

G A coronal section through the brain, cutting the medulla oblongata through the middle of the inferior olivary nucleus. Mulligan stain. x1.04

1 Central tegmental tract
2 Cerebellum
3 Dentate nucleus
4 Fourth ventricle
5 Hilum of inferior olivary nucleus
6 Inferior cerebellar peduncle
7 Inferior olivary nucleus
8 Medial accessory olivary nucleus
9 Medial lemniscus
10 Medulla oblongata
11 Occipital lobe
12 Olive
13 Pyramid

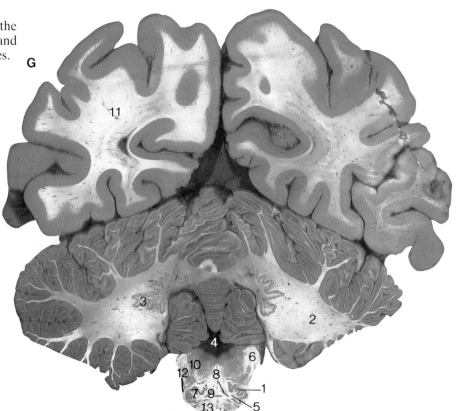

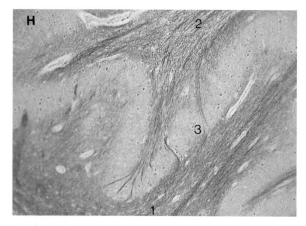

H An histological section to show the afferent and efferent fibres of the inferior olivary nucleus. Luxol fast blue stain. x57
1 Afferent fibres
2 Efferent fibres
3 Inferior olivary nucleus

CXWMS

I An histological section to show the cellular organization of part of the inferior olivary nucleus. Cresyl violet stain. x71
1 Blood vessel
2 Inferior olivary nucleus
3 Neuronal cell bodies

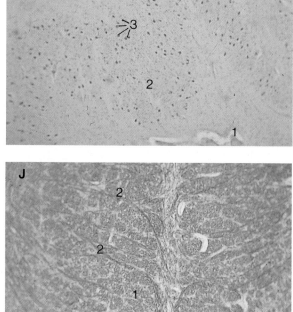

J A paraffin wax section to show olivocerebellar efferent fibres intersecting with the medial lemniscus. Luxol fast blue stain. x89
1 Medial lemniscus
2 Olivocerebellar fibres

K-N Sections to show the pathway from the cerebellum through the superior cerebellar peduncle to the red nucleus.

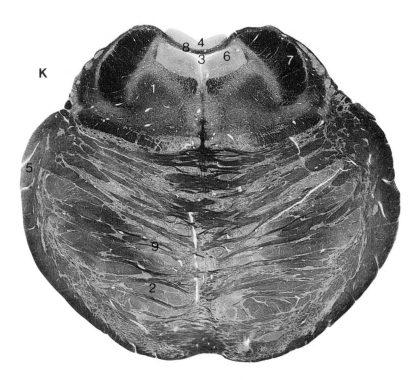

K A transverse section of pons passing through the superior and middle cerebellar peduncles. Weigert stain. x3.74

1 Central tegmental tract
2 Corticospinal fibres
3 Fourth ventricle
4 Lingula of cerebellum
5 Middle cerebellar peduncle
6 Periaqueductal grey matter
7 Superior cerebellar peduncle
8 Superior medullary velum
9 Transverse pontine fibres

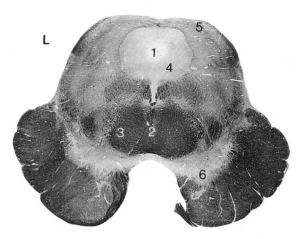

L A transverse section of the midbrain showing the decussation of the superior cerebellar peduncle. Weigert stain. x2.4

1 Cerebral aqueduct
2 Decussating fibres
3 Decussation of the superior cerebellar peduncle
4 Periaqueductal grey matter
5 Inferior colliculus
6 Substantia nigra

M An high magnification photomicrograph of decussating fibres from the decussation of the superior cerebellar peduncle. Luxol fast blue and cresyl violet stain. x120

1 Decussating fibres
2 Neuroglial cells

CXWMS

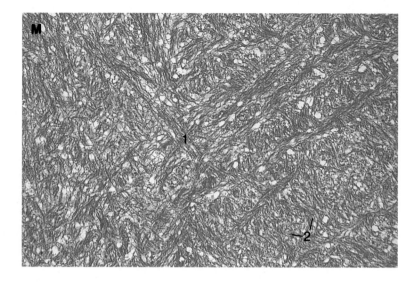

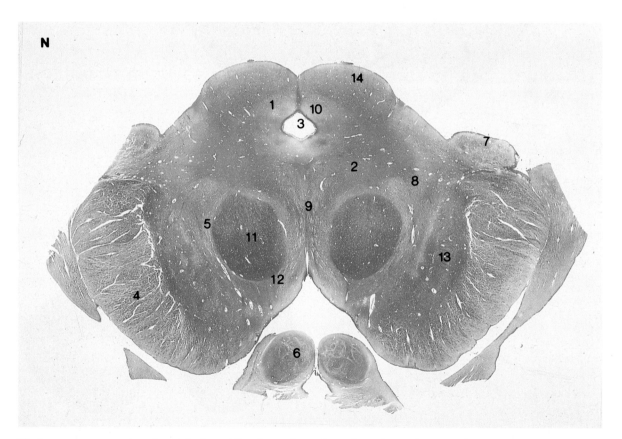

N A transverse section through the midbrain to show the red nucleus, dentatorubrothalamic fibres (from superior cerebellar peduncle) and the rubrospinal and central tegmental tracts. Luxol fast blue and acid fuchsin stain. x3.27

1 Central grey matter	6 Mamillary body	11 Red nucleus
2 Central tegmental tract	7 Medial geniculate body	12 Rubrospinal tract
3 Cerebral aqueduct	8 Medial lemniscus	13 Substantia nigra
4 Crus cerebri	9 Oculomotor nucleus	14 Superior colliculus
5 Dentatorubrothalamic tract	10 Periaqueductal grey matter	

The Thalamus in Movement Control

The ventral lateral nucleus of the thalamus is known as the motor thalamic nucleus because it is a component of several motor pathways. It receives afferent tracts from the cerebellum, either directly or via the red nucleus, from the substantia nigra, the globus pallidus and the corpus striatum. It projects efferent fibres to motor and premotor areas of the frontal lobe cortex. Thus it links subcortical structures having motor functions to the motor cortex. Through this link the subcortical structures can affect movement by influencing cortical function.

O-T Preparations to demonstrate structures in the basal ganglia and diencephalon which are involved in movement control.

O-P Histological sections to illustrate the parts of the thalamus involved in movement control.

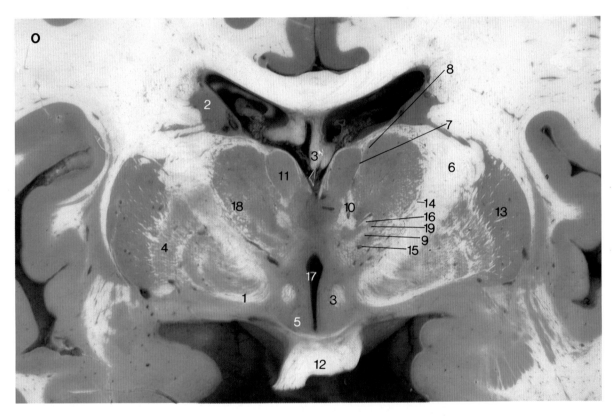

O A coronal thick slice through the thalamus and adjacent forebrain structures to show the subthalamus and the ventral lateral nucleus of the thalamus. Mulligan stain. x2.1

1 Ansa lenticularis	**8** Lateral dorsal thalamic nucleus	**14** Reticular nuclei of thalamus
2 Caudate nucleus	**9** Lenticular fasciculus or field	**15** Subthalamic nucleus
3 Fornix	H2 of Forel	**16** Thalamic fasciculus
4 Globus pallidus	**10** Mamillothalamic tract	(field H1 of Forel)
5 Hypothalamus	**11** Medial thalamic nuclei	**17** Third ventricle
6 Internal capsule	**12** Optic chiasma	**18** Ventral lateral thalamic nucleus
7 Internal medullary lamina	**13** Putamen	**19** Zona incerta

Dentatothalamic and rubrothalamic fibres adjacent to the red nucleus form field H of Forel or the prerubra area. They join with fibres from the globus pallidus to the thalamus to form the thalamic fasciculus, or field H1 of Forel.

● *Auguste H. Forel (1848-1931) was a Swiss neurophysiologist who described the areas in the subthalamus that bear his name.*

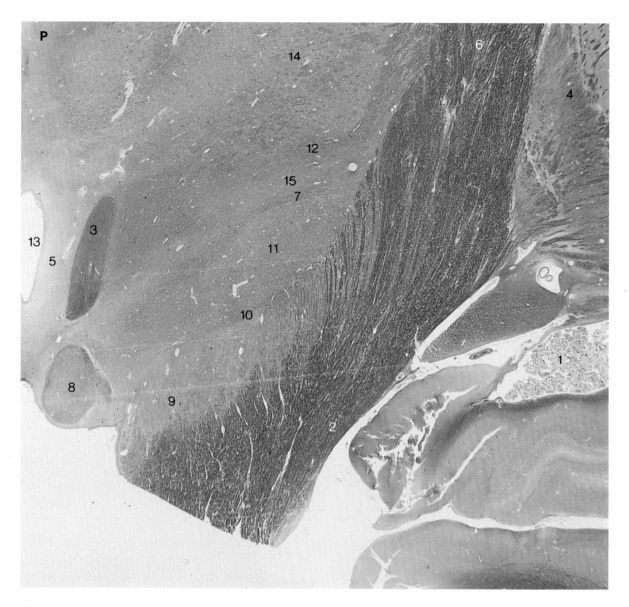

P Part of a coronal section through the diencephalon to illustrate the detailed anatomy of the subthalamic area. Light green and solochrome cyanin stain. x6.8

1 Choroid plexus
2 Crus cerebri
3 Fornix
4 Globus pallidus
5 Hypothalamus
6 Internal capsule
7 Lenticular fasciculus
8 Mamillary body
9 Substantia nigra
10 Subthalamic fasciculus
11 Subthalamic nucleus
12 Thalamic fasciculus
13 Third ventricle
14 Ventral lateral thalamic nucleus
15 Zona incerta

The Basal Ganglia in Movement Control

These are a group of nuclei which interact with each other and with the ventral thalamic nuclei and with motor and premotor areas of the frontal lobe cortex to facilitate smooth, controlled, voluntary movement by acting at cortical level.

The basal ganglia comprise the caudate nucleus, lentiform nucleus, subthalamic nucleus and substantia nigra. The lentiform nucleus has two parts, the putamen and the globus pallidus. Connecting fibres crossing the internal capsule link the caudate nucleus and putamen together as the corpus striatum.

Connecting pathways run through the basal ganglia and thalamus to form a loop-like circuit: firstly from cerebral cortex (particularly sensory and motor cortex) to the corpus striatum, secondly from the corpus striatum to the globus pallidus, thirdly from the globus pallidus to the ventral thalamic nuclei via the pallidothalamic tracts (ansa lenticularis, lenticular fasciculus), and fourthly from the ventral thalamic nuclei to the motor, premotor and supplementary motor areas of the cerebral cortex. This circuit may act as a feedback system through which cortical activity can be influenced.

The corpus striatum also has connections with the substantia nigra and direct pathways to the thalamus.

A second loop links the subthalamic nucleus of the diencephalon with the globus pallidus through the subthalamic fasciculus, which contains both afferent and efferent fibres. This enables the subthalamic nucleus to interact with other components of the basal ganglia. It is also connected to the substantia nigra. Commissural fibres connect left and right subthalamic nuclei.

The substantia nigra in the midbrain has extensive afferent and efferent connections with the corpus striatum, forming a loop through which it can influence striatal function. It is also connected to the ventral thalamic nuclei and the globus pallidus, and some links with the cerebral cortex and the red nucleus have been described.

● *The corpus striatum contains cholinergic and GABA—containing neurons. The latter are on pathways to the globus pallidus and substantia nigra. Both cell types, but chiefly the GABA-ergic cells, are depleted in Huntington's chorea.*

● *The substantia nigra is unpigmented at birth.*

● *Cells are lost and the transmitter, dopamine is diminished in the substantia nigra in Parkinson's disease.*

Diagram to illustrate the looped nature of connections between the cerebral cortex, corpus striatum and thalamus (shown in green), the corpus striatum and substantia nigra (shown in red) and the subthalamic nucleus and globus pallidus (shown in blue) on one side.

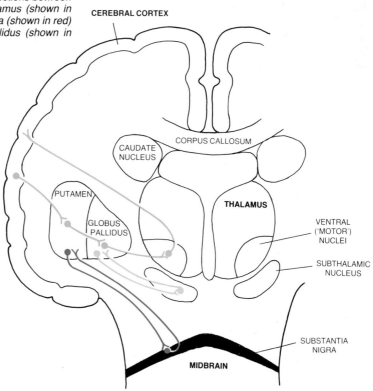

CEREBRAL CORTEX

CORPUS CALLOSUM

CAUDATE NUCLEUS

PUTAMEN

GLOBUS PALLIDUS

THALAMUS

VENTRAL ('MOTOR') NUCLEI

SUBTHALAMIC NUCLEUS

SUBSTANTIA NIGRA

MIDBRAIN

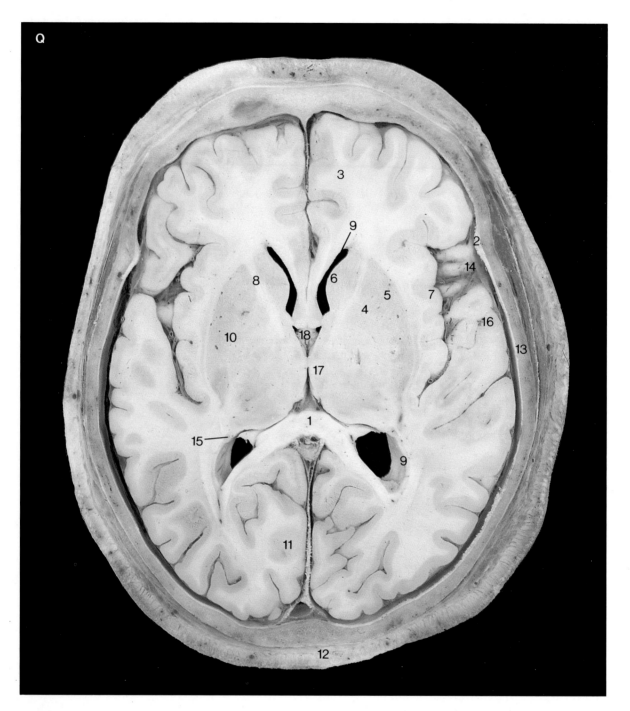

Q An horizontal section through the head passing through the caudate and lentiform nuclei. x.93

1 Corpus callosum
2 Dura mater
3 Frontal lobe
4 Globus pallidus ⎫
5 Putamen ⎬ Lentiform nucleus
6 Head of caudate nucleus
7 Insula

8 Internal capsule
9 Lateral ventricle
10 Lentiform nucleus
11 Occipital lobe
12 Scalp
13 Skull bones
14 Subarachnoid space

15 Tail of caudate nucleus
16 Temporal lobe
17 Thalamus
18 Third ventricle

UN

R A coronal section of the base of the forebrain to demonstrate connections between the caudate nucleus, putamen and globus pallidus. Phosphotungstic acid and haematoxylin stain. x3.3

1 Amygdaloid nucleus
2 Anterior thalamic nuclei
3 Claustrum
4 Connections between caudate nucleus and putamen
5 Connections between putamen and globus pallidus
6 Corpus callosum
7 External capsule
8 Extreme capsule
9 Fornix
10 Globus pallidus
11 Hypothalamus
12 Internal capsule
13 Lateral ventricle
14 Optic tract
15 Putamen

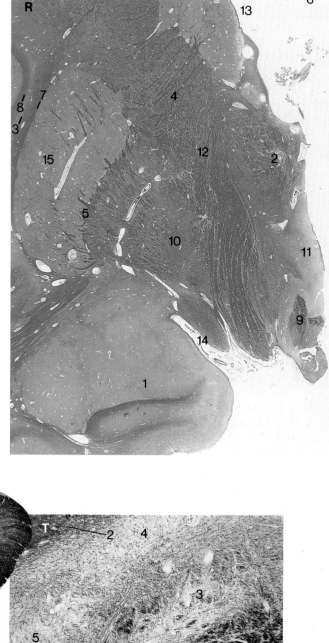

S–T Sections to illustrate the structure of the substantia nigra.

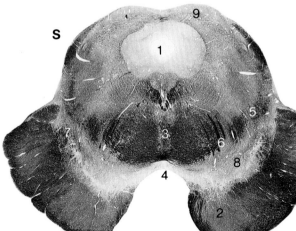

S A transverse section of midbrain showing the position of the substantia nigra and the pallidonigral and nigrostriatal connecting fibres. Weigert stain. x2.03

1 Cerebral aqueduct
2 Crus cerebri
3 Decussation of superior cerebellar peduncle
4 Interpeduncular fossa
5 Medial lemniscus
6 Oculomotor nerve fibres
7 Pallidonigral and nigrostriatal fibres
8 Substantia nigra
9 Superior colliculus

T Detail of the substantia nigra and the pallidonigral and nigrostriatal fibres. Weigert stain. x33

1 Crus cerebri
2 Medial lemniscus
3 Pallidonigral and nigrostriatal fibres
4 Pigmented neurons of substantia nigra
5 Substantia nigra

LIMBIC SYSTEM

The limbic system comprises a number of forebrain structures which are connected anatomically and have a common functional role in emotional aspects of behaviour. It is concerned both with subjective emotional experience and with changes in bodily functions associated with emotional states. Particularly, it is involved in aggressive, submissive and sexual behaviour, in pleasure, memory and learning, and in generating emotional responses, both subjective and physical, to external sensory stimuli.

These functions are based on the anatomy and connections of components of the limbic system. It contains both cortical and subcortical structures itself, and is connected to non-limbic, mainly sensory, parts of the cerebral cortex and to autonomic centres in the hypothalamus and brainstem.

Cortical components of the limbic system are the temporal pole and orbital gyri, the insula, cingulate gyrus, parahippocampal gyrus and the hippocampus or hippocampal formation. Except for the insula, the orbital gyri and temporal pole, they form a rim (limbus) on the medial side of the cerebral hemisphere, almost encircling the corpus callosum and diencephalon.

The cingulate gyrus is connected to the sensory association cortex and to thalamic anterior nuclei.

The insula is connected to olfactory, gustatory, auditory and somatic sensory areas of the cerebral hemisphere.

The parahippocampal gyrus has two-way connections with the olfactory system, blending with olfactory cortex at the uncus. It is connected to the hippocampus and to the sensory association cortex of all the sensory systems by afferent and efferent pathways.

The hippocampus is the inrolled medial border of the temporal lobe. It has a specialised three-layered allocortex. It has extensive afferent and efferent connections to the hypothalamus, especially the mamillary body, via its major tract, the fornix. It contains large amounts of acetylcholine, dopamine, serotonin and norepinephrine.

Subcortical limbic nuclei include the amygdaloid nucleus, the septal nuclei including the nucleus accumbens, the habenular nuclei, the hypothalamus particularly the mamillary body, and the thalamus, especially the anterior nuclei.

The amygdaloid nucleus lies in the temporal lobe. Although it is anatomically continuous with the caudate nucleus it belongs functionally with the limbic system, not with the basal ganglia in movement control. It is widely connected to the temporal lobe cortex and with the thalamus and hypothalamus. It contains many opiate receptors.

The nucleus accumbens underlies the paraterminal gyri of the frontal lobe and merges with the head of the caudate nucleus. Above it lies the septum pellucidum containing small septal nuclei. All are linked to the olfactory system and to the hippocampus. The septal nuclei are also connected to the thalamus and habenular nuclei.

Important limbic tracts are the fornix, between the hippocampus and the hypothalamus; the mamillothalamic tract, between the mamillary body and anterior thalamus; the cingulum, underlying the cingulate gyrus; and the stria terminalis, carrying amygdaloid efferent fibres and joining the medial forebrain bundle, which is the main longitudinal pathway of the hypothalamus.

The majority of the connections between components of the limbic system carry both efferent and afferent fibres, so there is no obligatory starting point for neural activity in the limbic system. There are many opportunities for interaction between cortical and subcortical parts.

One important connecting pathway forms a circuit known as the Papez circuit.

It connects:

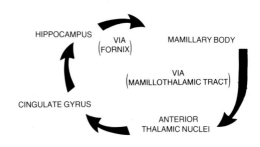

- *The name 'Ammon's horn', sometimes given to the hippocampal formation in a coronal section, refers to its resemblance to a ram's horn. Ammon was a ram-headed ancient Egyptian God.*

- *The hippocampal formation is so named because of an imagined resemblance to a seahorse (hippocampus) when viewed from above.*

- *In Alzheimer's disease, there is extensive cellular degeneration—especially in the hippocampus.*

- *Loss of the hippocampal formation by disease or injury causes severe anterograde amnesia.*

- *Surgical removal of the amygdaloid nucleus may reduce aggressive behaviour and violence.*

- *Stimulation of the septal area in conscious patients produces euphoria.*

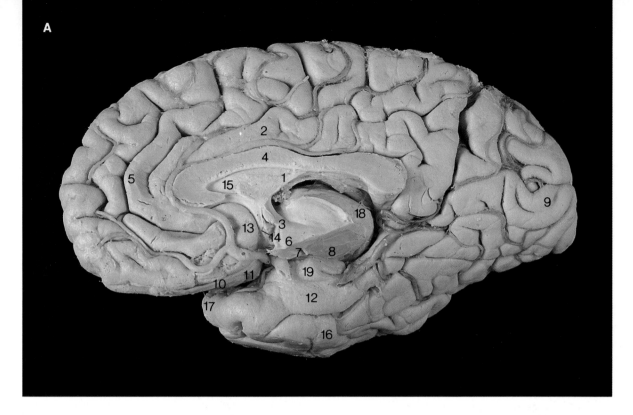

A The medial side of the brain with the brainstem sectioned through the midbrain to illustrate the components of the limbic system. x.78

1 Body of fornix	**8** Midbrain	**15** Septum pellucidum
2 Cingulate gyrus	**9** Occipital lobe	**16** Temporal lobe
3 Column of fornix	**10** Olfactory tract	**17** Temporal pole
4 Corpus callosum	**11** Orbital gyri	**18** Thalamus
5 Frontal lobe	**12** Parahippocampal gyrus	**19** Uncus
6 Hypothalamus	**13** Paraolfactory gyrus	
7 Mamillary body	**14** Paraterminal gyrus	

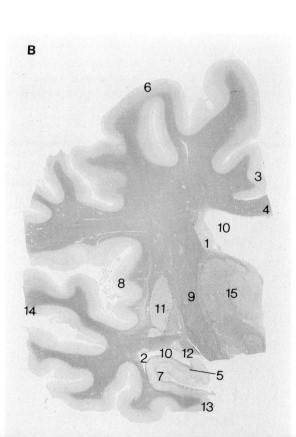

B A coronal section of a cerebral hemisphere and diencephalon to show the parahippocampal gyrus and the hippocampus. Solochrome cyanin and nuclear fast red stain. x.90

1 Caudate nucleus (head)
2 Caudate nucleus (tail)
3 Cingulate gyrus
4 Corpus callosum
5 Fimbria of fornix
6 Frontal lobe
7 Hippocampus
8 Insula
9 Internal capsule
10 Lateral ventricle
11 Lentiform nucleus
12 Optic tract
13 Parahippocampal gyrus
14 Temporal lobe
15 Thalamus

● *The hippocampus has a very complex structure of fibrous and cellular layers. The different regions have different names.*

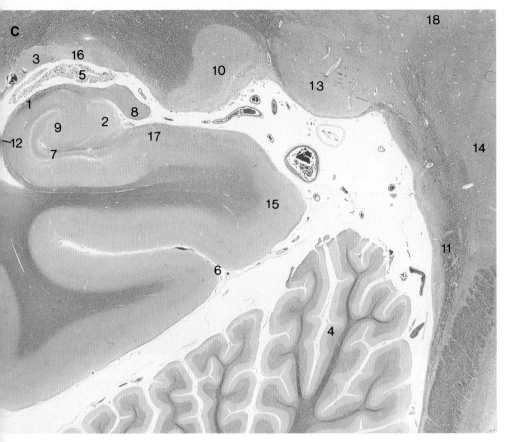

C A longitudinal section through the rostral end of the brainstem and the medial border of the temporal lobe to show the parts and relationships of the hippocampus (hippocampal formation). Solochrome cyanin and nuclear fast red stain. x6.6

1 Alveus of hippocampus
2 Ammon's horn of hippocampus
3 Caudate nucleus
4 Cerebellum
5 Choroid plexus of the lateral ventricle
6 Collateral sulcus
7 Dentate gyrus of hippocampus
8 Fimbria of fornix
9 Hippocampus (hippocampal formation)
10 Lateral geniculate body
11 Lateral lemniscus
12 Lateral ventricle
13 Medial geniculate body
14 Midbrain
15 Parahippocampal gyrus
16 Stria terminalis
17 Subiculum of hippocampus
18 Thalamus

● *At its rostral end the hippocampus widens into the pes hippocampi.*

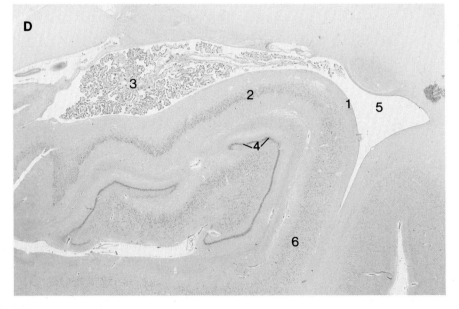

D A section through the pes hippocampi showing the dentate gyrus and Ammon's horn. Cresyl violet stain. x7.5

1 Alveus (nerve fibre layer)
2 Ammon's horn (pyramidal cells)
3 Choroid plexus of the lateral ventricle
4 Dentate gyrus (granular cells)
5 Lateral ventricle
6 Subiculum

E-F Histological sections to illustrate the structure of the dentate gyrus and Ammon's horn.

E A section showing the granular cells of the dentate gyrus. Cresyl violet stain. x89
1 Granular layer
2 Molecular layer
3 Polymorphic cell layer

CAM

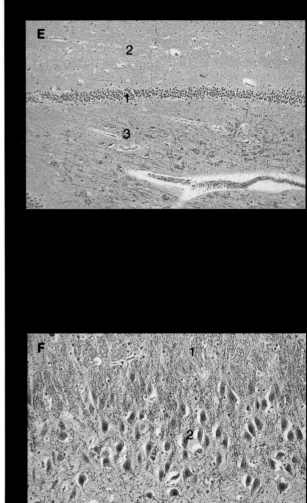

F A section showing the pyramidal cells of Ammon's horn. Cresyl violet stain. x223
1 Nerve fibres of alveus
2 Pyramidal neurons

CAM

• *The indusium griseum is a thin layer of grey matter on the superior surface of the corpus callosum which is continuous with the dentate gyrus of the hippocampus.*

G-H Histological sections to show the amygdaloid nucleus.

G A coronal section through one cerebral hemisphere to show the position and relationships of the amygdaloid nucleus. Carmine stain. x.98
  1 Amygdaloid nucleus
  2 Arachnoid mater
  3 Caudate nucleus
  4 Cingulate gyrus
  5 Cingulum
  6 Corpus callosum
  7 Frontal lobe
  8 Frontal operculum
  9 Hypothalamus
 10 Insula
 11 Internal capsule
 12 Lentiform nucleus
 13 Temporal lobe
 14 Temporal operculum

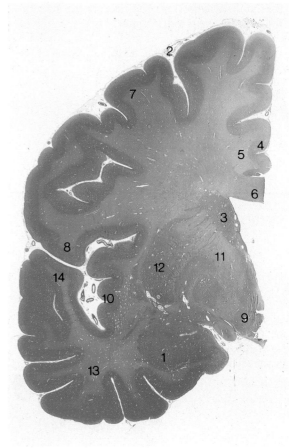

The amygdaloid nucleus is not a single nucleus but a complex consisting of several nuclei with different connections. The medial or corticomedial nuclei have olfactory connections. The lateral basal or basolateral nuclei have links to the hippocampus and indirectly to the cingulate gyrus and the orbital cortex of the frontal lobe. Left and right amygdaloid nuclei connect via the anterior commissure.

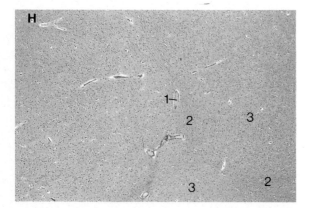

H A medium power photomicrograph of the amygdaloid nucleus showing the separation of individual nuclei within it by nerve fibre bundles. Phosphotungstic acid and haematoxylin stain. x22
  1 Blood vessel
  2 Fibre bundle
  3 Nucleus

• *Porpoises have an extremely reduced or absent sense of smell and the corticomedial portion of their amygdaloid nucleus is small.*

I-K Diencephalic components of the limbic system.

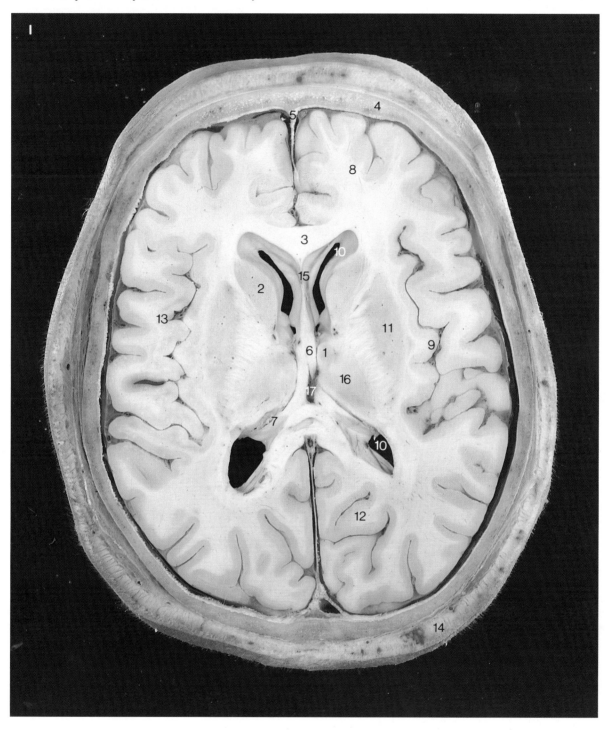

I Horizontal section of the brain *in situ* showing the anterior thalamus and the fornix. x.95

1 Anterior thalamic nucleus	**7** Fornix (crus)	**13** Parietal operculum
2 Caudate nucleus	**8** Frontal lobe	**14** Scalp
3 Corpus callosum	**9** Insula	**15** Septum pellucidum
4 Cranium	**10** Lateral ventricle	**16** Thalamus
5 Falx cerebri	**11** Lentiform nucleus	**17** Third ventricle
6 Fornix (body)	**12** Occipital lobe	

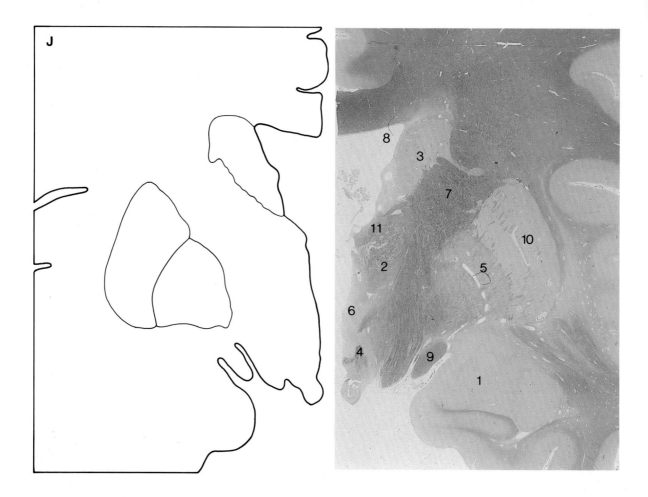

J Part of a coronal section through the forebrain at the level of the interventricular foramen to show the anterior thalamic nucleus, amygdaloid nucleus, stria terminalis, and the fornix passing through the hypothalamus. Weil stain. x1.7

1 Amygdaloid nucleus
2 Anterior thalamic nucleus
3 Caudate nucleus (head)
4 Column of fornix

5 Globus pallidus
6 Hypothalamus
7 Internal capsule
8 Lateral ventricle

9 Optic tract
10 Putamen
11 Stria terminalis

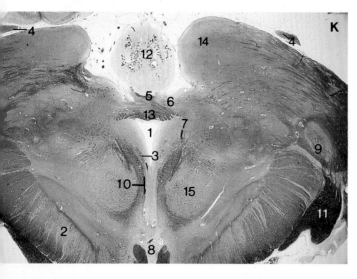

K A coronal section of the caudal end of the diencephalon showing the habenular nucleus and associated tracts. x1.9

1 Cerebral aqueduct becoming third ventricle
2 Crus cerebri
3 Dorsal longitudinal fasciculus
4 Fornix
5 Habenular commissure
6 Habenular nucleus
7 Habenulopeduncular tract or fasciculus retroflexus
8 Hypothalamus
9 Lateral geniculate body
10 Mamillotegmental tract
11 Optic tract
12 Pineal organ
13 Posterior commissure
14 Pulvinar of thalamus
15 Red nucleus

MHMS

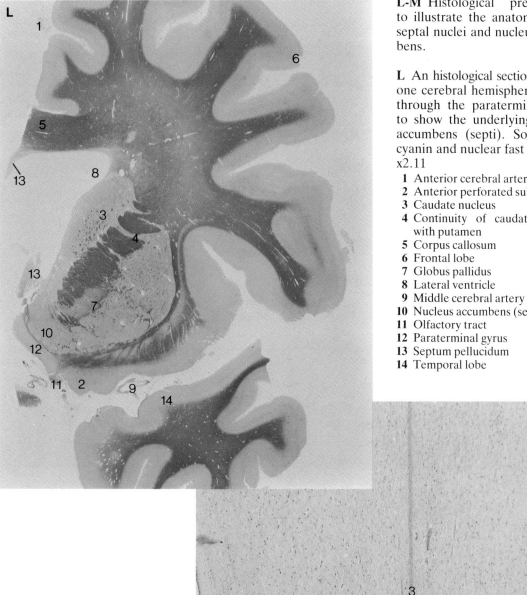

L An histological section through one cerebral hemisphere passing through the paraterminal gyrus to show the underlying nucleus accumbens (septi). Solochrome cyanin and nuclear fast red stain. x2.11

1 Anterior cerebral artery
2 Anterior perforated substance
3 Caudate nucleus
4 Continuity of caudate nucleus with putamen
5 Corpus callosum
6 Frontal lobe
7 Globus pallidus
8 Lateral ventricle
9 Middle cerebral artery
10 Nucleus accumbens (septi)
11 Olfactory tract
12 Paraterminal gyrus
13 Septum pellucidum
14 Temporal lobe

M A vertical histological section through the septum pellucidum, to show how it is formed by fusion of the septa pellucida of the two cerebral hemispheres. Cresyl violet stain. x45

1 Blood vessel
2 Ependyma
3 Fusion of left and right septa pellucida
4 Septum pellucidum

N-R Dissections and histological preparations showing the fornix, mamillary body, mamillothalamic tract, stria terminalis and medial forebrain bundle.

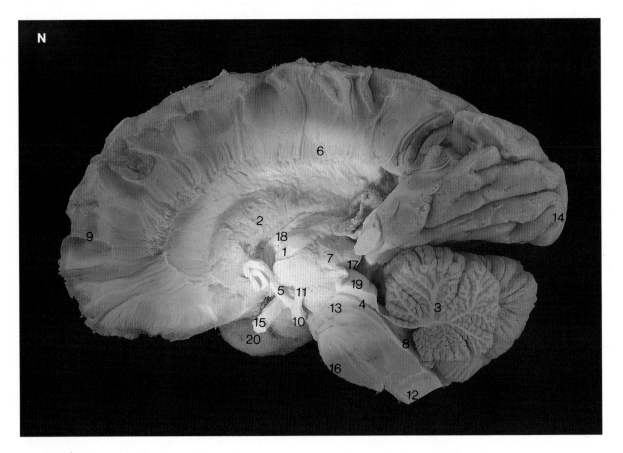

N Brain dissected from the medial side to show the fornix, mamillothalamic tract and stria terminalis. The mamillothalamic tract and the columns of the fornix are embedded in the hypothalamus. x.87

1 Anterior thalamic nuclei	**8** Fourth ventricle	**15** Optic nerve
2 Caudate nucleus	**9** Frontal lobe	**16** Pons
3 Cerebellum	**10** Mamillary body	**17** Pulvinar of thalamus
4 Cerebral aqueduct	**11** Mamillothalamic tract	**18** Stria terminalis
5 Column of fornix	**12** Medulla oblongata	**19** Tectum
6 Corona radiata	**13** Midbrain	**20** Temporal lobe
7 Dorsomedial thalamic nucleus	**14** Occipital lobe	

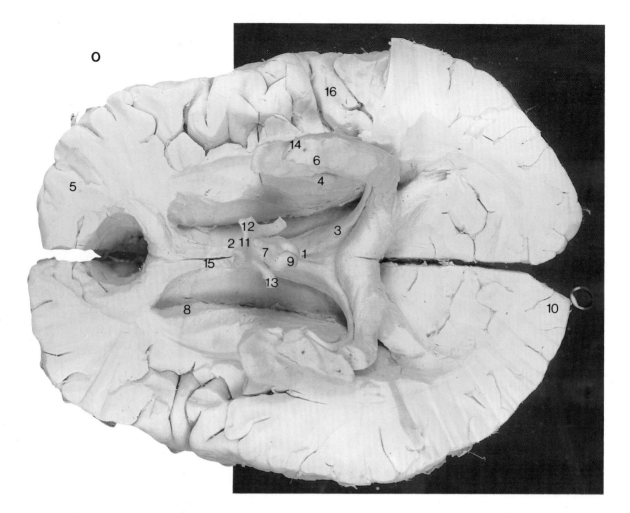

O The brain viewed from below and dissected to show the hippocampus and the fimbria, crura and body of the fornix. x1

1 Body of fornix	**5** Frontal lobe	**9** Mamillary body	**13** Optic tract
2 Corpus callosum	**6** Hippocampus	**10** Occipital lobe	**14** Parahippocampal gyrus
3 Crus of fornix	**7** Hypothalamus	**11** Optic chiasma	**15** Septum pellucidum
4 Fimbria of fornix	**8** Lateral ventricle	**12** Optic nerve	**16** Temporal lobe

OXF

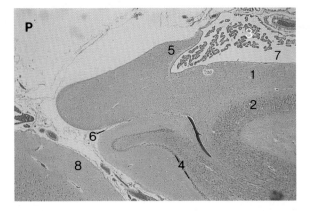

P Histological section of the hippocampus showing the alveus, a superficial layer of nerve fibres and the fimbria of the fornix, into which these fibres aggregate. Cresyl violet stain. x22

1 Alveus
2 Ammon's horn
3 Choroid plexus of lateral ventricle
4 Dentate gyrus
5 Fimbria
6 Hippocampal sulcus
7 Lateral ventricle
8 Subiculum

CAM

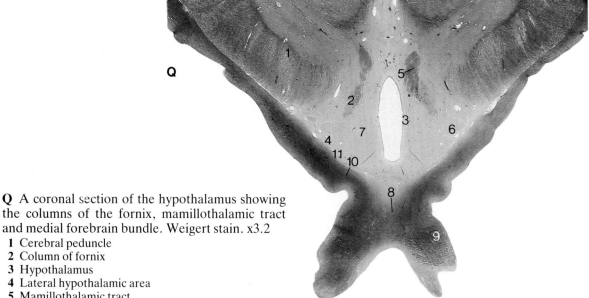

Q A coronal section of the hypothalamus showing the columns of the fornix, mamillothalamic tract and medial forebrain bundle. Weigert stain. x3.2

1 Cerebral peduncle
2 Column of fornix
3 Hypothalamus
4 Lateral hypothalamic area
5 Mamillothalamic tract
6 Medial forebrain bundle
7 Medial hypothalamic area
8 Optic chiasma
9 Optic nerve
10 Optic tract
11 Supraoptic nucleus of hypothalamus

R A section showing the fibres of the fornix surrounding the mamillary body. Luxol fast blue and acid fuchsin stain. x26

1 Fibres of fornix
2 Nucleus of mamillary body

CXWMS

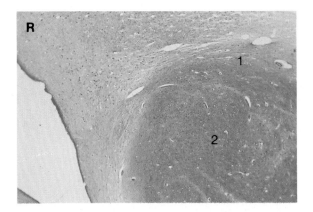

● *The fornix contains approximately one million fibres.*

● *The medial forebrain bundle is poorly myelinated and hence is difficult to see in histological sections.*

The student can perform a simple examination of the formalin and alcohol-fixed brain by following the sequence given in photographs **A-I**. Protective gloves should be worn during this study.

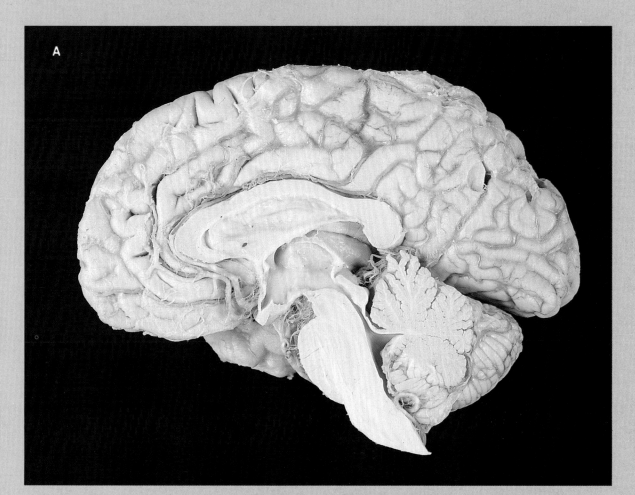

A Make a sagittal cut through the brain and identify the following structures. x.87

1 Cerebellum
2 Corpus callosum
3 Gyrus
4 Fourth ventricle
5 Frontal lobe
6 Hypothalamus
7 Inferior colliculus
8 Infundibulum
9 Interventricular foramen

10 Mamillary body
11 Medulla oblongata
12 Midbrain
13 Occipital lobe
14 Olfactory bulb and tract
15 Optic chiasma
16 Parietal lobe
17 Pia-arachnoid membranes
18 Pineal stalk

19 Pons
20 Posterior commissure
21 Septum pellucidum
22 Sulcus
23 Superior colliculus
24 Thalamus
25 Third ventricle

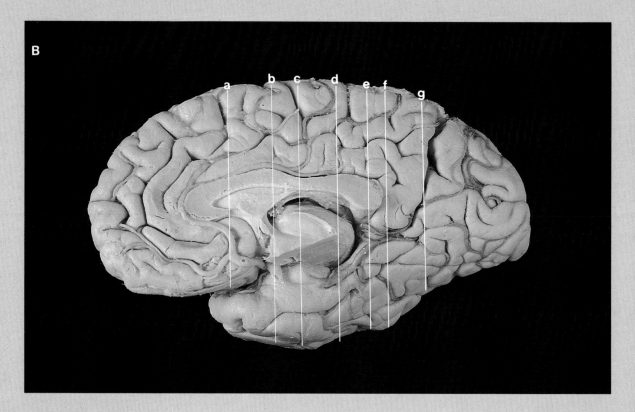

B Cut through the midbrain and remove the cerebellum and brainstem. This photograph illustrates the right hemisphere following removal of the cerebellum and brainstem. Make the incision shown at **a.** x.76

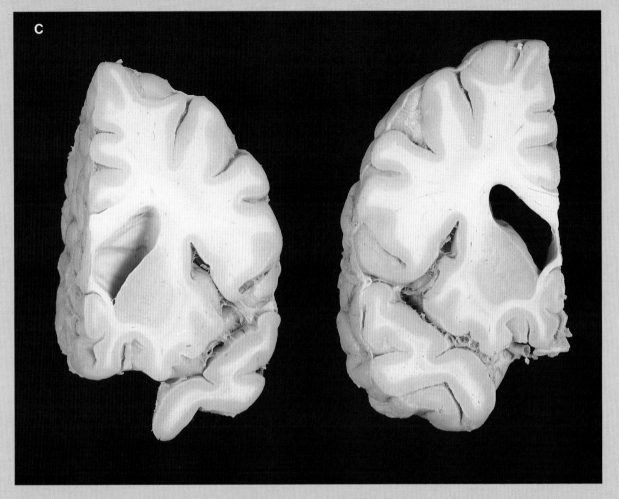

C Identify the following landmarks in the section at
a. The frontal pole of the cerebral hemisphere is on
the left. x.99

1 Anterior cerebral artery
2 Caudate nucleus
3 Cerebral cortex
4 Claustrum
5 Corpus callosum
6 External capsule
7 Insula
8 Lateral sulcus (with middle cerebral vessels)
9 Lateral ventricle (anterior horn)
10 Lentiform nucleus
11 Temporal lobe
12 White matter

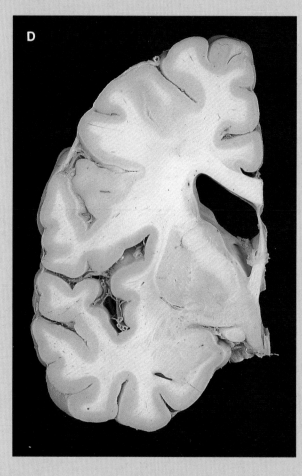

D The section at **b.** Identify the following structures. x1.1

1 Amygdaloid nucleus
2 Caudate nucleus
3 Choroid plexus of lateral ventricle
4 Corpus callosum
5 External capsule
6 Insula
7 Internal capsule
8 Lateral sulcus
9 Lateral ventricle (body)
10 Lentiform nucleus
11 Optic nerve
12 Septum pellucidum
13 Temporal lobe

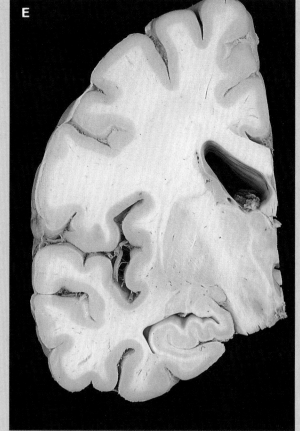

E The section cut at **c.** Identify the following landmarks. x1

1 Claustrum
2 Corpus callosum
3 External capsule
4 Hippocampus
5 Hypothalamus
6 Insula
7 Internal capsule
8 Lateral ventricle (body and inferior horn)
9 Third ventricle

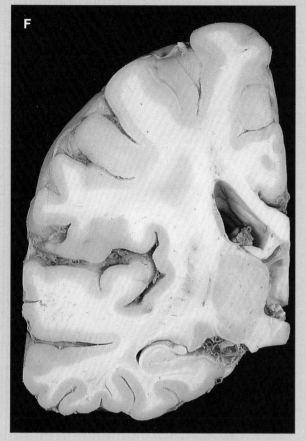

F The section cut at position **d.** The following landmarks should be identified. x1
1 Corpus callosum
2 Hippocampus
3 Insula
4 Internal capsule
5 Lateral geniculate body
6 Lateral ventricle (with choroid plexus)
7 Lentiform nucleus
8 Parahippocampal gyrus
9 Thalamus

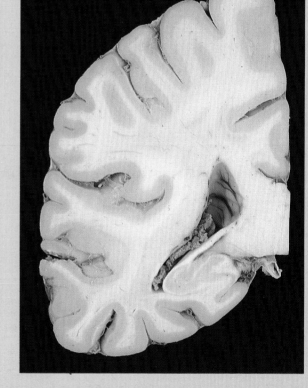

G The section cut at position **e.** The following structures should be identified. x.95
1 Corpus callosum (splenium)
2 Lateral ventricle (inferior and posterior horns)
3 Posterior cerebral artery
4 Temporal lobe

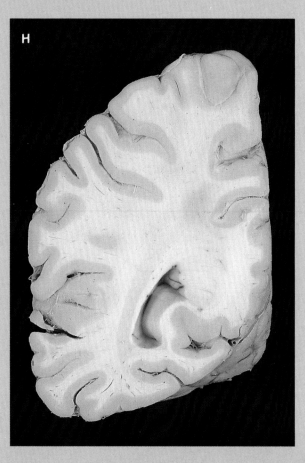

H The section at **f.** Identify these landmarks. x1
1 Lateral ventricle (posterior horn)
2 Occipital lobe
3 Parietal lobe

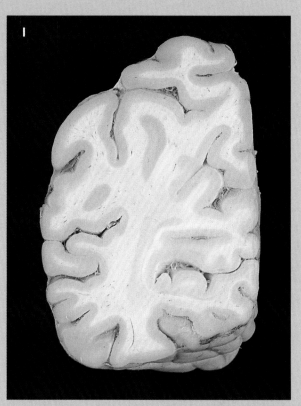

I The final section has been cut. Examine the section at
g and identify these landmarks. x1.2
1 Calcarine sulcus
2 Grey matter
3 Occipital lobe
4 Primary visual cortex
5 White matter

Glossary

Abducens nerve	6th cranial nerve (VI)
Accessory nerve	11th cranial nerve (XI)
Afferent	Towards (sensory if towards the central nervous system)
Angiogram	Display of blood vessels *in vivo* for diagnostic purposes, by using contrast medium and x-rays
Arachnoid (mater)	Middle layer of meninges
Ascending tract	Central sensory pathway, usually from spinal cord to brain
Association fibres	Fibres connecting parts of the same cerebral hemisphere
Autonomic nervous system	Visceral innervation; sympathetic and parasympathetic divisions
Axon	Process of a nerve cell, usually long and generally conducts impulses away from the cell body
Basal ganglia (nuclei)	Nuclei involved in modification of motor control, the caudate and lentiform nuclei, the sub-thalamus and the substantia nigra
Basilar artery	One of the arteries supplying the brain
Brainstem	Medulla, pons and midbrain (some authors include the diencephalon)
CAT or CT scan	Computerized axial tomography: a diagnostic imaging technique
Cauda equina	'Horse's tail': the lower lumbar, sacral, and coccygeal spinal nerves as they lie in the vertebral canal
Caudal	Towards the tail, or hindmost part of neuraxis
Caudate nucleus	One of the basal ganglia forming part of the corpus striatum
Cell body	Part of neuron containing nucleus
Central nervous system	Brain and spinal cord
Cerebellar hemisphere	One of two lateral components of the cerebellum
Cerebellar peduncle	Inferior, middle and superior, fibre tracts linking cerebellum and brainstem
Cerebellum	'Little brain', a dorsal outgrowth from the embryonic hindbrain
Cerebral aqueduct (of Sylvius)	Passage through midbrain, part of ventricular system
Cerebral hemisphere	One half of the cerebrum
Cerebral peduncle	One crus cerebri plus one half of the midbrain tegmentum
Cerebrospinal fluid	Fluid in ventricle (CSF) and in subarachnoid space
Cerebrum	Largest part of the brain, consists of two hemispheres
Cervical	Referring to the neck region
Chorda tympani	Part of the 7th cranial nerve (VII) (see facial nerve)
Choroid plexus	Vascular structure secreting CSF into ventricles
Circle of Willis	Anastomosis between internal carotid and basilar arteries around hypophysis
Cisterna	Expanded portion of subarachnoid space
Claustrum	Grey matter superficial to external capsule
CNS	Abbreviation for 'central nervous system'
Colliculi	Parts of tectum, sensory/motor integration centres: auditory (inferior colliculi) and visual (superior colliculi)
Commissure	Connection of fibres between similar points on left and right sides of the brain
Contralateral	On the opposite side
Corpus callosum	The largest commissure, connects the two cerebral hemispheres
Corpus striatum	Caudate, putamen, and globus pallidus, nuclei inside cerebral hemisphere
Cortex	Superficial layer of grey matter covering the cerebrum, midbrain (colliculi), and cerebellum

Corticobulbar tract	Descending tract connecting motor cortex with motor cranial nerve nuclei	*Falx cerebri*	Fold of dura mater between cerebral hemispheres
Corticospinal tract	Descending tract, from motor cortex to anterior (ventral) horn cells of the spinal cord	*Fasciculus*	A tract or bundle of nerve fibres
Cranial nerve nuclei	Collections of cells in brainstem giving rise to or receiving fibres from cranial nerves, may be sensory or motor	*Fasciculus cuneatus*	Ascending tract for conscious proprioception and discriminating touch above T6 segment of the spinal cord
Cranial nerves	12 pairs of nerves arising from the brain	*Fasciculus gracilis*	Ascending tract for conscious proprioception and discriminating touch below T6 segment of the spinal cord
Crus cerebri (basis pedunculi)	Basal part of cerebral peduncle of midbrain, containing corticospinal and corticobulbar tracts	*Flocculus*	Part of cerebellum
CSF	Cerebrospinal fluid	*Folium*	A flat leaflike fold on the surface of the cerebellum
Decussation	Crossing over of fibres	*Foramen*	An opening, aperture
Dendrite	Receptive process of a neuron, normally conducts impulses towards cell body	*Foramen of Luschka*	Lateral foramen (of fourth ventricle)
Descending tract	Central motor pathway from brain to spinal cord	*Foramen of Magendie*	Median foramen (of fourth ventricle)
Diencephalon	The posterior part of the embryonic forebrain; made up of the thalamus, hypothalamus and epithalamus of adult	*Forebrain*	Anterior division (vesicle) of embryonic brain; cerebrum and diencephalon of adult
Dorsal columns	Fasciculus gracilis and fasciculus cuneatus, pathways for fine touch, and conscious proprioception	*Fornix*	Arch-like tract below corpus callosum
		Fourth ventricle	Cavity in hindbrain, containing CSF
Dorsal root	Afferent sensory component of spinal nerve	*Frontal lobe*	Part of cerebral hemisphere
Dura (mater)	Outermost layer of meninges	*Funiculus*	A large aggregation of white matter in the spinal cord, may contain several tracts
Dural venous sinuses	Large venous channels for draining blood from the brain; run in dura mater	*Ganglion*	Swelling on nerve or nerve root, contains cell bodies, e.g. dorsal root or sympathetic ganglion
Effector	A neuron functioning in producing a response to a stimulus, innervating a muscle or gland	*Geniculate bodies*	Lateral and medial parts of thalamus, relay centres on visual (lateral) and auditory (medial) pathway respectively
Efferent	Away from (motor if away from the central nervous system)	*Glial cell (neuroglial cell)*	Supporting cell in central nervous system
External capsule	White matter superficial to lentiform nucleus	*Globus pallidus*	Part of lentiform nucleus
Extrapyramidal motor pathways	Descending tracts (motor pathways) other than the corticospinal tract	*Glossopharyngeal nerve*	9th cranial nerve (IX)
		Grey/Gray matter	Nervous tissue, mainly nerve cell bodies
Facial nerve	7th cranial nerve (VII) (see chorda tympani)	*Gyrus*	A convoluted fold on a cerebral hemisphere
Falx cerebelli	Fold of dura mater between cerebellar hemispheres	*Hindbrain*	Posterior division of the embryonic brain; pons and medulla oblongata and cerebellum of adult

Hippocampus or hippocampal formation	Specialised area of phylogenetically old cortex in floor of inferior horn of lateral ventricle, in temporal lobe, part of limbic system	Midbrain	The middle division of the embryonic brain, also part of the adult brainstem
Hypoglossal nerve	12th cranial nerve (XII)	Motor	To do with movement or response
Innervation	Nerve supply, sensory or motor	Myelin sheath	Covering of nerve fibre, part of Schwann cell or oligodendrocyte
Insula	Buried portion of cerebral hemisphere below lateral sulcus	Nerve fibre	Neuronal cell process, plus sheathing cells, plus myelin if present; if in peripheral nervous system enclosed in basal lamina
Internal capsule	White matter between lentiform nucleus and thalamus and head of caudate nucleus		
Internal carotid artery	One of the arteries supplying the brain	Neuraxis	The straight longitudinal axis of the embryonic or primitive neural tube, bent in later evolution and development
Interventricular foramen	Opening from lateral into 3rd ventricle		
Ipsilateral	On the same side	Neuron	Nerve cell
Lacunae	Irregularly-shaped venous 'lakes' or channels draining into the superior sagittal sinus	Neuropil	A complex meshwork of axon terminals, dendrites and neuroglial processes
Lateral foramen	Foramen of Luschka, opening in roof of 4th ventricle for escape of CSF into subarachnoid space surrounding the brain	NMR	Nuclear magnetic resonance, also known as magnetic resonance image (MRI); a diagnostic imaging method
Lateral ventricle	Cavity in cerebral hemisphere	Node of Ranvier	Gap in myelin sheath between two successive Schwann cells or oligodendrocytes
Lemniscus	A band-like bundle of nerve fibres e.g. medial lemniscus		
Lentiform nucleus	Part of corpus striatum, composed of putamen and globus pallidus	Nucleus	An aggregation of nerve cells within the CNS
		Nucleus cuneatus	Nucleus at upper end of fasciculus cuneatus
Leptomeninges	Arachnoid and pia mater	Nucleus gracilis	Nucleus at upper end of fasciculus gracilis
Limbic system	Part of brain associated with emotional behaviour	Occipital lobe	Part of cerebral hemisphere
Lower motor neurons	Anterior horn cells and their axons of spinal cord or cell in motor cranial nerve nucleus	Oculomotor nerve	3rd cranial nerve (III)
		Olfactory nerve	1st cranial nerve (I)
Lumbar	Referring to the lower back region	Operculum	Frontal, parietal and temporal folds of cerebral hemisphere covering and so concealing the insula
Medial lemniscus	Brainstem portion of sensory pathway for fine touch and conscious proprioception, after synapse in nucleus gracilis and nucleus cuneatus		
		Optic chiasma	X-shaped union between optic nerves, with fibre decussation
		Optic nerve	2nd cranial nerve (II)
Median foramen	Foramen of Magendie, opening from 4th ventricle into cisterna magna of subarachnoid space for escape of CSF surrounding the brain	Pachymeninx	The dura mater
		Parietal lobe	Part of cerebral hemisphere
		Pathway	A chain of functionally interconnected neurons making a connection between one region of CNS and another, a tract or tracts and nuclei connected e.g. visual pathway
Medulla oblongata	Narrow caudal part of the hindbrain		
Meninges	Covering layers of the central nervous system		

Peduncle	A thick stalk or stem, bundle of nerve fibres
Peripheral nervous system	Nerve roots, nerves and ganglia outside the CNS
Pia (mater)	Innermost layer of meninges
Pons	Enlarged middle portion of the brainstem, part of hindbrain
Proprioception	The sense of body position (conscious or unconscious)
Putamen	Part of lentiform nucleus
Pyramidal tract	Corticospinal tract. Pyramidal system is the corticospinal and corticobulbar tracts
Receptor	Sense organ
Red nucleus	Structure in the midbrain, red in fresh material
Reticular formation	Diffuse nervous tissue in brainstem
Rostral	Towards the nose, or the most anterior end of the neuraxis
Rubrospinal tract	Descending tract from red nucleus of midbrain to spinal cord
Sacral	Referring to the pelvic region
Schwann cell	Sheathing cell of peripheral nerve fibres
Secretor	Motor nerve supply to a gland
Sensory	To do with receiving information from the environment
Septum pellucidum	Two layers of thin membranes separating the anterior horns of the lateral ventricles
Somatic senses	Touch, pain, temperature, pressure, proprioception, vibration
Special senses	Sight, hearing, balance, taste (gustatory) and smell (olfactory)
Spinocerebellar tracts	Ascending tracts for unconscious proprioception
Spinothalamic tracts	Ascending tracts for pain, temperature, nondiscriminative touch, pressure
Subarachnoid space	Space between arachnoid and pia mater
Subcortical	Not in the cerebral cortex, i.e. at a functionally or evolutionarily 'lower' level in the central nervous system
Substantia nigra	Area in midbrain, appears dark in fresh material
Sulcus	Groove between adjacent gyri
Synapse	Area of structural and functional specialisation between neurons where transmission occurs
Tectum	Roof of midbrain
Tegmentum	The dorsal portion of the medulla oblongata and pons and the part of the midbrain between the tectum and crus cerebri. Contains nuclei, tracts and reticular formation
Telencephalon	Rostral part of embryonic forebrain; primarily cerebral hemisphere of adult
Temporal lobe	Part of cerebral hemisphere
Tentorium cerebelli	Fold of dura mater overlying cerebellum
Third ventricle	Cavity in diencephalon, containing CSF
Thoracic	Referring to the chest region
Tract	A bundle of nerve fibres within the CNS, with a common origin and destination, e.g. optic tract
Trigeminothalamic tracts	Ascending tracts for sensations from the face
Trigeminal nerve	5th cranial nerve (V)
Trochlear nerve	4th cranial nerve (IV)
Upper motor neuron	Cell in motor cortex or other motor area in the brain, connected by descending tract to lower motor neurons
Vagus	10th cranial nerve (X)
Ventral root	Efferent motor component of mixed spinal nerve
Ventricles	Cerebrospinal fluid-filled cavities inside the brain
Vermis	Unpaired midline portion of cerebellum between hemispheres
Vertebral artery	An artery supplying spinal cord and brainstem
Vestibulocochlear or acoustic nerve	8th cranial nerve (VIII)
Vestibulospinal tract	Descending tract from vestibular nuclei of medulla to spinal cord
Visceral	Referring to internal organs
White matter	Nervous tissue made up mainly of nerve fibres

Suggestions for Further Reading

Barr, M.L. and Kiernan, J.A. (1988) *The Human Nervous System—An Anatomical Viewpoint,* Philadelphia, J.B. Lippincott Company.

Carpenter, M.B. (1985) *Core Text of Neuroanatomy* 3rd edition, London, Williams and Wilkins Company.

Fitzgerald, M.J.T. (1985) *Neuroanatomy Basic and Applied*, London, Ballière Tindall.

Kahle, W., Leonhardt, H. and Platzer, W. (1986) *Color Atlas and Textbook of Human Anatomy,* Vol. 3 Nervous System and Sensory Organs, New York, Georg Thieme Verlag Thieme Inc.

Liebman, M. (1987) *Neuroanatomy Made Easy and Understandable* 3rd edition, Aspen Publishers U.S.A.

Snell, R.S. (1980) *Clinical Neuroanatomy for Medical Students,* 2nd revised edition Boston, Little, Brown and Company.

Suggestions for Further Reference

Gluhbegovic, N. and Williams, T.H. (1980) *The Human Brain: a photographic guide* Philadelphia, Harper and Row.

Young, J.Z. (1978) *Programs of the Brain Based on the Gifford Lectures, 1975-1977,* Oxford, Oxford University Press.

Index

This index is not meant to be exhaustive; many terms used infrequently in the book have not been included. To find illustrations of a particular item readers should look first at the page shown below and then at the remaining pages of that particular section. Many parts of the brain and spinal cord are also illustrated in additional sections.

All numbers refer to page numbers.

D

E

subcortical limbic nuclei, 258
taste impulses, 229

I

L

M